Healthcare Informatics Innovation Post-COVID-19 Pandemic

"This book is essential reading for those in healthcare informatics, as well as healthcare administrators, clinicians, and regulators, as they navigate the evolving landscape of healthcare post-pandemic."
—**Dr. Steven D. Berkshire**, professor and director of the Doctor of Health Administration Program, Central Michigan University

The coronavirus disease 2019 (COVID-19) pandemic brought unprecedented challenges to global healthcare systems, revealing vulnerabilities and pushing the boundaries of healthcare informatics. In response, the rapid adoption of digital tools and innovative technologies reshaped the way healthcare is delivered, managed, and analyzed. This transformation has not only revolutionized patient care but also underscored the importance of adopting new strategies to ensure data security, interoperability, and equitable access to healthcare services.

Healthcare Informatics Innovation Post-COVID-19 Pandemic explores the lasting impact of these innovations on the healthcare sector. The book examines the key lessons learned from the pandemic, as well as the challenges and opportunities that have emerged in its wake. It covers a broad range of topics, including telehealth, artificial intelligence (AI), the Internet of Things (IoT), and cybersecurity, and examines the critical role each plays in transforming healthcare delivery.

Highlights include:

- Bridging the digital divide with telehealth
- AI in post-pandemic healthcare
- Navigating post-pandemic mental health challenges with AI
- Genomics and personalized medicine
- Ethics, privacy, and security in healthcare informatics

The book's chapters were written by contributors from diverse academic and professional backgrounds. Together, they share their expertise in healthcare, information technology, and policy. Through their insights, the book provides a comprehensive overview of the current state of healthcare informatics and offers a roadmap for future advancements. This book was written to address the growing recognition that healthcare systems worldwide must be resilient, adaptable, and equipped with cutting-edge tools to navigate future public health crises. As healthcare professionals, academics, policymakers, and technologists work together, it is crucial to share knowledge and collaborate on innovative solutions that can sustain the progress made during the pandemic.

Healthcare Informatics Innovation Post-COVID-19 Pandemic

Edited by
Philip Eappen and Narasimha Rao Vajjhala

CRC Press
Taylor & Francis Group
Boca Raton London New York

CRC Press is an imprint of the
Taylor & Francis Group, an **informa** business

AN AUERBACH BOOK

Cover image: Shutterstock

First edition published 2025
by CRC Press
2385 NW Executive Center Drive, Suite 320, Boca Raton FL 33431

and by CRC Press
4 Park Square, Milton Park, Abingdon, Oxon, OX14 4RN

CRC Press is an imprint of Taylor & Francis Group, LLC

ISBN: 978-1-032-77540-1 (hbk)
ISBN: 978-1-032-77969-0 (pbk)
ISBN: 978-1-003-48562-9 (ebk)

DOI: 10.1201/9781003485629

Typeset in Times
by Apex CoVantage, LLC

Contents

Foreword vii
Steven D. Berkshire

Preface..ix
Philip Eappen and Narasimha Rao Vajjhala

Acknowledgments...xv
About the Editors xvii
About the Contributors...xix

Chapter 1 Healthcare Informatics Innovation Post-COVID-19: Lessons,
Challenges, and Opportunities 1

Philip Eappen and Narasimha Rao Vajjhala

Chapter 2 Lessons Learned: COVID-19 and the Future of Healthcare Informatics 9

Khaldoun M. Aldiabat and Mohamad Musa

Chapter 3 Telehealth Revolution: Bridging the Digital Divide....................................24

Ruiling Guo, Christopher Thompson, and Myllissa Reyes

Chapter 4 Artificial Intelligence in Post-Pandemic Healthcare................................... 41

*Sarad Pawar Naik Bukke, Venkatesh Chandrakala, Anupam Maity,
Chandrashekar Thalluri, Narayana Goruntla, Tadele Mekuriya Yadesa,
and Soosamma John*

Chapter 5 Navigating Post-Pandemic Mental Health Challenges: Unleashing
the Potential of Artificial Intelligence..55

Abilash K, Sindhuja Manisha Kamini P, and Ruchi Joshi

Chapter 6 Leveraging Digital Health Technologies in Health Care Teams:
A Discussion of Policy and Practice in Canada 65

Charlotte Hruczkowski, Ryan Brown, and Tim Konoval

Chapter 7 How Data-Driven Insights Can Improve Patient Outcomes, Public Health
Strategies, and Decision-Making 83

Rafiqul Chowdhury and Sahand Ashtab

Chapter 8 Genomics and Personalized Medicine: An Insight from the Healthcare
Perspective..98

*Tabsum Chhetri, Saurav Kumar Mishra, Anagha Balakrishnan, Sneha Roy,
Kusum Gurung, and John J. Georrge*

Chapter 9   Preferences and Selection of Vaccines by Healthcare Consumers 110

                    Antonio Pesqueira, Andréia de Bem Machado, and Maria José Sousa

Chapter 10   Innovation Management Practices in Kazakhstan's Healthcare Sector.................. 135

                    Rajasekhara Mouly Potluri, Karina Kim, and Bissultan Omirbayev

Chapter 11   Advancing Healthcare Informatics in Fluorescence Microscopy Using
                    Computational Imaging Techniques 145

                    Suman Kumar Maji and Jerome Boulanger

Chapter 12   Global Healthcare Informatics: Structural Considerations and Workforce
                    Training Challenges and Solutions 160

                    *Philip Eappen, Karen Parker Davidson, Matthew MacLeod, Alex Cousins,
                    and Virginia Gunn*

Chapter 13   Ethics, Privacy, and Security in Healthcare Informatics 180

                    Azamat Ali

Chapter 14   Cybersecurity Challenges in Healthcare Informatics 198

                    Smitha Shivshankar, Neeraj Makhija, and Premkumar Mathusudhanan

Chapter 15   Impact of Cybersecurity and Artificial Intelligence on Healthcare
                    Operations 215

                    Lola A. Osawe and Benjamin A. Osawe

Chapter 16   Healthcare Cyberattacks over the 2014–2023 Period: Trends, Lessons
                    Learned, and Potential Paths Forward 231

                    David J. Ranney

Chapter 17   Intelligent Transportation System for Healthcare Improvement...........................243

                    *Angayarkanni S.A., Rajaram V, Pandimurugan V,
                    Balakiruthiga B, Umamageswaran C., and Rajesh Babu*

Chapter 18   COVID-19: Predicting Daily Caseload and Mortality during Multiple Waves of
                    the Epidemic in Different Countries 259

                    *M. I. M. Wahab, Azam Dekamin, Nades Palaniyar, Mohamad Y. Jaber,
                    and Horace Chan*

Index...277

Foreword

The integration of healthcare informatics post-pandemic represents one of the most significant advancements in the medical field in recent history. As we navigate the complexities of modern medicine, the demand for innovative informatics solutions to improve patient outcomes, streamline operations, and reduce costs has become increasingly paramount. Healthcare informatics, with its ability to manage vast amounts of patient data, identify patterns, and provide insights, is reshaping traditional healthcare paradigms, making it an indispensable tool for healthcare providers, researchers, and policymakers.

This book delves into the exciting innovations brought about by the growing influence of healthcare informatics. These technological advancements in diagnosing, monitoring, and treating diseases have transformed the healthcare landscape, especially in the aftermath of the COVID-19 pandemic. The pandemic necessitated a re-evaluation of healthcare delivery and management, much like how it impacted work patterns, education, and personal relationships worldwide. Innovations in healthcare informatics have spanned both developed and developing economies, allowing healthcare systems to adapt and evolve in response to global challenges.

Various chapters examine these innovations, from the application of healthcare informatics to advancements in telemedicine, remote monitoring, and cybersecurity, to organizational learning and the ethical challenges associated with technology-driven healthcare. Healthcare informatics plays a crucial role in enhancing healthcare delivery, improving diagnostics, personalizing treatment plans, and safeguarding patient data—particularly in an era where major cyber threats have exposed sensitive patient information.

The use of healthcare informatics is poised to transform medicine by offering unprecedented opportunities for enhancing diagnostic accuracy, personalizing treatment, improving patient management, and streamlining administrative processes. However, realizing the full potential of healthcare informatics requires careful consideration of ethical, legal, and regulatory challenges. As we continue to explore these advancements, the focus must remain on leveraging technology to improve patient care, ensuring that the benefits of healthcare informatics translate into tangible improvements for patients and healthcare professionals alike.

This book is essential reading for those in healthcare informatics, as well as for healthcare administrators, clinicians, and regulators, as they navigate the evolving landscape of healthcare post-pandemic.

Steven D. Berkshire, EdD, MHA, FACHE
Central Michigan University, Mount Pleasant, Michigan, USA

Preface

The coronavirus disease 2019 (COVID-19) pandemic brought unprecedented challenges to global healthcare systems, revealing vulnerabilities and pushing the boundaries of healthcare informatics. In response, the rapid adoption of digital tools and innovative technologies reshaped the way healthcare is delivered, managed, and analyzed. This transformation has not only revolutionized patient care but also underscored the importance of adopting new strategies to ensure data security, interoperability, and equitable access to healthcare services.

This book, *Healthcare Informatics Innovation Post-COVID-19 Pandemic*, was conceived with the intention of exploring the lasting impact of these innovations on the healthcare sector. This book examines the key lessons learned from the pandemic, as well as the challenges and opportunities that have emerged in its wake. The chapters within this book cover a broad range of topics, including telehealth, artificial intelligence (AI), the Internet of Things (IoT), and cybersecurity—each playing a critical role in transforming healthcare delivery.

The contributors to this volume come from diverse academic and professional backgrounds, bringing together expertise in healthcare, information technology, and policy. Through their insights, we hope to provide a comprehensive overview of the current state of healthcare informatics and offer a roadmap for future advancements. Our motivation for compiling this book stems from the growing recognition that healthcare systems worldwide must be resilient, adaptable, and equipped with cutting-edge tools to navigate future public health crises. As healthcare professionals, academics, policymakers, and technologists work together, it is crucial to share knowledge and collaborate on innovative solutions that can sustain the progress made during the pandemic.

In the first chapter—Healthcare Informatics Innovation Post-COVID-19: Lessons, Challenges, and Opportunities—the authors state that the COVID-19 pandemic has had a transformative effect on global healthcare systems, forcing a rapid adoption of digital tools and technologies to manage patient care, data, and operations more effectively. This chapter explores the innovations that emerged during this crisis, focusing on the pivotal role of artificial intelligence (AI), machine learning (ML), telehealth, and the Internet of Things (IoT) in reshaping healthcare delivery. It provides a thorough examination of the advantages these technologies have brought, such as enhanced patient care and operational efficiency, while also addressing challenges like interoperability issues, patient privacy concerns, and unequal access to digital healthcare services. Looking forward, the chapter offers insights into the future of healthcare informatics, emphasizing the need for continued research to overcome the existing barriers and make healthcare systems more resilient and equitable. The authors propose strategies for optimizing healthcare informatics, including enhancing data security, improving digital infrastructure, and addressing ethical considerations. As healthcare becomes increasingly digitalized, the lessons learned from the pandemic will serve as a roadmap for building a more robust and inclusive healthcare environment.

In the second chapter—Lessons Learned: COVID-19 and the Future of Healthcare Informatics—the authors examine the crucial role that healthcare informatics played during the COVID-19 pandemic, with a focus on technology-enabled rapid response systems for crisis management and public health decision-making. Informatics tools were essential for disease surveillance, resource allocation, and data reporting, allowing healthcare providers to quickly process information and provide care. Despite the successes, the pandemic also highlighted several vulnerabilities within healthcare IT infrastructure, particularly regarding the interoperability and security of data systems. In response to these challenges, the chapter suggests key areas for improvement, such as investing in cloud-based platforms, strengthening cybersecurity, and adopting common data standards across jurisdictions. The authors also examine issues of data privacy and ethics, especially in light of the extensive data collection during the pandemic. They stress the importance of modernizing IT infrastructure, enhancing digital literacy among healthcare providers, and fostering cross-sector collaboration to prepare for future health crises.

In the third chapter—Telehealth Revolution: Bridging the Digital Divide—the authors emphasize that the rapid expansion of telehealth during the COVID-19 pandemic played a critical role in ensuring healthcare accessibility during lockdowns and social distancing measures. This chapter provides a detailed analysis of how telehealth technologies bridged the digital divide, allowing patients to receive care remotely while minimizing exposure to the virus. The authors highlight the numerous benefits telehealth provided, such as improved patient access, timely consultations, and the overall reduction of healthcare burdens during the pandemic. However, challenges remain in telehealth's full-scale implementation. The chapter addresses issues such as limited broadband infrastructure, digital literacy gaps, and concerns over data privacy and security. Looking beyond the pandemic, the chapter recommends strategies for expanding telehealth capabilities, improving training for healthcare professionals and patients, and ensuring equitable access to these technologies, particularly in underserved communities.

In the fourth chapter—Artificial Intelligence in Post-Pandemic Healthcare—the authors emphasize that AI played a pivotal role in managing the COVID-19 pandemic by aiding in disease prediction, data analysis, and resource management. This chapter explores the various applications of AI during the pandemic, including the use of ML and deep learning (DL) algorithms to predict disease spread, manage healthcare workers' workloads, and enhance drug discovery. AI's integration with the IoT (AI-IoT) also helped healthcare systems streamline real-time data analysis, contact tracing, and patient management. Post-pandemic, AI continues to offer promising solutions for personalized healthcare, improving diagnosis, and treatment for conditions like cancer, hypertension, and diabetes. The chapter highlights how AI has the potential to transform tele-pharmacy and other digital health services, ultimately reducing the burden on healthcare workers. By examining AI's contributions during and after the pandemic, the chapter offers insights into the future role of AI in enhancing healthcare delivery.

In the fifth chapter—Navigating Post-Pandemic Mental Health Challenges: Unleashing the Potential of Artificial Intelligence—the authors highlight that the mental health crisis brought on by the COVID-19 pandemic highlighted the need for innovative solutions to support mental health services. This chapter investigates the role of AI in addressing the growing demand for mental health care, particularly through AI-driven solutions like predictive modeling, sentiment analysis, and virtual assistants. The authors discuss how AI can revolutionize mental health diagnosis and treatment by enabling remote monitoring, teletherapy, and digital interventions, making mental health care more accessible. Additionally, the chapter examines the ethical considerations and privacy concerns surrounding AI in mental healthcare. While AI offers promising tools for mental health services, maintaining a human-centric approach remains essential to ensure that AI complements rather than replaces the human touch in mental healthcare. The chapter also calls for increased transparency, privacy protections, and ethical frameworks to guide AI-enabled mental healthcare in the post-pandemic era.

In the sixth chapter—Leveraging Digital Health Technologies in Healthcare Teams: A Discussion of Policy and Practice in Canada—the authors explore how the COVID-19 pandemic accelerated the adoption of digital health technologies (DHT) in healthcare teams across Canada. With technologies such as electronic health records, telemedicine, and wearable devices, healthcare providers were able to improve patient outcomes and accessibility to care. The authors examine the critical role of DHT in fostering interprofessional collaboration within healthcare teams, particularly through the lens of the Canadian Interprofessional Health Collaborative's Competency Framework. The chapter provides case studies of Canadian digital health initiatives, emphasizing the importance of virtual care in reshaping healthcare practices during and after the pandemic. In addition to examining the successes, the chapter also discusses the policy barriers and enablers of DHT integration. It highlights how patients have evolved into active partners in their healthcare journey, driven by access to digital health tools. The authors recommend policy reforms to ensure that DHT can be fully integrated into clinical practices, creating a more efficient and patient-centered healthcare system. By advocating for further research and policy support, this chapter offers insights into the future of digital health in Canada and beyond.

In the seventh chapter—How Data-Driven Insights Can Improve Patient Outcomes, Public Health Strategies, and Decision-Making—the authors posit that the increasing reliance on data-driven approaches in healthcare decision-making has revolutionized patient care and public health strategies. This chapter explores how the analysis of high-quality healthcare data, particularly longitudinal data, has helped healthcare providers improve patient outcomes by enabling a better understanding of disease progression and treatment effectiveness. By using data from the Health and Retirement Study (HRS) in the United States, the authors demonstrate the value of longitudinal data analysis in guiding public health decision-making. The chapter also emphasizes the importance of data-driven insights in shaping broader healthcare policies and public health interventions. As data collection and analysis become more integrated into healthcare systems, they provide actionable information for both individual care and population-level health strategies. By illustrating the potential of data-driven approaches through case studies, the chapter outlines the benefits of leveraging data for informed healthcare decision-making and improved patient outcomes.

In the eighth chapter—Genomics and Personalized Medicine: An Insight from the Healthcare Perspective—the authors explore how the integration of genomics and personalized medicine is transforming the healthcare landscape. Personalized medicine offers tailored treatment strategies based on an individual's genetic makeup, marking a significant shift from the traditional one-size-fits-all approach to medical care. Genomic technologies, such as next-generation sequencing and genome-wide association studies, have provided healthcare providers with the tools to better understand genetic variants and their impact on disease susceptibility, drug responses, and treatment outcomes. While personalized medicine has the potential to revolutionize healthcare by reducing unnecessary diagnostics and improving treatment precision, the chapter also addresses the challenges of integrating genomic data into clinical practice. These challenges include the need for specialized knowledge to interpret genetic data and the resources required to implement these advancements widely. The authors provide a comprehensive overview of how genomics is reshaping the healthcare industry and highlight the benefits and obstacles of adopting personalized medicine in clinical settings.

In the ninth chapter—Preferences and Selection of Vaccines by Healthcare Consumers—the authors examine the complex dynamics of healthcare consumers' (HC's) preferences and decision-making processes, focusing specifically on vaccine selection. Understanding the various factors that influence vaccine choice—ranging from cognitive attitudes to purchasing behaviors—is essential for optimizing distribution strategies and improving vaccination rates. The authors analyze how predictive technologies, such as AI and managerial dynamic capabilities (MDC), can be employed to forecast HC's behaviors and refine healthcare decision-making. Using the Theory, Context, Characteristics, and Methods (TCCM) methodology, the chapter presents case studies to illustrate the relationships between predictive technologies and healthcare organizations' strategic approaches. By examining these connections, the authors offer insights into how healthcare systems can improve vaccine distribution strategies through better prediction models. This chapter provides a framework for both future research and the practical implementation of predictive technologies to support sustainable and efficient healthcare operations.

In the tenth chapter—Innovation Management Practices in Kazakhstan's Healthcare Sector—the authors state that Kazakhstan's healthcare system has made strides in embracing innovation, but it faces unique challenges in fully realizing its potential. This chapter investigates the current state of healthcare innovation management in Kazakhstan, focusing on the strategies, opportunities, and obstacles the system faces. Using a multiple-method approach, the authors draw on qualitative data from literature reviews and governmental sources, alongside quantitative data from a targeted questionnaire, to present a comprehensive analysis of Kazakhstan's healthcare innovation landscape. The chapter identifies key governmental initiatives aimed at fostering innovation in healthcare, but it also highlights significant barriers, such as resource allocation challenges and limited access to up-to-date medical technologies. By offering recommendations for enhancing Kazakhstan's healthcare innovation ecosystem, the chapter provides valuable insights for both policymakers and healthcare practitioners. Although the findings are specific to Kazakhstan, the authors suggest that the lessons learned could be applicable to other former USSR countries with similar healthcare challenges.

In the eleventh chapter—Advancing Healthcare Informatics in Fluorescence Microscopy Using Computational Imaging Techniques—the authors emphasize that fluorescence microscopy is a vital tool in healthcare informatics, allowing for high-contrast visualization and analysis of biological samples. However, the limitations of fluorescence microscopy—such as photobleaching and phototoxicity—create challenges in accurately imaging living tissues. This chapter explores the role of computational deconvolution techniques in overcoming these obstacles by enhancing image clarity and resolution beyond the diffraction limit. The chapter provides an in-depth review of the computational algorithms developed for fluorescence microscopy, offering experimental analyses of their performance. These advancements have significantly improved diagnostic and therapeutic applications of microscopy in healthcare. By highlighting the progress made in computational imaging and its impact on healthcare diagnostics, the authors present a comprehensive look at the future potential of fluorescence microscopy in medical informatics.

In the twelfth chapter—Global Healthcare Informatics: Structural Considerations and Workforce Training Challenges and Solutions—the authors examine the structural and educational challenges faced by global healthcare systems in implementing healthcare informatics (HI) in a post-pandemic world. The authors focus on the complexities of training a diverse healthcare workforce to effectively use HI tools and technologies. Several key challenges are identified, including insufficient and fragmented training programs, a lack of integration of HI into health curricula, and varied reception among healthcare workers regarding the adoption of digital technologies. To address these challenges, the chapter proposes several solutions, including sustained investment in workforce training, stronger legislative frameworks, and the development of standardized infrastructures to support the integration of healthcare technologies across systems. By analyzing current best practices and recent research, the chapter offers recommendations for policymakers, educators, and healthcare managers. These strategies aim to equip healthcare systems with the necessary skills and infrastructure to fully leverage the benefits of HI in the future.

In the thirteenth chapter—Ethics, Privacy, and Security in Healthcare Informatics—the authors state that with the increasing reliance on digital technologies for patient data management and medical procedures, a comprehensive examination of the ethical, privacy, and security concerns in HI is required. The authors explore the delicate balance between utilizing technological advancements to improve healthcare outcomes and adhering to ethical principles that protect patient rights and dignity. They discuss the risks associated with the large-scale collection of sensitive medical data, such as data breaches and unauthorized access, which pose significant challenges for healthcare systems. The chapter also highlights the robust security measures that are essential to safeguarding patient data from cyber threats. It concludes with practical recommendations for healthcare providers, IT professionals, and policymakers, proposing a framework that fosters ethical practices, enhances privacy protection, and implements stringent security protocols. By addressing these key concerns, the chapter underscores the importance of maintaining trust and integrity in the use of digital technologies within the healthcare sector.

In the fourteenth chapter—Cybersecurity Challenges in Healthcare Informatics—the authors focus on the critical role of cybersecurity in healthcare, emphasizing its importance in maintaining the safety and integrity of healthcare systems. Drawing an analogy to personal hygiene, the authors argue that cybersecurity requires consistent and proactive practices to protect healthcare organizations from potential threats. As healthcare becomes increasingly digitalized through e-healthcare systems, the risk of cyberattacks, particularly the theft of protected health information (PHI), has grown significantly. The chapter offers practical solutions for mitigating cybersecurity risks, such as conducting regular risk assessments, adopting advanced encryption techniques, and implementing multilayered security protocols. By reviewing various cybersecurity applications—such as secure data-sharing platforms and intrusion detection systems—the authors provide a roadmap for healthcare organizations to adopt standardized security practices. These measures will ensure that e-healthcare systems are protected against evolving cyber threats, thus safeguarding patient data and the operational efficiency of healthcare organizations.

In the fifteenth chapter—Impact of Cybersecurity and Artificial Intelligence in Healthcare Operations—the authors state that COVID-19 pandemic exposed significant vulnerabilities in healthcare systems, particularly in terms of cybersecurity and the lack of integrated information technology platforms. This chapter explores the profound impact that cybersecurity and AI have had on healthcare operations, both in the United States and globally. The authors highlight the challenges faced by public health entities, private medical groups, and hospital systems in managing the healthcare crisis, and they emphasize the need for innovation to meet the evolving needs of communities worldwide. By examining the role of advanced technologies like AI and secure information systems, the chapter identifies opportunities for improving healthcare delivery. The authors stress the importance of adopting robust cybersecurity measures to protect patient data from cyberattacks. Furthermore, they explore how AI can be responsibly integrated into healthcare operations to enhance efficiency, optimize resources, and ensure a resilient healthcare system in the post-pandemic era.

In the sixteenth chapter—Healthcare Cyberattacks over the 2014–2023 Period: Trends, Lessons Learned, and Potential Paths Forward—the authors state that over the past decade, cyberattacks in the healthcare sector have evolved in both complexity and impact. While the number of attacks has decreased, their financial and operational costs to healthcare organizations have risen. This chapter examines the trends in cyberattacks on healthcare organizations from 2014 to 2023, focusing on the growing expertise of cybercriminals who have become subject matter experts in exploiting the vulnerabilities of healthcare systems. The chapter provides a detailed analysis of how healthcare organizations have responded to these attacks and the lessons learned over the years. The authors offer insights into the tactics used by cybercriminals and propose strategies to strengthen cybersecurity programs. By examining real-world case studies, the chapter presents actionable recommendations for healthcare decision-makers to build more resilient and secure cybersecurity systems to protect against future threats.

In the seventeenth chapter—Intelligent Transportation System for Healthcare Improvement—the authors explore how intelligent transportation systems (ITS) are revolutionizing emergency healthcare response and public health outcomes. The integration of sophisticated algorithms and computational power has enabled the development of vehicular networks that enhance communication between vehicles and healthcare infrastructure. The authors focus on the role of vehicular ad-hoc networks (VANETs), which facilitate real-time coordination of critical information such as accident reports and health data, improving the efficiency of healthcare services in emergencies. The chapter also discusses how VANETs, when integrated with smart city infrastructure, can optimize the flow of emergency vehicles, such as ambulances, by dynamically managing traffic. By creating a unified network of hospitals, blood banks, and roadside assistance services, ITS frameworks ensure better resource allocation and personnel coordination during emergencies. The authors highlight how these systems ultimately save lives by streamlining emergency response efforts.

In the last chapter of this book—COVID-19: Predicting Daily Caseload and Mortality during Multiple Waves of the Epidemic in Different Countries—the authors emphasize that accurately predicting the progression of COVID-19 has been essential for managing the pandemic, particularly as countries experienced multiple waves of infection. This chapter introduces a modified diffusion model that utilizes real-time data from the Johns Hopkins University Center for Systems Science and Engineering to predict daily case numbers and mortality rates during different waves of the pandemic. The model successfully forecasts critical features of the epidemic curve, including the peak of daily cases and the timing of each wave's conclusion in countries such as the United States, Canada, Germany, Italy, and Spain. In addition to the diffusion model, the chapter presents a multivariate prophet approach to accurately predict COVID-19-related deaths. By training the model on different segments of the epidemic curve, the authors demonstrate how these predictive tools can inform public health strategies and improve pandemic response efforts globally. The chapter offers valuable insights into managing future waves of the pandemic and highlights the importance of predictive models in improving public health outcomes.

We are grateful to all the authors who contributed their time, expertise, and passion to this project. Their dedication has been instrumental in shaping this book. We would also like to extend our appreciation to the institutions and organizations that supported the development of this work. This book would not have been possible without their encouragement and resources.

In presenting this volume, we hope to provide valuable insights to healthcare professionals, researchers, policymakers, and students who are navigating the evolving landscape of healthcare informatics. As we look to the future, we believe that the lessons learned during the pandemic will continue to inform and inspire innovation in healthcare, ensuring that systems are prepared to meet the demands of tomorrow.

We invite readers to explore the chapters that follow, each offering a unique perspective on the critical role of HI in the post-pandemic world.

Editors:
Philip Eappen
Narasimha Rao Vajjhala

Acknowledgments

I would like to express my deep gratitude to all those who contributed to this project. To my co-editor, Dr. Narasimha Rao Vajjhala, your collaboration and shared vision have been invaluable. I am also immensely thankful to every one of the esteemed authors who authored the chapters within this book. Your time, expertise, and dedication have shaped a valuable resource that will provide insights into the post-pandemic evolution of healthcare informatics. Without your contributions, this book would not have been possible.

I extend my heartfelt thanks to the institutions and organizations that supported this endeavor. Your encouragement and resources were critical in making this project a reality.

Finally, I would like to acknowledge the unwavering support of my family and thank my wife, Figgi; my son, Evan; and my mom, Baby—your love, patience, and belief in my work have been a constant source of motivation. More importantly, I also wish to honor the memory of my late dad Eappen, who passed during this work and whose values, wisdom, and guidance inspire me daily. This book stands as a testament to our collective effort to enhance and innovate in healthcare for the betterment of patients and systems worldwide.

Dr. Philip Eappen

About the Editors

Dr. Philip Eappen is an assistant professor of healthcare management at Cape Breton University. He also served as the director of clinical services and transition to community at the Breton Ability Center. With over a decade of experience in hospital and healthcare management operations, Dr. Eappen has a solid academic background. Before joining Cape Breton University, he taught healthcare management at the University of Toronto, the Southern Alberta Institute of Technology, and Fanshawe College. Dr. Eappen also worked as a director of Health Services and chief administrator of Healthcare Operations at the American University of Nigeria. Additionally, he has served as a faculty member at the American University and other universities and colleges.

Dr. Eappen holds a doctorate in healthcare administration from Central Michigan University in the United States, a Master of Business Administration in Healthcare Management, a Bachelor of Nursing, and a postgraduate certificate in International Health.

Dr. Eappen is a board director on various boards, including the American College of Healthcare Executives, Myeloma Canada, and the Aplastic Anemia and Myelodysplasia Association of Canada. Dr. Eappen is also a long-serving member of the American College of Healthcare Executives and the Canadian College of Health Leaders. His research interests are focused on healthcare innovations, particularly healthcare informatics, and he has published various articles, book chapters, and books on the subject in recent years.

Dr. Narasimha Rao Vajjhala currently serves as the dean of the Faculty of Engineering and Architecture at the University of New York Tirana in Albania. He previously held the position of chair for the Computer Science and Software Engineering programs at the American University of Nigeria. Dr. Vajjhala is a senior member of both the Association for Computing Machinery (ACM) and Institute of Electrical and Electronics Engineers (IEEE). He is the editor-in-chief of the *International Journal of Risk and Contingency Management* (IJRCM) and a member of the Risk Management Society (RIMS) and the Project Management Institute (PMI). With over 23 years of experience, Dr. Vajjhala has taught programming and database-related courses across Europe and Africa at both graduate and undergraduate levels. He has also worked as a consultant for technology firms in Europe and participated in EU-funded projects. Dr. Vajjhala holds a doctorate in Information Systems and Technology from the United States, a Master of Science in Computer Science and Applications from India, and a Master of Business Administration specializing in Information Systems from Switzerland.

Dr. Eappen and Dr. Vajjhala have diverse international backgrounds and played important roles in shaping their disciplines through teaching, research, and professional service. These distinguished professionals have substantially contributed to their respective fields, combining strong academic credentials with practical leadership and international experience. Their work continues to impact healthcare management and technology in academic settings and through their involvement with professional organizations and industry projects.

About the Contributors

Abilash K is an assistant professor of psychology at CHRIST (Deemed to be University), Bengaluru, and holds a PhD in clinical psychology from Amity University, Jaipur. His research focuses on character strengths, environmental ethics, and the impact of AI on mental health. Dr. Kasi has published several book chapters, including in Scopus-indexed publications, and has presented at national and international conferences. He recently contributed to the books *The Climate Change Crisis and Its Impact on Mental Health* and *Emotional AI and Human–AI Interactions in Social Networking*. Dr. Kasi is also the founder of The Sanguine Minds psychology clinic, where he offers psychological assessment, diagnosis, and therapy. He actively engages in academic research, mentorship, and community service and has completed certifications from prestigious institutions, including the University of Pennsylvania and Stanford University.

Khaldoun M. Aldiabat is a faculty member at the School of Nursing at Cape Breton University in Sydney, NS, Canada, where he serves as the assistant dean of Research and Scholarship and is an associate professor in Community and Mental Health Nursing. He is the founder and editor-in-chief of the *Canadian Journal of Multidisciplinary Qualitative Research* (CJMQR) and a co-developer and associate editor of the *International Journal of Nursing Student Scholarship*, the first Canadian and international peer-reviewed open-access journal dedicated to showcasing outstanding and innovative work by nursing and health sciences students. Dr. Aldiabat's research focuses on nursing education in Cape Breton, mental health and addiction management, cancer care, and other health and nursing issues. His broader interests include community and population health nursing, chronic diseases, gerontology, and the intersection of culture, immigration, and health. In addition to his academic roles, Dr. Aldiabat is a scientist and research affiliate with Nova Scotia Health, the Centre of Excellence in Healthy Aging, and the Strategy for Patient-Oriented Research—Maritime SPOR Support Unit (SPOR-MSSU), and a member of Sigma Theta Tau.

Azamat Ali is an assistant professor in the School of Liberal and Creative Arts (Journalism and Mass Communication) at Lovely Professional University, Phagwara, Punjab. He holds an MPhil and PhD from the Central University of Gujarat, Gandhinagar; a BSc in physics (Hons.) from Aligarh Muslim University; an MSc in science communication from Devi Ahilya University, Indore; and a PG Diploma in broadcast technology from Jamia Millia Islamia, New Delhi. His research interests include emerging technologies, development communication, and health and science communication. With over 7 years of teaching experience, he has published more than 20 research papers in reputed journals, attended numerous Indian and international conferences, and successfully supervised 7 PhD scholars to the award of their degrees.

Angayarkanni S.A. is an assistant professor in the Department of Networking and Communication, with a total teaching experience of 16.8 years. She obtained her BTech (information technology) and ME (wireless technologies) from Anna University in 2005 and 2008, respectively. She scored 91.89 percentile in the GATE-IT 2006 examination. She completed her PhD in 2021 from Anna University. Her research domain is intelligent transportation systems. Her areas of interest include networking, wireless technologies, and intelligent road traffic systems for Indian roads. She has published 14 Scopus-indexed papers in international journals and conferences, of which three are Science Citation Indexed (SCI). She is a lifetime member of The Institution of Engineers (India)—IEI—and the Indian Society of Technical Education (ISTE).

Sahand Ashtab received his Industrial and Manufacturing Systems Engineering doctorate from the University of Windsor, Canada. He is currently an associate professor and chair of the Department of Management Science at Cape Breton University. Dr. Ashtab has been involved in several applied research projects and has won the Canadian Operational Research Society (CORS) Practice Prize. His research areas include short food supply chains, circular economy, closed loop supply chains, and healthcare management.

Rajesh Babu currently serves as an associate professor in the School of Computing Science and Engineering, boasting a comprehensive teaching experience spanning over 15 years. His affiliation with Galgotias University dates back to October 2023. Driven by a profound belief in productivity and efficiency, he upholds an unwavering work ethic and can thrive in a fast-paced, time-sensitive environment. As a dedicated educator, he views teaching not merely as the transmission of course concepts but also as a means to cultivate critical thinking and assess alternative problem-solving approaches. Dr. Rajesh Babu is committed to the holistic development of his students. Specializing in network engineering, he holds a 5G core design doctorate.

Balakiruthiga B has a distinguished academic career, beginning as an assistant professor in the Department of Computer Science and Engineering at Kalasalingam Academy of Research and Education (KARE), Virudhunagar, Tamil Nadu, where she served from July 2011 to October 2022. Since November 2022, she has contributed her expertise as an assistant professor in the Department of Networking and Communications in the School of Computing, Faculty of Engineering and Technology at SRM Institute of Engineering and Technology, Kattankulathur, Tamil Nadu. She earned her Doctor of Philosophy with a dissertation titled "Design of Traffic Optimization Schemes for Software Defined Data Center" under the guidance of Dr. P. Deepalakshmi, the dean of the School of Computing and the director of Accreditation and Ranking at KARE. Dr. Balakiruthiga is also an active reviewer for several prestigious journals, reflecting her deep engagement with the academic community. With 13 years of teaching experience, she has significantly impacted her students and field. Her educational journey began with a Bachelor of Engineering in Computer Science and Engineering from Maharaja Engineering College, affiliated with Anna University, Chennai, Tamil Nadu, in 2009. She completed her Master of Technology in Network Engineering from KARE in 2011. Dr. Balakiruthiga's broad research interests include networks, distributed computing, software-defined networks, network routing and traffic management, distributed intelligence, and federated learning for IoT-based cloud applications. Currently, she is guiding several student projects in cutting-edge areas such as federated learning for IoT applications, digital twin applications in 5G and 6G, and quality of service optimization in data center networks.

Anagha Balakrishnan completed her postgraduation degree in biology in 2020 from the Indian Institute of Science Education and Research (IISER), Tirupati, India. She worked as a junior research fellow at the Female Reproduction and Metabolic Syndrome Laboratory, Rajiv Gandhi Centre for Biotechnology. She is currently pursuing PhD at the Department of Bioinformatics, University of North Bengal. Her research interest is in designing novel drug candidates against cancer.

Steven D. Berkshire serves as a professor and director of the Doctor of Health Administration program at Central Michigan University. Dr. Berkshire has a half-century of healthcare experience, ranging from being a hospital CEO to a healthcare government relations professional, consulting in the field and academia. Dr. Berkshire teaches healthcare policy, organizational behavior, leadership, and management and mentors many doctoral dissertation students.

Jerome Boulanger received a PhD (2007) in telecommunication and signal processing from the University of Rennes I, France. He joined the French National Centre for Scientific Research as a researcher at the Institut Curie, Paris, France, in 2011. Since 2015, he has been an investigator scientist at the Laboratory of Molecular Biology at the Medical Research Council in Cambridge, United Kingdom.

Ryan Brown is a paramedic who has undergone clinical training, is an educator, and is a researcher passionate about interprofessional education (IPE) and collaborative person-centered care. Ryan holds a Master of Public Health and an Executive Master of Business Administration, and has been a Fellow of the Royal Society for Public Health. He is also an alumnus of the Keystones Simulation Certification from Simulation Canada. Ryan has held numerous educational, operational, regulatory, and research leadership positions throughout his career, and he has extensive experience in interprofessional (IP) simulation and curriculum design and delivery, spanning entry-to-practice, continuing education, online education, and university-based learning. He is currently a professional practice leader with Nova Scotia Health and an assistant adjunct professor in the Department of Emergency Medicine, Faculty of Medicine at Dalhousie University. Ryan's research interests include the delivery of primary and emergency care by IP teams, evidence synthesis, health policy, and IPE utilizing simulation. His primary area of expertise is in novel primary care delivery models utilizing allied health professionals, specifically looking at treating ambulatory care-sensitive conditions. He has presented his work both within his native Canada and internationally.

Sarad Pawar Naik Bukke is working as an associate professor and research coordinator in the Department of Pharmaceutics and Pharmaceutical Technology at Kampala International University, Western Campus, Uganda, Africa. He holds a PhD from Sun Rise University (SRU), Alwar, Rajasthan, in 2018, with a postgraduation from Sri Venkateshwara University, Tirupati, Andhra Pradesh, in 2011 and his undergraduation from Sri Padmavathi School of Pharmacy (SPSP), Tirupati, Andhra Pradesh, in 2009, and a teaching experience of 13 years. He gained many accolades as a presenter of research papers in national symposia in India and Uganda. He has published more than 25 research and review publications in various reputed journals and attended more than 20 conferences and workshops. He has 2 patents and has published one book and several book chapters. He is a reviewer of several journals viz., *Annals of Medicine and Surgery*, Bentham Publishers, BP International, and *Tropical Journal of Natural Product Research* and a serving member of *International Journal of Health & Medical Research* and *Global Scientific Journals*. He has been awarded Dr. Sarvepalli Radhakrishnan Eminent Associate Professor & Researcher Award 2024 in Pharmaceutical Sciences. He has expertise in the area of formulation and evaluation of novel controlled Drug Delivery Systems and the development of various nanocarriers like solid lipid nanoparticles, nanodispersions, nanoemulsions, liposomes, niosomes, transferosomes, and ethosomes for the targeted delivery of drugs, formulation of transdermal drug delivery systems, and enhancement of solubility and dissolution rate of BCS class II drugs. He guides 17 postgraduate students and 36 undergraduate students who have completed their thesis work. He is a lifetime member of the Indian Pharmaceutical Association (IPA).

Horace Chan graduated from Toronto Metropolitan University in 2022 with an MASc in Mechanical and Industrial Engineering. His research focuses on the intersection of data analytics and supply chain management. His fields of interest include sales forecasting, inventory management, weather, healthcare, and machine learning.

Venkatesh Chandrakala earned her Bachelor of Pharmacy from the Government College of Pharmacy in Bangalore, Karnataka. She further pursued her Master of Pharmacy in Pharmaceutics from the same institution, qualifying GATE with a 96th percentile score. Dr. Chandrakala completed her PhD at VIT, Vellore. Currently, she serves as the head of the Department and a professor in the Department of Pharmaceutics at East Point College of Pharmacy, Bidarahalli, Bangalore, Karnataka, with over 16 years of academic and research experience. She has published over 30 research and review articles in reputable national and international journals. She has also authored three book chapters, and her contributions to the field have been recognized with the granting of two patents and two design patents. Her mentorship extends to guiding over 15 undergraduate and 20 postgraduate students. Actively engaged in research, Dr Chandrakala focuses on nanoparticles and bioadhesive drug delivery systems and has received a grant from the university.

Tabsum Chhetri is involved in drug target identification, transcriptomics data analysis, and novel inhibitor identification for pathogens-related research. She is also intensely interested in genomics profiles and their impact on disease understating via advanced computational bioinformatics approaches.

Rafiqul Chowdhury received his PhD in biostatistics from the Institute of Statistical Research and Training (ISRT), Dhaka University, Bangladesh. After that, he completed a postdoctoral research fellowship in the Department of Mathematics and Statistics of the University of New Brunswick, Canada. He is an assistant professor at the Shannon School of Business at Cape Breton University, Sydney, NS, Canada. Previously, he taught at the Department of Mathematics and Statistics, University of Fraser Valley (UFV), Abbotsford, BC; School of Mathematical and Computational Sciences, University of Prince Edward Island (UPEI), Charlottetown, PE; Department of Health Information Administration (HIA), FAHSN, Kuwait University, Kuwait; and Computer and Information Technology Institute (currently Institute of Information Technology), Jahangirnagar University, Savar, Dhaka, Bangladesh. His current research interest is in developing statistical and machine learning models/frameworks to analyze big data and trajectory risk prediction collected longitudinally. His research interests include covariate-dependent Markov models, repeated measure data, joint modeling, and models for extensive data analysis, among others.

Alex Cousins is currently a researcher at Cape Breton University. Alex's graduate work was in philosophy and political science, with research focused on education and training for medical professionals, ethics in mental health, and political philosophy. Alex is passionate about interdisciplinary work that bridges the gap between theory and practice, particularly in bringing rich insights from one field into another. Alex's work aims to integrate the depth of philosophical inquiry into practical applications, such as informing policy with a more profound understanding of underlying principles. Alex is committed to translating academic knowledge into actionable insights for practitioners, enhancing their professional development and enabling them to approach their work with a deeper, more informed perspective.

Karen Parker Davidson is a global expert in nasal function, data interpretation, AI methods, and the medical devices used to capture data. In this field, she has numerous copyrights and pending patents. For more than three decades, she has held several positions in the medical device industry and various clinical nursing positions, and has specialty certifications in the private sector and time in the US Air Force Reserves as a flight nurse and critical care nurse. He is a respected educator, subject matter expert (SME), and adjunct professor at Liberty University and Central Michigan University.

She is the vice president at GM Instruments, Ltd.; founder of FACT Healthcare Consulting Group, LLC; and the co-founder of Reliant Biomedical Technologies. She is an executive board member and president at the Healthcare Navigation Project 501(c)(3), an editorial board member for *Dental Sleep Practice* (DSP) magazine, a peer reviewer for medical journals, currently serving a 4-year term on the Commission on Dental Accreditation (CODA) Review Committee, and a member of the American College of Healthcare Executives (ACHE).

Her research discussing nasal function and breathing disorders can be found in various medical journals, magazines, books, and academic textbooks. She is the author of *Breathe through Your Nose, Don't Pay through It: The Impact the Healthcare Industry Has on Nasal Function and How We Breathe*; the creator and author of the *My Little Nose* series of children's books; a contributing author to *Growing into Breathing Problems: The Quest for Collaborative Lifetime Solutions* (2024), *Health Informatics and Patient Safety in Times of Crisis* (2023), *The Clinician's Handbook for Dental Sleep Medicine* (2nd ed.; 2024), and *Healthcare Informatics Innovation Post-COVID-19 Pandemic* (2025); and a coauthor of future releases The Power of the Tongue In the Beginning, We

Were All Tongue Tied and Sleep Apnea and Pregnancy: The Female Response to Sleep Breathing Disorders. She is a member of speaker bureaus and a guest lecturer at university residency programs and professional academy meetings at the national and international levels.

Her work has been awarded and recognized by Women We Admire as one of the top 50 women leaders in the Washington, DC for 2022; she has been identified as a 2023 Carolina Nursing Alumni Award nominee for outstanding contributions to the field of nursing and research and is a recipient of a National Science Foundation award as a team member in the development of a medical device for improved manual ventilation in airway emergencies. She is also recognized by the Speaker of the House, US House of Representatives, in a congratulatory letter of recognition. She holds a Doctor of Health Administration degree with a focus on health policy; three master's degrees in administration, nursing, and education; and a bachelor's degree in nursing; and is currently pursuing a PhD in Business Administration with an emphasis in international business. She is a member of the ACHE.

Azam Dekamin holds a PhD from Toronto Metropolitan University, Canada. She is a lecturer at Cape Breton University and a freelance data science consultant focused on developing cutting-edge artificial intelligence (AI) and analytics products. Her research interests include data analytics, AI, predictive modeling, causal inference, and medical decision-making.

John J. Georrge is an associate professor at the Department of Bioinformatics, University of North Bengal, Darjeeling, West Bengal, India. He is also one of the executive council members of the University of North Bengal and a member of a governing body of the Salesian College, Sonada and Siliguri (autonomous), as a University of North Bengal representative. Formerly, for about two decades, he served as an assistant professor and head at the Department of Bioinformatics, Christ College, affiliated with Saurashtra University, Rajkot. Besides that, he served as a bioinformatics nodal officer of Gujarat State Biotechnology Mission (GSBTM, Government of Gujarat) and a coordinator of the Department of Biotechnology (DBT), and Government of India sponsored postgraduate diploma in the computational biology course. He has received the Best Teacher Award twice from the Gujarat Science Academy and William Research Center, Kanyakumari, India. He is a visiting researcher at the Indian Institute of Science (IISc), Bangalore. He is also a former research associate at the Institute of Biochemistry and Molecular Biology, University of Bonn, Germany, where he researched novel drug target identifications through proteomics approaches. Under his supervision, three students completed their PhD, and two PhD students are expected to complete it soon. He has been a resource person for over 65 international and national symposia, workshops, seminars, etc., and has published over 100 research papers and chapters in internationally reputed journals and books. He holds master's degrees in various subjects such as biotechnology, bioinformatics, law, and PhD, and many diplomas. He is a highly dynamic teacher, researcher, and academic administrator.

Narayana Goruntla received his Bachelor of Pharmacy (2006) and Master of Pharmacy in pharmacy practice in 2008 from Annamalai University, Chidambaram, Tamil Nadu. He joined the Raghavendra Institute of Pharmaceutical Education & Research (RIPER), Jawaharlal Nehru Technological University Anantapur, where he teaches courses dealing with professional practice and patient care as assistant professor and hospital in-charge in the Department of Pharmacy Practice since 2009. He has been a scientific co-coordinator of International Society for Pharmacoeconomics & Outcome Research (ISPOR), Andhra Pradesh—regional chapter—India since February 2009 and director of ISPOR AP chapter since 2015. He was skilled in various areas of pharmacovigilance, including the detection, assessment, and monitoring of adverse drug reactions. His research interests include pharmacovigilance, therapeutic drug monitoring (TDM), and medication therapy management (MTM) services, as well as patient counseling and community educational programs. He participated in conferences and seminars at both national and international levels. He organized a "one-day national symposium on pharmacoeconomics and outcome research" at RDT Hospital, Bathalapalli. Currently, he works as an associate professor in the Department of Clinical Pharmacy and Pharmacy Practice at Kampala International University (KIU), Western Campus, Ishaka, Uganda. He has expertise in pharmacoepidemiology and pharmacoeconomics/clinical epidemiology/community medicine. He has vast experience in teaching and research guidance in pharmaceutical care, pharmacovigilance, pharmacoeconomics, and rational drug use. He is recognized as a supervisor/guide for undergraduate/postgraduate students and as a visiting professor/subject matter expert/evaluator/examiner for universities.

Virginia Gunn is an assistant professor at the School of Nursing at Cape Breton University, NS, Canada, and an affiliate researcher at the Institute of Environmental Medicine, Karolinska Institute, Sweden. She completed her PhD and master's studies at the University of Toronto and acquired cross-disciplinary academic and research training in health and social sciences. Dr. Gunn is currently involved in several international AI projects involving multidisciplinary teams of researchers from Sweden, Finland, the Netherlands, Spain, Australia, and the United States. Specific research areas include algorithmic management (AM) and its impact on workers' health and well-being, the application of AM to healthcare, and the training of the workforce in healthcare informatics.

Ruiling Guo is a professor of healthcare administration at Idaho State University's College of Business. She holds a Doctor of Health Administration (DHA) from Central Michigan University, a Master of Library and Information Science (MLIS) from McGill University, and a Master of Public Health (MPH) from Idaho State University. Dr. Guo has extensive working and teaching experience in academia and international healthcare systems. Her current research interests focus on evidence-based management in healthcare, population health, healthcare policy, comparative health systems, and health information science. Dr Guo teaches both graduate and undergraduate courses in healthcare administration. She holds a graduate faculty position at Idaho State University's Graduate School. The courses she has taught include the US Health System and Policy, Business of Healthcare, Health Care Policy, Health Information System, Health Informatics, Managerial Epidemiology, Population Health, Health Services Management, AI and IT in Healthcare, and Administration and Management of Healthcare Organizations. Dr. Guo serves as a board member of the Association of the University Programs in Health Administration (AUPHA), an editorial board member of the ACHE, a fellow of the Center for Evidence-Based Management, a distinguished member of the Academy of Health Information Professionals (AHIP), a member of the ACHE, and a reviewer for the AUPHA certification committees and peer-reviewed journals in healthcare administration and medicine/health sciences. She has received numerous research grants and awards and published over 25 peer-reviewed articles.

Kusum Gurung is a postgraduate student. She is interested in and has worked in fields like pharmacogenomics, trends of AI in healthcare, automation in healthcare, and personalized medicines. She is passionate about modifying the healthcare sector with advanced technologies, making diagnosis and treatments easier, and increasing the success rate.

Charlotte Hruczkowski completed a Bachelor of Science in nursing and a Master of Nursing in teaching and is currently a PhD candidate in educational psychology. As an educator across the health professions, she has taught various courses in online and in-person environments. Her students have praised her ability to teach and support their learning using simulation and technology, which was demonstrated by her receiving a nomination for the Jaye Fredrickson Award for Teaching Excellence in 2018. She is also proud of developing training courses for health providers in various clinical settings.

Mohamad Y. Jaber is a professor of Industrial Engineering at Toronto Metropolitan University (formerly Ryerson University). His PhD is in manufacturing and operations management from the

University of Nottingham, UK. Dr. Jaber has published many papers in peer-reviewed journals and conferences and a few edited books and has supervised many postdoctoral fellows and doctoral and master's students. He is an editor for *Applied Mathematical Modeling, Computers & Industrial Engineering*, and Information Systems and Operational Research (INFOR) and a member of the editorial boards for several journals. Dr. Jaber received research funding from Canadian federal agencies. He has served on several committees and is a member of several professional societies. Dr. Jaber is an adjunct faculty at the University of Dalhousie, Canada, and a member of the PhD program board in Energy Transition and Sustainable Production Systems at the University of Brescia, Italy.

Soosamma John is an associate professor at the Department of Pharmacognosy, East Point College of Pharmacy, Bengaluru, Karnataka. She graduated with a BPharm from JSS College of Pharmacy, Rocklands, Ooty, in 1992 and an MPharm (pharmacognosy) in 2007 from Al-Ameen College of Pharmacy, Bangalore. She has 11 years of industrial experience and 17 years of teaching experience. She has attended various national and international conferences conducted by multiple institutions. She has over 15 national and international papers in her account and two patents in her credit.

Ruchi Joshi, assistant professor at Manipal University, Jaipur, is an academician, researcher, and RCI-certified rehabilitation counsellor. She has completed her master's in clinical psychology from Jai Narayan Vyas University, a doctorate from Rajasthan University, a postgraduate diploma in child guidance and counseling from Kota Open University, and an advanced diploma in child guidance and counselling from Jai Narayan Vyas University, Jodhpur. She has 10 years of experience in counseling, research, and teaching in various parts of the country. She has been associated with organizations of repute like Mohan Lal Sukhadia University, Udaipur; Poornima Group of Colleges, Jaipur; Maharana Mewar Public School, Udaipur; and Amity University, Rajasthan. She has several national and international publications to her credit, including UGC CARE, Taylor and Francis Index, and publication houses. She has presented papers at several international-, national-, and regional-level conferences, seminars, workshops, etc. She has been invited as a resource person and panelist in workshops, panel discussions, seminars. and webinars on issues related to mental health and physical and sexual violence.

Sindhuja Manisha Kamini P is a consultant psychologist and former assistant professor at CHRIST (deemed to be university) in Bengaluru. She holds a PhD in clinical psychology from Amity University Jaipur, with her research focusing on menstrual experiences and psychosocial attributes among adolescent girls. In addition to her academic role, she serves as the director of The Sanguine Minds Psychology Clinic in Tamil Nadu, where she provides psychological assessments and therapy. Dr. Sindhuja is an active researcher with numerous publications and presentations in national and international forums, and she is dedicated to advancing mental health awareness and education. She is a project scientist I for the ICMR_Granthon—2022 at St. John's Medical College.

Karina Kim is a researcher from the Business School of the Kazakh-British Technical University of Almaty, Kazakhstan. Karina's research interests are marketing and consumer behavior, brand management, entrepreneurship, and innovation management.

Tim Konoval is an interdisciplinary health assistant professor at the College of Health Sciences, University of Alberta. Tim holds a BSc in kinesiology, a master's in sport management, and a PhD in sociocultural studies. Tim has taught and developed several undergraduate and graduate courses in sports, physical activity, and health throughout his academic years. Tim's diverse degree areas have led to a deep interest in interdisciplinarity. His research intersects teams, leadership, equity, and culture. Moving from sports to health system studies has changed his focus to collaborative care and examining how health professionals can work better together. In his current role, Tim is teaching IP health courses and leading the development of a new undergraduate health sciences degree program.

Andréia de Bem Machado has a PhD in engineering and knowledge management. She is a post-doctoral fellow at the Federal University of Santa Catarina and an evaluator of the National Institute of Educational Studies and Research Anísio Teixeira (Ministry of Education Brazil). She is an ad hoc evaluator of national and international journals, an evaluator in the PNLD Infantile Education program, and a consultant in the production of low-vision UNESCO teaching material. She has been working in the education field for over 25 years. She is part of the scientific committee of national and international journals. Currently, her areas of study are innovation in the public sector, entrepreneurship, smart cities, education, special education, and digital pedagogical models. She likes to innovate in the art of researching and disseminating knowledge.

Matthew MacLeod is a research assistant at Cape Breton University, working on several projects focused on AM, including a scoping review of applications of AM in healthcare and a scoping review of interventions addressing the impact of AM on workers and work environments. Matthew's research interests include AM bias and how AM perpetuates discriminatory attitudes against specific population groups. He is currently applying to graduate school and planning on studying applied psychology with a focus on forensic psychology.

Anupam Maity is an assistant professor in East Point College of Pharmacy, Bangalore, Karnataka. He has completed his BPharm from Dr. B. C. Roy College of Pharmacy & Allied Health Sciences, Durgapur, WB, and his MPharm from Rajiv Gandhi University of Health Sciences, Bangalore, Karnataka. He qualified for the Graduate Pharmacy Aptitude Test (GPAT) in 2021 with an All-India Rank of 1509. He has published one review paper. He is a registered pharmacist under the West Bengal Pharmacy Council. He has a keen interest in novel drug delivery systems and nanoformulations to improve the solubility and bioavailability of anticancer drugs.

Suman Kumar Maji received his PhD in computer science from INRIA Bordeaux, France, in 2014 following a postgraduate degree in telecommunication networks from the Indian Institute of Technology Kharagpur, India, in 2008. From 2014 to 2015, he worked as a research engineer with the Institute of Hematology, University Paris 7, and INSERM. He is an assistant professor at the Department of Computer Science and Engineering, Indian Institute of Technology Patna, India. His research interests include medical imaging, bioinformatics, machine learning, and image processing. Dr. Maji has authored several conferences and journal papers and was a recipient of various research fellowships and awards such as the European CORDIS Doctoral Fellowship, Region Aquitaine OPTAD Research Fellowship, FRM Research Fellowship, SERB Early Career Research Award, and SERB CRG Research Grant.

Neeraj Makhija has extensive experience managing technology teams and large projects in organizations such as GE Healthcare, Sonar Technologies, Alfred Imaging, and Scan Connect. Neeraj has over 20 years of industry experience designing and supporting systems for central banks, hospitals, HIMS, and PACS & RIS-based systems. He has been instrumental in project-managing deployments of large PACS and RIS installations in Australia. As technical director of Scan Connect, Neeraj played a critical role in defining the technology roadmap for Scan Connect, "A health Solutions Company with a vision of one diagnostic network," and drove the innovation of solutions for major healthcare providers and users. He has also been the acting CIO for AHSconnect, a significant provider of services in the healthcare IT field, dealing mainly with radiology and associated sciences. Neeraj now leads 'Scan@ptics' as the CEO. Scan@ptics is the first-of-its-kind cloud provider on RIS/PACS and EDI solution suite for radiology providers.

Premkumar Mathusudhanan has experience working as a system administrator and has been involved in setting up and managing RIS/PACS support for radiology providers while working with Alfred Imaging. Premkumar was a part of the technical team that set up, managed, and maintained the radiology support systems for AHS and Scan Connect. He is currently the systems and application support for Scan@ptics, the first-of-its-kind cloud provider on RIS/PACS and EDI solution suite for radiology providers.

Saurav Kumar Mishra does research in miRNAs, immunoinformatics, computational biology, molecular biology, and host–pathogen interaction analysis.

Mohamad Musa is an assistant professor and founding faculty member in the Department of Social Work at Cape Breton University. Mohamad received his PhD in social work from the University of Windsor. His area of research is mental illness perceptions and mental health education among migrant populations from the Middle East. Mohamad is focused on engaging service users and providers to enhance the existing mental health systems in Atlantic Canada. Mohamad's other research areas include social work education, the scholarship of teaching and learning, and child welfare. Mohamad has extensive clinical practice experience as a clinical supervisor and clinical therapist in postsecondary institutions, youth health, youth mental health, and youth justice agencies in Canada.

Bissultan Omirbayev is a business disciplines researcher from the Business School of Kazakh-British Technical University of Almaty, Kazakhstan. Bissultan's research interests are entrepreneurship, small business management, and innovation management.

Benjamin A. Osawe is the founder and president of Clarity Advisory Services LLC, a boutique advisory practice specializing in information technology services, including cybersecurity, IT administration, and strategic planning. He is a seasoned project management executive with over 25 years of technology and operations management experience. He has held positions in various aspects of technology, including information management services, telecommunications, project management, engineering services, and operations management for multinational companies. He is an experienced and versatile technology leader with attention to detail, customer service, and oral communication skills, and is strong in vendor management, business development, project planning, and problem-solving. His areas of expertise include project management, reverse engineering, vulnerability analysis, network analysis, assembly, network protocols like Agile and scrum, Oracle database design, and software requirements gathering using unified modeling language (UML). He started his career as an engineer and has a BEng in mechanical engineering from the University of Ilorin, Nigeria. He has completed his MSc in computer science at the University of Bradford, United Kingdom. Since relocating to the United States, he has completed his DM in Information Systems & Technology at the University of Phoenix, AZ, and MSc in cybersecurity at the University of Delaware, DE. Due to his keen interest in cybersecurity as a consultant, he is completing his DEng in cybersecurity at George Washington University, Washington, DC. He is married with three children and lives in Maryland, USA. He is an active member of the Institute of Electrical and Electronics Engineers (IEEE) and the Project Management Institute (PMI).

Lola A. Osawe is an innovative and well-rounded executive with over 25 years of leadership experience. She has successfully managed programs and facilities, leading diverse military, private, and public teams. Her most recent leadership roles include starting Clarity Advisory Services, an IT company, with her husband as co-founder; serving as a CEO of a privately held medical group; service-line leadership as director of cancer services for the regional health system; management consultant in physician services; and leading a joint venture ambulatory surgery center. Her professional interests include practice management, health information technology, digital health, organizational transformation, and the use of digital platforms, including AI in healthcare delivery optimization. Dr. Osawe is double board certified as a Fellow of the ACHE (FACHE) and a Fellow of the American College of Medical Practice Executives (FACMPE). She received her DHA and postgraduate certificate in international health from Central Michigan University, Michigan. She also received her

Master of Health Services Administration from Central Michigan University, a second master's in military operational art and leadership from Air University and her bachelor's degree in biological sciences from the University of Delaware. She has served on healthcare boards as a national board member, the Medical Group Management Association (MGMA), former chair of the Higher Education Network Committee, ACHE, and various state-level leadership roles throughout her career. Before her civilian career, she served on active duty in various leadership roles in military treatment facilities, including leading health information systems; managed care operations; and served as a line officer before her medical service officer appointment as a management engineer, ensuring adequate workforce and resource allocation for warfighters. She continues her military service in the reserves (current grade Colonel) in the Air Force Medical Service (AFMS), supporting medical operations for Unites States Space Force personnel at the office of the Air Force Surgeon General. She is married with three kids and lives in Maryland.

Nades Palaniyar received a PhD in molecular biology and genetics at the University of Guelph, Canada. As a postdoctoral fellow, he studied DNA/RNA and immune systems at the University of Cincinnati, USA; University of Oxford, UK; and Harvard Medical School, USA. He continues to conduct research work on the innate immune system, neutrophils, rare pediatric lung diseases (e.g., cystic fibrosis, alveolar proteinosis, respiratory distress, surfactants, MUC5B deficiency, and neuroendocrine system), COVID-19, and other infectious and inflammatory diseases. Dr. Palaniyar and his research lab made 78 original discoveries, and he has authored more than 100 scientific publications and made more than 200 conference presentations. For the last 15 years, he has been the chair of the Technological Advances in Science, Medicine, and Engineering (TASME) international conference and helped increase participation from 7 to 700. For his research work, leadership, and dedication, TASME awarded him a "Lifetime Scientific Achievement Award" and a "Visionary Leader" title and named an award the "Nades Palaniyar Award."

Pandimurugan V is an associate professor of computer science and engineering at the Acharya Institute of Technology, Bangalore, India. He completed his BE (EEE) and ME (CSE) at Anna University in 2005 and 2008, respectively. He completed his PhD (CSE) in 2019 from Manonmaniam Sundaranar University (MSU) Tirunelveli, Tamil Nadu. He has 15 years of teaching experience and has published 24 Scopus-indexed papers, which include 8 SCI papers. His research interests include health informatics, AI, and IoT. He has published principles of communication, Python, and three Scopus-indexed book chapters. He has three granted and two published patents in his credit.

Antonio Pesqueira is a healthcare commercial leader specializing in life sciences, a university professor, and a research fellow at ISCTE/Instituto Universitário de Lisboa (IUL). The current areas of his research interest are digital technologies, healthcare data management, blockchain, innovation, and business management. Among his other activities are having served as the chair of the Pharmaceutical Supply Chain & Security World Forum and a regular keynote speaker at the Pharma Track & Trace, Serialization & Labeling Summit.

In addition to coauthoring more than 20 articles and book chapters, Antonio has published in several scientific journals (such as the *Journal of Business Research*, *Future Generations Computer Systems*, *Journal of Medical Systems*, *Journal of Knowledge Management*, *WSEAS Transactions on Business and Economics*, and *Information Systems Frontiers*) and peer-reviewed international conferences. Furthermore, he holds certifications in data science and agile coaching.

Rajasekhara Mouly Potluri is a seasoned academician and researcher with an illustrious career spanning 33 years in industry and academia across ten countries. He is currently serving as a professor of marketing at the Business School of Kazakh-British Technical University in Almaty, Kazakhstan, and holds a PhD and MPhil in management/marketing from Shivaji University. He also earned an MBA in marketing and an MCom in banking from Andhra University, India. He has made significant contributions to scholarly literature with over a 120 publications, including research articles, books, book chapters, and case studies. His work appears in prestigious peer-reviewed journals indexed in Scopus, Australian Business Deans Council (ABDC), Social Sciences Citation Index (SSCI), IEEE, KCI, and international conferences. He has been honored with over 20 Best Research Paper Awards and Academic Service Excellence Awards, underscoring his impactful research contributions. His research interests encompass marketing, Islamic marketing, corporate social responsibility (CSR) and sustainability, human resource management (HRM) and organizational behavior (OB), and entrepreneurship. He continues to enrich the academic community with his extensive knowledge and research contributions, aiming to advance understanding and practices in his areas of expertise globally.

Rajaram V is currently an assistant professor in the Department of Networking and Communication, School of Computing, SRM Institute of Science and Technology, Kattankulathur. He completed his doctorate from Anna University, Chennai, and has 13 years of teaching experience. He has published several research papers in international journals and conferences. His research areas include wireless sensor networks and IoT.

David J. Ranney is an accomplished author specializing in healthcare-related topics. He holds an MBA from Regis University and a Master of International Management from Whitworth University. David earned his DHA from Central Michigan University. His graduate fellowship was conducted through Yale University and the Clinton Foundation in Ethiopia, focusing on international healthcare. David is spearheading efforts to bridge the knowledge gap between universities and healthcare organizations in Africa. He is crucial in establishing Africa's College of Healthcare Administrators (AfCHCA) and actively contributes to the Global Health Executive Mentoring (GHEM) program.

Myllissa Reyes is a distinguished Air Force veteran who served with honor and dedication, contributing significantly to national defense and security. After her military service, Myllissa pursued higher education, earning a BSc from Boise State University. Her commitment to advancing her knowledge and skills led her to further her education at Idaho State University, where she obtained a master's in healthcare administration. Myllissa's unique combination of military experience and academic achievement positions her as a competent and knowledgeable professional in the healthcare administration field. Her leadership skills, enhanced in the Air Force, complement her in-depth understanding of healthcare systems, making her a valuable asset in improving healthcare delivery and policy. Myllissa is dedicated to using her expertise to enhance the quality of care and operational efficiency within healthcare organizations. She is a member of the ACHE.

Sneha Roy is a dedicated student in the field of chemoinformatics, with a focus on drug discovery, personalized drug development, network pharmacology, and plant-derived natural products using advanced computational and bioinformatics approaches.

Smitha Shivshankar is the associate dean (academic) at the Australian International Institute of Higher Education, Sydney, NSW, Australia. At the heart of her profile is a commitment to empowering the next generation of IT professionals. She has actively participated in the pivotal processes that uphold the quality of education, and this experience has equipped her with a profound understanding of the standards and expectations of the modern-day academic landscape. She is currently focused on critical areas of research in teaching and learning, the impact of AI on teaching and learning, and cybersecurity and AI in healthcare. She is passionate about understanding AI as cutting-edge technology and advancing research collaborations. She is collaborating with Scanaptics, a leading RIS–PACS–EDI provider, to explore the transformative potential of AI.

Maria José Sousa is a pro-rector for the Development of Distance Learning and a professor and a research fellow at ISCTE/IUL. She is also an expert in digital education and digital skills, as she assumed a postdoc position from 2016 to 2018, researching that field, with several publications in journals with high impact factors (*Journal of Business Research, Journal of Grid Computing, Future Generation Computer Systems*, and others). She worked as an expert on a European Commission project to create a new category regarding digital skills to be integrated with the European Innovation Scoreboard (EIS). She was a member of the Coordinator Committee of the PhD in management at Universidade Europeia. She was also a senior researcher at GEE (Research Office) in the Portuguese Ministry of Economy, where she was responsible for innovation, research, and entrepreneurship policies. She was a knowledge and competencies manager at American Medical Association (AMA), IP, and Public Reform Agency (Ministry of the Presidency and the Ministers Council). She was also a project manager at the Ministry of Labor and Employment, responsible for innovation, evaluation, and development of qualification projects. Her current research interests are public policies on innovation and education. She is a best-seller author in research methods, information and communication technologies (ICT), and people management; and has coauthored over 100 articles and book chapters in high-level journals (such as the *European Planning Studies, Information Systems Frontiers, Systems Research, Behavioral Science, Computational and Mathematical Organization Theory*, and *Future Generation Computer Systems*); and is the guest-editor of more than 5 special issues from Elsevier and Springer.

Chandrashekar Thalluri is an associate professor at the Faculty of Pharmaceutical Science, Assam Downtown University, Assam, India. He earned his postgraduate degree in pharmaceutics from the Tamil Nadu Dr. M.G.R. Medical University, Chennai, India, in 2009 and his PhD in pharmaceutical science from Jawaharlal Nehru Technological University Anantapur, Andhra Pradesh, India, in 2016. Dr. Thalluri is a prolific researcher and academician, having authored three books and published sixteen articles. He actively participates in scientific research and is a peer reviewer for national and international journals. He has presented over 20 scientific papers at various seminars and conferences. As a mentor, Dr. Thalluri supervises six PhD scholars and has guided 14 postgraduate students through their research projects. He is also involved with several journal editorial boards and professional bodies in India. Balancing his extensive academic responsibilities with ongoing scholarly activities, Dr. Thalluri continues to contribute significantly to the field of pharmaceutical science through his research and participation in educational seminars.

Christopher Thompson is an emergency medicine resident physician at Dignity Health East Valley in Chandler, Arizona. He holds a Doctor of Osteopathic Medicine (DO) from the Idaho College of Osteopathic Medicine, is a current candidate for a Master of Healthcare Administration (MHA) from Idaho State University and received his Bachelor of Science (BS) in exercise science from Brigham Young University. Dr. Thompson completed medical school at the Idaho College of Osteopathic Medicine. While there, he pursued a concurrent degree of a MHA from Idaho State university. He is intensely interested in the medical and business aspects of the current US healthcare system. He recently began his emergency medicine residency training at Dignity Health East Valley in Chandler, Arizona. Dr. Thompson continues to be heavily engaged in undergraduate medical education at the Idaho College of Osteopathic Medicine by serving as a lead tutor and medical student advisor for undergraduate medical students. He has also received many prestigious awards, including Student Leader of the Year, Sterling F. Welch Scholar Award, and ultimately the Class of 2024 President's Award. Dr. Thompson is a member of the American College of Emergency Physicians (ACEP), the American College of Osteopathic Medicine Physicians (ACOEP), the Emergency Medicine Residents' Association (EMRA), and the American College of Physicians (ACP). He has also published medical research in the *Journal of Ultrasound in Medicine*.

Umamageswaran C is an assistant professor in the Department of Computer Science Engineering at Amrita School of Computing, Amrita Vishwa Vidyapeetham. He completed his BTech in Information Technology in 2005 from Vel Tech Engineering College (Anna University), Chennai, and his ME in Computer Science and Engineering in 2010 from Vel Tech Multi Tech Dr. RR Dr. SR Engineering College (Anna University), Chennai. He obtained his PhD in Information and Communication Engineering from Anna University, Chennai, in 2023. He has 16 years of teaching experience and has presented and published many national and international conferences and journals.

M. I. M. Wahab received a BSc (Eng) in mechanical engineering from the University of Moratuwa, Sri Lanka, in 1995; an MEng in industrial engineering from the Asian Institute of Technology, Bangkok, Thailand, in 1999; and a PhD in industrial engineering from the University of Toronto, Canada, in 2006. He is currently a professor of industrial engineering and an associate chair of the Mechanical and Industrial Engineering Department at Ryerson University, Toronto, ON, Canada. He has published several journal and conference papers and book chapters. His research interests lie in intersections between operations research and finance. He has actively carried out research in the areas of supply chain management, service management, and manufacturing systems. He is a registered professional engineer in the Province of Ontario, Canada. While pursuing a master's degree at the Asian Institute of Technology in Thailand, Sri Lanka-born Mohamed Wahab received a unique recognition: He was awarded a scholarship from the King of Thailand. "The experience illustrated that remarkable things happen when you strive for excellence," says Wahab. Moving to Canada to pursue doctoral studies in industrial engineering, Wahab went on to specialize in helping organizations improve their operations and decision-making. With expertise in operational research and finance engineering, Wahab works across diverse industries, including healthcare, energy, supply chain, marketing, and finance. The projects he leads are as diverse as the industries he serves. He has worked with marketing firms to improve their process of introducing new products to market, built a model for a major grocery store chain to predict how changes in weather impact the demand for coffee, and designed a first-of-its-kind financial model that enables a major auto manufacturer to assess the cost of purchasing a flexible manufacturing system. "The common theme in my work is helping organizations become more efficient and effective," he says. "I love combining theory and application to find ways to make better decisions.

Tadele Mekuriya Yadesa is an academician, researcher, and clinical pharmacist consultant. Dr. Tadele completed his BPharm (2010) and MSc in clinical pharmacy (2014), both from Jimma University, Ethiopia. He received his PhD in medication safety in 2023 from Mbarara University of Science and Technology, Uganda. Dr. Tadele also completed a postdoctoral fellowship under Lancet Global Commission in Medical Oxygen Security at Makerere University, Uganda. He has worked as a senior lecturer in five different universities in Ethiopia and Uganda since 2014. He has various experiences, and a skill mix in teaching and research across different pharmacy, medicine, and public health areas. Dr. Tadele has supervised more than 24 master's students to graduation. In addition, he has extensive experience as a clinical pharmacy practitioner and clinical tutor to undergraduate and postgraduate pharmacy students. Dr. Tadele has authored about 45 articles in peer-reviewed journals, coauthored several book chapters in reputable publishers, and edited a book for Elsevier Science publishers.

1 Healthcare Informatics Innovation Post-COVID-19
Lessons, Challenges, and Opportunities

Philip Eappen and Narasimha Rao Vajjhala

1.1 INTRODUCTION

The coronavirus disease 2019 (COVID-19) pandemic has brought significant changes to healthcare and acted as a pivotal force for innovation and transformation. The pandemic highlighted the strengths and vulnerabilities of healthcare systems, leading to an accelerated adoption of digital technologies and a redefined, crucial role for healthcare informatics (HI) in the post-pandemic era. As healthcare systems transition into this new era, integrating HI advancements is critical in enhancing resilience, efficiency, and quality of care (Yogesh & Karthikeyan, 2022).

The pandemic pointed out several critical lessons for the future of HI. The need for real-time data analysis, technology integration, and quicker responses to health threats became more evident and allowed policymakers to make necessary changes. These new lessons have informed the development of innovative practices to improve healthcare systems' efficiency and resilience (Glette et al., 2023). Many countries utilized this opportunity, and many healthcare systems across the globe have successfully implemented digital transformation strategies, including using more and more electronic health records (EHRs) and telemedicine platforms, enhancing healthcare delivery and addressing existing healthcare challenges (Senbekov et al., 2020).

Moreover, the transition characterized by integrating medical Internet of Things (MIoT) technologies revolutionizes patient monitoring and remote diagnostics (Li et al., 2024). IoT devices made the monitoring easier for healthcare professionals and made it more comfortable for their patients. Many IoT devices had emerged during the pandemic, and many were better refined to suit the needs of patients and healthcare professionals after the pandemic. However, this shift brings significant privacy challenges, necessitating robust strategies to protect patient data (Pool et al., 2024). The widespread adoption of interconnected health devices across the globe requires a careful balance between innovation and privacy protection (Yadav, 2024).

The pandemic also brought in many devices such as remote applications for detecting hearing loss, and they have gained prominence, offering accessible diagnostic services for patients in rural areas and others with less access (Irace et al., 2020). Pandemic also brought and refined systems capable of monitoring oxygen saturation, blood pressure, temperature, and so on from a distance and providing accurate feedback on time to their assigned professionals. These technologies have proven effective in diagnosing and managing hearing loss remotely, particularly during the pandemic when in-person visits were limited. Post-pandemic world has accepted and started using such technologies more often than before, and it has helped provide care much easier than earlier.

DOI: 10.1201/9781003485629-1

1.2 REVIEW OF LITERATURE

Artificial intelligence (AI) has emerged as a transformative force in managing post-pandemic healthcare needs in various parts of the globe (Eappen, 2022). AI applications, ranging from predictive analytics to personalized treatment plans, have significantly improved disease prediction, patient management, and operational efficiency across different continents, especially in high- and medium-income countries (Alowais et al., 2023). AI in healthcare has changed into a tremendous tool in addressing mental health challenges by offering digital tools and virtual therapy solutions to patients from a distance during the pandemic, and it has turned into a common practice post-pandemic as well (Alowais et al., 2023). Similarly, the contemporary healthcare landscape is becoming more intricate, requiring more innovative approaches to maintain a balance among efficiency, effectiveness, and care quality (Vajjhala & Eappen, 2024).

Machine learning (ML) has been instrumental in identifying and managing health crises during the pandemic (Malik et al., 2020). Various models have been applied to predict outbreaks, monitor disease progression, and analyze health data, providing valuable insights for crisis management across the globe. ML techniques have paved the way for more effective health responses, reassuring us about the potential of ML in future pandemics and for future healthcare operations. Moreover, large datasets created during the pandemic have helped the advancements make more accurate predictions compared to pre-pandemic. During and after the pandemic, ML has emerged as a significant field of study due to its ability to address a wide range of complex and challenging healthcare issues (Sharma et al., 2023). By leveraging large datasets and powerful computational techniques, ML has been applied successfully in various domains, including healthcare and many more. Development and access to sophisticated algorithms during the pandemic through deep learning, reinforcement learning, and unsupervised learning have further enhanced the capabilities of ML and made it capable enough to tackle issues that were unresolved pre-pandemic (Syeda et al., 2021).

Furthermore, integration of AI, ML in fluorescence microscopy, and computational imaging has revolutionized healthcare research and diagnostics by enhancing precision, efficiency, and accuracy in data analysis (Quazi, 2022). AI and ML have become essential tools for disease detection, personalized treatment, and predictive analytics, analyzing large datasets to uncover patterns and improve patient outcomes (Alowais et al., 2023). Concurrently, advancements in fluorescence microscopy, such as super-resolution and live-cell imaging, have significantly increased the ability to study biological processes at the molecular level with higher clarity (Chen et al., 2024). Computational imaging further amplifies these capabilities by improving image quality and enabling detailed analysis through algorithms and AI. Moreover, it is evident that the advancements post-pandemic and consistent usage of technologies have led to more reliable diagnostics and better treatment options, and ultimately improved healthcare outcomes (Yeung et al., 2023).

In addition, public health strategies during the pandemic have turned to data-driven insights for improving health outcomes and refining decision-making processes. By depending on comprehensive data, public health professionals can identify trends, assess risks, and allocate resources efficiently, which will lead to more impactful and targeted interventions. Datasets that track health-related variables over extended periods are valuable in this context, and they enable the analysis of long-term trends and identification of emerging health threats. Moreover, public health professionals can gain a deeper understanding of the factors influencing health outcomes and adjust strategies by examining changes over time within populations (Braveman & Gottlieb, 2014). The use of longitudinal data supports the design and implementation of effective public health initiatives and plays a critical role in monitoring their impact over time. Similarly, observing the long-term effects of lifestyle interventions on chronic diseases helps refine public health guidelines to prevent and manage chronic conditions. Emphasis on data-driven decision-making creates confidence in both the public and professionals.

Rapid evolution of HI during and after the pandemic presents new challenges for workforce training. Continuous education and skill development are essential for healthcare professionals to keep pace with technological advancements (Lera et al., 2020). Strategies for managing these training challenges include curriculum development, professional development programs, and certification initiatives designed to equip the workforce with the necessary skills. In addition, digital health technologies have transformed how healthcare teams collaborate and deliver care by integrating these technologies. However, integration requires careful consideration of policies and practices to ensure effective implementation and coordination within healthcare teams (Yogesh & Karthikeyan, 2022).

HI has certainly fixed some gaps that existed earlier by using telehealth as a vital component of modern healthcare, bridging the digital divide and improving access to care (Eappen & Olujinmi, 2022). The expansion of telehealth services during the pandemic has highlighted its potential to address disparities in healthcare access, particularly in underserved populations (Franciosi et al., 2021). Moreover, proliferation of 5G networks helped make HI works better due to their better speed and brought significant potential for their faster implementation (Vajjhala & Eappen, 2023). In addition, intelligent transportation systems (ITS) offer significant potential for improving healthcare delivery by optimizing logistics and patient access. These systems enhance patient transportation, emergency response, and logistical coordination, improving healthcare outcomes (Ardakani et al., 2023).

Despite all the merits, there are demerits to consider as well. Expansion of HI made the ethical, privacy, and security concerns become more important. Best practices for protecting sensitive health information and ensuring compliance with regulatory standards are very critical to maintain the trust of patients (Tariq & Hackert, 2023). Moreover, healthcare professionals have the moral responsibility to hold the ethics, privacy, and security of patient data very high to keep the trust of patients toward innovations in healthcare. In addition, cybersecurity remains a critical challenge in HI, and the rise in current cyberattacks on healthcare organizations highlights the need for robust security measures. Analyzing trends and strategies for improving cybersecurity is necessary to protect against emerging threats and for keeping patient trust and confidence in the healthcare system and its professionals.

1.3 CHALLENGES IN HI INNOVATION POST-PANDEMIC

The post-pandemic era of HI is marked by numerous challenges, especially in the context of innovation. One of the primary challenges is integrating the vast array of digital tools and technologies that emerged during the COVID-19 crisis (Al Knawy et al., 2022; Brahmbhatt et al., 2022; Guggenberger et al., 2021). While the pandemic accelerated the adoption of electronic health records (EHRs), telemedicine, and real-time data analytics, the difficulty lies in ensuring that these tools are effectively interoperable across different healthcare systems (Katehakis & Kouroubali, 2021; Wang et al., 2021). The lack of interoperability not only hampers the efficiency of healthcare delivery but also introduces potential risks related to data accuracy and continuity of care. Healthcare organizations must navigate the complexities of digital integration to fully leverage the benefits of these innovations.

Another significant challenge involves the balance between innovation and patient privacy (Newlands et al., 2020; Shachar et al., 2020). The widespread use of Internet of Things (IoT) devices for remote monitoring and diagnostics, while enhancing patient care, raises critical concerns about the security of personal health data (Awotunde et al., 2021; Jagadeeswari et al., 2018). The potential for data breaches and unauthorized access to sensitive health information presents a significant obstacle in the adoption of new technologies (Luna et al., 2016; Slepchuk et al., 2022). Healthcare institutions must develop robust cybersecurity frameworks that can mitigate the risks posed by interconnected health devices, ensuring that innovation does not come at the expense of patient privacy and trust (Okafor et al., 2023). A further challenge relates to the sustainability of telehealth services because the pandemic saw a rapid rise in the use of telemedicine, which helped bridge healthcare gaps, particularly in rural and underserved areas (Blandford et al., 2020; Thomas et al.,

2022). However, as healthcare systems move beyond the pandemic, the question remains whether telehealth can be integrated into mainstream healthcare in a sustainable way (Caffery et al., 2022; Kaundinya & Agrawal, 2022). There are ongoing concerns regarding reimbursement policies, patient access to digital tools, and the ability of healthcare providers to deliver quality care remotely (Ftouni et al., 2022; Omboni et al., 2022). Addressing these issues requires long-term policy planning and infrastructure development to prevent a digital divide in healthcare delivery.

The training and development of the healthcare workforce also pose challenges in this rapidly evolving technological landscape (Wang et al., 2021). As HI becomes more complex with the integration of AI, ML, and other digital tools, healthcare professionals must continuously update their skills (Stanfill & Marc, 2019). The challenge lies in designing effective training programs that not only equip the workforce with technical skills but also emphasize digital literacy and the ethical implications of technology use in healthcare (Faghy et al., 2022). This includes training on how to use AI and ML tools for predictive analytics, disease management, and personalized care. Another challenge is the ethical use of AI in healthcare decision-making (Arunagiri & Udayaadithya, 2022; Borda et al., 2022). AI and ML have proven to be transformative in disease prediction, diagnostics, and treatment plans (Govindaraj et al., 2024; Noorbakhsh-Sabet et al., 2019). However, the lack of transparency in AI algorithms and the potential for biases in decision-making processes raise concerns about the ethical use of these technologies (Lysaght et al., 2019; Zhang & Zhang, 2023). Healthcare systems must develop frameworks that ensure AI-driven decisions are transparent, unbiased, and aligned with ethical healthcare standards, ensuring patient safety and fairness (Williamson & Prybutok, 2024).

Data management and analysis represent additional challenges in the post-pandemic healthcare landscape (Olorunsogo et al., 2024; Omaghomi et al., 2024). The vast amounts of data generated during the pandemic, from patient records to public health surveillance, present an opportunity for improved healthcare outcomes (Wang et al., 2021; Ye, 2020). However, the challenge lies in effectively managing, storing, and analyzing these data to extract meaningful insights. Healthcare organizations need advanced data infrastructure and analytic capabilities to transform raw data into actionable knowledge while ensuring compliance with data privacy regulations (Rehman et al., 2022; Wang et al., 2018). Furthermore, HI innovation faces significant regulatory challenges. The rapid pace of technological advancement often outpaces existing regulatory frameworks, creating uncertainty around the approval, implementation, and oversight of new healthcare technologies. Policymakers must work to develop agile regulatory frameworks that can keep pace with innovation while ensuring patient safety, ethical standards, and accountability in healthcare delivery.

A critical challenge post-pandemic is addressing the healthcare disparities that were exacerbated during the crisis (Benfer et al., 2021). While digital health technologies have the potential to reduce gaps in healthcare access, particularly for underserved populations, they can also widen these disparities if not implemented equitably (Purnell et al., 2016). Factors such as digital literacy, access to the Internet, and the availability of devices play a significant role in determining who benefits from healthcare innovations (Bodie & Dutta, 2008; Senbekov et al., 2020). Therefore, healthcare systems must prioritize equitable access to digital health technologies to avoid perpetuating or worsening healthcare inequalities (Kepper et al., 2024). The financial constraints imposed by the pandemic also present challenges to healthcare innovation (Sharma et al., 2020). Many healthcare institutions, especially in low-resource settings, are grappling with the financial aftermath of the crisis. This limits their ability to invest in new technologies, upgrade infrastructure, and provide the necessary training for staff. Overcoming these financial barriers requires innovative funding models and partnerships that can support the continued growth of HI while ensuring that advancements are accessible to all healthcare providers, regardless of their financial situation (Sharma et al., 2020).

Finally, the challenge of maintaining innovation momentum in the face of healthcare system fatigue cannot be overlooked. The pandemic placed unprecedented strain on healthcare professionals and systems, leading to burnout and resource depletion (Franc-Guimond & Hogues, 2021). As healthcare systems transition out of the crisis, maintaining the drive for innovation while addressing these human and systemic challenges is crucial. Healthcare leaders must encourage a culture of resilience and adaptability, where innovation is seen as a tool for strengthening healthcare systems, rather than an additional burden.

1.4 FUTURE RESEARCH DIRECTIONS

First, there is a need for more extensive studies on the integration of artificial AI and ML into healthcare systems. While the pandemic has already accelerated the adoption of these technologies, future research should examine deeper into optimizing AI and ML for personalized care, predictive analytics, and improving operational efficiency. Investigating the long-term impact of these technologies on patient outcomes and healthcare cost reduction would also be a valuable area of exploration. Furthermore, research can explore how AI and ML tools can be integrated into low-resource healthcare systems to improve access to care and bridge the gap between high- and low-income countries.

Second, the role of cybersecurity in HI must be prioritized, especially given the increased use of digital health tools during the pandemic. With the rise of telehealth and remote patient monitoring, the protection of sensitive health information has become a significant concern. Future studies should focus on developing more robust cybersecurity frameworks tailored specifically to the healthcare sector. This could involve exploring advanced encryption methods, data anonymization techniques, and secure data-sharing protocols to mitigate the risks of cyberattacks. Additionally, research can investigate how healthcare organizations can balance innovation with privacy protection, ensuring patient trust in digital health solutions.

Another key area of research is the sustainability of telehealth services beyond the pandemic. While telehealth proved invaluable during COVID-19, questions remain about its long-term integration into mainstream healthcare. Future research should focus on the effectiveness of telehealth in managing chronic diseases, improving patient engagement, and reducing healthcare disparities, particularly for underserved populations. Moreover, studies should investigate the regulatory and reimbursement policies needed to support the sustainable use of telehealth, ensuring equitable access and preventing a digital divide in healthcare delivery.

Further research should also examine the potential of emerging technologies such as the IoT in revolutionizing patient monitoring and care. While IoT devices have demonstrated value during the pandemic, future studies could investigate how these technologies can be further refined to enhance patient outcomes, particularly in remote areas. Researchers should also explore the ethical implications of IoT adoption, including data privacy concerns and the need for policies that balance innovation with patient rights. This research could help establish best practices for integrating IoT devices into healthcare workflows and ensuring their safe and effective use.

Lastly, future research should address workforce training and development in response to rapid technological advancements in HI. As digital tools become integral to healthcare systems, healthcare professionals must adapt to these changes. Studies could explore the most effective training programs for healthcare workers, focusing on continuous education, digital literacy, and competency in using AI, ML, and telehealth technologies. Additionally, research should explore how healthcare organizations can foster a culture of innovation and collaboration, ensuring that technology adoption enhances care quality without overwhelming the workforce.

1.5 CONCLUSION

The COVID-19 pandemic has acted as a catalyst for unprecedented advancements in HI, reshaping the landscape of patient care, data management, and healthcare delivery. While the rapid integration of AI, ML, telehealth, and IoT has enhanced operational efficiency and patient outcomes, significant challenges remain. Issues such as data privacy, cybersecurity, interoperability, and equitable access to digital healthcare must be addressed to ensure that the benefits of these innovations are realized across all healthcare systems. Moreover, the need for continuous workforce training, ethical AI implementation, and robust data infrastructure is critical for sustaining these advancements. As healthcare systems navigate the post-pandemic era, a balanced approach that prioritizes innovation, patient safety, and system resilience will be essential. Future research must focus on overcoming these challenges to fully harness the potential of HI in improving global healthcare outcomes.

REFERENCES

Al Knawy, B., McKillop, M. M., Abduljawad, J., Tarkoma, S., Adil, M., Schaper, L., Chee, A., Bates, D. W., Klag, M., & Lee, U. (2022). Successfully implementing digital health to ensure future global health security during pandemics: a consensus statement. *JAMA Network Open, 5*(2), e220214–e220214.

Alowais, S. A., Alghamdi, S. S., Alsuhebany, N., Alqahtani, T., Alshaya, A. I., Almohareb, S. N., Aldairem, A., Alrashed, M., Saleh, K. B., Badreldin, H. A., Yami, M. S. A., Harbi, S. A., & Albekairy, A. M. (2023). Revolutionizing healthcare: the role of artificial intelligence in clinical practice. *BMC Medical Education, 23*(1). https://doi.org/10.1186/s12909-023-04698-z

Ardakani, E. S., Larimi, N. G., Nejad, M. O., Hosseini, M. M., & Zargoush, M. (2023). A resilient, robust transformation of healthcare systems to cope with COVID-19 through alternative resources. *Omega, 114*, 102750. https://doi.org/10.1016/j.omega.2022.102750

Arunagiri, A., & Udayaadithya, A. (2022). Governing artificial intelligence in post-pandemic society. In *Global Pandemic and Human Security: Technology and Development Perspective* (pp. 413–433). Springer.

Awotunde, J. B., Jimoh, R. G., Folorunso, S. O., Adeniyi, E. A., Abiodun, K. M., & Banjo, O. O. (2021). Privacy and security concerns in IoT-based healthcare systems. In *The Fusion of Internet of Things, Artificial Intelligence, and Cloud Computing in Health Care* (pp. 105–134). Springer.

Benfer, E. A., Bhandary-Alexander, J., Cannon, Y., Makhlouf, M. D., & Pierson-Brown, T. (2021). Setting the health justice agenda: addressing health inequity & injustice in the post-pandemic clinic. *Clinical Letter Review, 28*, 45.

Blandford, A., Wesson, J., Amalberti, R., AlHazme, R., & Allwihan, R. (2020). Opportunities and challenges for telehealth within, and beyond, a pandemic. *The Lancet Global Health, 8*(11), e1364–e1365.

Bodie, G. D., & Dutta, M. J. (2008). Understanding health literacy for strategic health marketing: eHealth literacy, health disparities, and the digital divide. *Health Marketing Quarterly, 25*(1–2), 175–203.

Borda, A., Molnar, A., Neesham, C., & Kostkova, P. (2022). Ethical issues in AI-enabled disease surveillance: perspectives from global health. *Applied Sciences, 12*(8), 3890.

Brahmbhatt, D. H., Ross, H. J., & Moayedi, Y. (2022). Digital technology application for improved responses to health care challenges: lessons learned from COVID–19. *Canadian Journal of Cardiology, 38*(2), 279–291.

Braveman, P., & Gottlieb, L. (2014). The social determinants of health: It's time to consider the causes of the causes. *Public Health Reports, 129*(1_suppl2), 19–31. https://doi.org/10.1177/00333549141291s206

Caffery, L. A., Muurlink, O. T., & Taylor-Robinson, A. W. (2022). Survival of rural telehealth services post-pandemic in Australia: a call to retain the gains in the 'new normal'. *Australian Journal of Rural Health, 30*(4), 544–549.

Chen, H., Yan, G., Wen, M. H., Brooks, K. N., Zhang, Y., Huang, P. S., & Chen, T. Y. (2024). Advancements and practical considerations for biophysical research: navigating the challenges and future of super-resolution microscopy. *Chemical & Biomedical Imaging, 2*(5), 331–344. https://doi.org/10.1021/cbmi.4c00019

Eappen, P. (2022). Healthcare informatics during the COVID-19 pandemic. In *Advances in Logistics, Operations, and Management Science Book Series* (pp. 193–209). https://doi.org/10.4018/978-1-6684-5279-0.ch010

Eappen, P., & Olujinmi, T. D. (2022). Telemedicine and digital public health in pandemic times. In *Advances in Healthcare Information Systems and Administration Book Series* (pp. 118–137). https://doi.org/10.4018/978-1-6684-5499-2.ch007

Faghy, M. A., Arena, R., Babu, A. S., Christle, J. W., Marzolini, S., Popovic, D., Vermeesch, A., Pronk, N. P., Stoner, L., & Smith, A. (2022). Post pandemic research priorities: a consensus statement from the HL-PIVOT. *Progress in Cardiovascular Diseases, 73*, 2–16.

Franc-Guimond, J., & Hogues, V. (2021). Burnout among caregivers in the era of the COVID-19 pandemic: insights and challenges. *Canadian Urological Association Journal, 15*(6 Suppl 1), S16.

Franciosi, E. B., Tan, A. J., Kassamali, B., Leonard, N., Zhou, G., Krueger, S., Rashighi, M., & LaChance, A. (2021). The impact of telehealth implementation on underserved populations and no-show rates by medical specialty during the COVID-19 pandemic. *Telemedicine Journal and e-Health, 27*(8), 874–880. https://doi.org/10.1089/tmj.2020.0525

Ftouni, R., AlJardali, B., Hamdanieh, M., Ftouni, L., & Salem, N. (2022). Challenges of telemedicine during the COVID-19 pandemic: a systematic review. *BMC Medical Informatics and Decision Making*, *22*(1), 207.

Glette, M. K., Ludlow, K., Wiig, S., Bates, D. W., & Austin, E. E. (2023). Resilience perspective on healthcare professionals' adaptations to changes and challenges resulting from the COVID-19 pandemic: a meta-synthesis. *BMJ Open*, *13*(9), e071828. https://doi.org/10.1136/bmjopen-2023-071828

Govindaraj, M., Khan, P., Krishnan, R., Gnanasekaran, C., & Lawrence, J. (2024). Revolutionizing healthcare: The transformative impact of artificial intelligence. In *Revolutionizing the Healthcare Sector with AI* (pp. 54–78). IGI Global.

Guggenberger, T., Lockl, J., Röglinger, M., Schlatt, V., Sedlmeir, J., Stoetzer, J.-C., Urbach, N., & Völter, F. (2021). Emerging digital technologies to combat future crises: learnings from COVID-19 to be prepared for the future. *International Journal of Innovation and Technology Management*, *18*(04), 2140002.

Irace, A. L., Sharma, R. K., Reed, N. S., & Golub, J. S. (2020). Smartphone-based applications to detect hearing loss: a review of current technology. *Journal of the American Geriatrics Society*, *69*(2), 307–316. https://doi.org/10.1111/jgs.16985

Jagadeeswari, V., Subramaniyaswamy, V., Logesh, R. t. a., & Vijayakumar, V. (2018). A study on medical internet of things and big data in personalized healthcare system. *Health Information Science and Aystems*, *6*(1), 14.

Katehakis, D. G., & Kouroubali, A. (2021). The EHR as an Instrument for Effective Digital Transformation in the Post COVID-19 Era. SWH@ ISWC.

Kaundinya, T., & Agrawal, R. (2022). Unpacking a telemedical takeover: recommendations for improving the sustainability and usage of telemedicine post-COVID-19. *Quality Management in Healthcare*, *31*(2), 68–73.

Kepper, M. M., Fowler, L. A., Kusters, I. S., Davis, J. W., Baqer, M., Sagui-Henson, S., Xiao, Y., Tarfa, A., Yi, J. C., & Gibson, B. (2024). Expanding a behavioral view on digital health access: drivers and strategies to promote equity. *Journal of Medical Internet Research*, *26*, e51355.

Lera, M., Taxtsoglou, K., Frantzana, A., & Kourkouta, L. (2020). Nurses' attitudes toward lifelong learning via new technologies. *Asian/Pacific Island Nursing Journal*, *5*(2), 89–102. https://doi.org/10.31372/20200502.1088

Li, C., Wang, J., Wang, S., & Zhang, Y. (2024). A review of IoT applications in healthcare. *Neurocomputing*, *565*, 127017. https://doi.org/10.1016/j.neucom.2023.127017

Luna, R., Rhine, E., Myhra, M., Sullivan, R., & Kruse, C. S. (2016). Cyber threats to health information systems: a systematic review. *Technology and Health Care*, *24*(1), 1–9.

Lysaght, T., Lim, H. Y., Xafis, V., & Ngiam, K. Y. (2019). AI-assisted decision-making in healthcare: the application of an ethics framework for big data in health and research. *Asian Bioethics Review*, *11*, 299–314.

Malik, Y. S., Sircar, S., Bhat, S., Ansari, M. I., Pande, T., Kumar, P., Mathapati, B., Balasubramanian, G., Kaushik, R., Natesan, S., Ezzikouri, S., Zowalaty, M. E. E., & Dhama, K. (2020). How artificial intelligence may help the Covid-19 pandemic: pitfalls and lessons for the future. *Reviews in Medical Virology*, *31*(5), 1–11. https://doi.org/10.1002/rmv.2205

Newlands, G., Lutz, C., Tamò-Larrieux, A., Villaronga, E. F., Harasgama, R., & Scheitlin, G. (2020). Innovation under pressure: implications for data privacy during the Covid-19 pandemic. *Big Data & Society*, *7*(2), 2053951720976680.

Noorbakhsh-Sabet, N., Zand, R., Zhang, Y., & Abedi, V. (2019). Artificial intelligence transforms the future of health care. *The American Journal of Medicine*, *132*(7), 795–801.

Okafor, C. M., Kolade, A., Onunka, T., Daraojimba, C., Eyo-Udo, N. L., Onunka, O., & Omotosho, A. (2023). Mitigating cybersecurity risks in the US healthcare sector. *International Journal of Research and Scientific Innovation (IJRSI)*, *10*(9), 177–193.

Olorunsogo, T. O., Balogun, O. D., Ayo-Farai, O., Ogundairo, O., Maduka, C. P., Okongwu, C. C., & Onwumere, C. (2024). Reviewing the evolution of US telemedicine post-pandemic by analyzing its growth, acceptability, and challenges in remote healthcare delivery during global health crises. *World Journal of Biology Pharmacy and Health Sciences*, *17*(1), 075–090.

Omaghomi, T. T., Akomolafe, O., Ogugua, J. O., Daraojimba, A. I., & Elufioye, O. A. (2024). Healthcare management in a post-pandemic world: lessons learned and future preparedness-a review. *International Medical Science Research Journal*, *4*(2), 210–223.

Omboni, S., Padwal, R. S., Alessa, T., Benczúr, B., Green, B. B., Hubbard, I., Kario, K., Khan, N. A., Konradi, A., & Logan, A. G. (2022). The worldwide impact of telemedicine during COVID-19: current evidence and recommendations for the future. *Connected Health*, *1*, 7.

Pool, J., Akhlaghpour, S., Fatehi, F., & Burton-Jones, A. (2024). A systematic analysis of failures in protecting personal health data: a scoping review. *International Journal of Information Management*, *74*, 102719. https://doi.org/10.1016/j.ijinfomgt.2023.102719

Purnell, T. S., Calhoun, E. A., Golden, S. H., Halladay, J. R., Krok-Schoen, J. L., Appelhans, B. M., & Cooper, L. A. (2016). Achieving health equity: closing the gaps in health care disparities, interventions, and research. *Health Affairs, 35*(8), 1410–1415.

Quazi, S. (2022). Artificial intelligence and machine learning in precision and genomic medicine. *Medical Oncology, 39*(8). https://doi.org/10.1007/s12032-022-01711-1

Rehman, A., Naz, S., & Razzak, I. (2022). Leveraging big data analytics in healthcare enhancement: trends, challenges and opportunities. *Multimedia Systems, 28*(4), 1339–1371.

Senbekov, M., Saliev, T., Bukeyeva, Z., Almabayeva, A., Zhanaliyeva, M., Aitenova, N., Toishibekov, Y., & Fakhradiyev, I. (2020). The recent progress and applications of digital technologies in healthcare: a review. *International Journal of Telemedicine and Applications, 2020*(1), 1–18. https://doi.org/10.1155/2020/8830200

Shachar, C., Engel, J., & Elwyn, G. (2020). Implications for telehealth in a postpandemic future: regulatory and privacy issues. *Jama, 323*(23), 2375–2376.

Sharma, H. B., Vanapalli, K. R., Cheela, V. S., Ranjan, V. P., Jaglan, A. K., Dubey, B., Goel, S., & Bhattacharya, J. (2020). Challenges, opportunities, and innovations for effective solid waste management during and post COVID-19 pandemic. *Resources, Conservation and Recycling, 162*, 105052.

Sharma, S., Gupta, Y. K., & Mishra, A. K. (2023). Analysis and prediction of COVID-19 multivariate data using deep ensemble learning methods. *International Journal of Environmental Research and Public Health, 20*(11), 5943. https://doi.org/10.3390/ijerph20115943

Slepchuk, A. N., Milne, G. R., & Swani, K. (2022). Overcoming privacy concerns in consumers' use of health information technologies: a justice framework. *Journal of Business Research, 141*, 782–793.

Stanfill, M. H., & Marc, D. T. (2019). Health information management: implications of artificial intelligence on healthcare data and information management. *Yearbook of Medical Informatics, 28*(01), 056–064.

Syeda, H. B., Syed, M., Sexton, K. W., Syed, S., Begum, S., Syed, F., Prior, F., & Yu, F. (2021). Role of machine learning techniques to tackle the COVID-19 crisis: systematic review. *JMIR Medical Informatics, 9*(1), e23811. https://doi.org/10.2196/23811

Tariq, R. A., & Hackert, P. B. (2023, January 23). *Patient Confidentiality*. StatPearls—NCBI Bookshelf. https://www.ncbi.nlm.nih.gov/books/NBK519540/

Thomas, E. E., Haydon, H. M., Mehrotra, A., Caffery, L. J., Snoswell, C. L., Banbury, A., & Smith, A. C. (2022). Building on the momentum: sustaining telehealth beyond COVID–19. *Journal of Telemedicine and Telecare, 28*(4), 301–308.

Vajjhala, N. R., & Eappen, P. (2023). The role of 5G networks in healthcare applications. In *CRC Press eBooks* (pp. 87–98). https://doi.org/10.1201/9781003227861–5

Vajjhala, N. R., & Eappen, P. (2024). Data envelopment analysis in healthcare management. In *Advances in Business Information Systems and Analytics Book Series* (pp. 245–260). https://doi.org/10.4018/979-8-3693-0255-2.ch011

Wang, Q., Su, M., Zhang, M., & Li, R. (2021). Integrating digital technologies and public health to fight Covid-19 pandemic: key technologies, applications, challenges and outlook of digital healthcare. *International Journal of Environmental Research and Public Health, 18*(11), 6053.

Wang, Y., Kung, L., & Byrd, T. A. (2018). Big data analytics: understanding its capabilities and potential benefits for healthcare organizations. *Technological Forecasting and Social Change, 126*, 3–13.

Williamson, S. M., & Prybutok, V. (2024). Balancing privacy and progress: a review of privacy challenges, systemic oversight, and patient perceptions in AI-driven healthcare. *Applied Sciences, 14*(2), 675.

Yadav, S. (2024). Transformative frontiers: A comprehensive review of emerging technologies in modern healthcare. *Cureus*. https://doi.org/10.7759/cureus.56538

Ye, J. (2020). The role of health technology and informatics in a global public health emergency: practices and implications from the COVID-19 pandemic. *JMIR Medical Informatics, 8*(7), e19866.

Yeung, A. W. K., Torkamani, A., Butte, A. J., Glicksberg, B. S., Schuller, B., Rodriguez, B., Ting, D. S. W., Bates, D., Schaden, E., Peng, H., Willschke, H., Van Der Laak, J., Car, J., Rahimi, K., Celi, L. A., Banach, M., Kletecka-Pulker, M., Kimberger, O., Eils, R., . . . Atanasov, A. G. (2023). The promise of digital healthcare technologies. *Frontiers in Public Health, 11*. https://doi.org/10.3389/fpubh.2023.1196596

Yogesh, M. J., & Karthikeyan, J. (2022). Health informatics: engaging modern healthcare units: a brief overview. *Frontiers in Public Health, 10*. https://doi.org/10.3389/fpubh.2022.854688

Zhang, J., & Zhang, Z.-m. (2023). Ethics and governance of trustworthy medical artificial intelligence. *BMC Medical Informatics and Decision Making, 23*(1), 7.

2 Lessons Learned
COVID-19 and the Future of Healthcare Informatics

Khaldoun M. Aldiabat and Mohamad Musa

2.1 INTRODUCTION

2.1.1 LESSONS LEARNED: COVID-19 AND THE FUTURE OF HEALTHCARE INFORMATICS

At the end of 2019, the outbreak of coronavirus disease 2019 (COVID-19), caused by severe acute respiratory syndrome coronavirus 2, occurred in Wuhan, China. For 2 years, from the beginning of 2020 until the end of 2021, the World Health Organization (WHO) declared the outbreak of COVID-19 an international public health emergency and a pandemic (Aldiabat et al., 2022). COVID-19 had extremely high mortality and morbidity rates worldwide, and almost all countries enforced quarantines for their populations in their homes because of the contagious nature of this disease. In addition to home quarantines, lockdowns, raising awareness, social distancing, wearing of face masks, school closures, restrictions on social gatherings and traveling, partial closures of workplaces, mandatory online work and education, and hand sanitizing measures were recommended by the WHO as the best COVID-19 transmission prevention strategies (Afrin et al., 2022; Flahault, 2020; Ganjali et al., 2022). Subsequently, the Pfizer COVID-19 vaccine was authorized, and the first person injected with the vaccine was a UK citizen ([BBC], December 8, 2020).

Government lockdowns, travel restrictions, and home quarantine (self-isolation) were the most restrictive strategies, and they hindered people from carrying on with their everyday lives or accessing healthcare services physically (Jassim et al., 2021). Although individuals struggled to deal with the pandemic, policymakers also struggled to adapt to the ever-changing guidance from public health authorities (Dixon & Holmes, 2021). Therefore, health authorities in every country had to adjust their plans to their respective countries' needs and make collective arrangements based on WHO recommendations to deploy innovative alternative solutions to manage the pandemic.

According to Worldometers.info (April 2, 2024), globally, the COVID-19 pandemic has affected more than 704,606,481 individuals worldwide, and more than 7,009,333 deaths have been attributed to the pandemic. Tracking and recording the morbidity and mortality rates of COVID-19 and vaccine distribution during different waves of the pandemic placed health authorities under pressure due to a lack of medical equipment, shortage of medical staff due to increased intensive care unit admissions, and crowded emergency rooms. It is imperative to prevent, treat, and control the pandemic according to global and local public health authorities' protocols. Amidst the challenging global situation, health informatics was one of the critical solutions utilized by healthcare providers, administrators, and public health authorities in managing patients, resources, and populations (Dixon & Holmes, 2021; Eappen, 2022).

Although COVID-19 has not yet been entirely eradicated, the Centers for Disease Control and Prevention (CDC) announced that May 11, 2023, was the end date of the federal COVID-19 public health emergency declaration (CDC, September 12, 2023). Furthermore, the United States and other countries announced that they were empowered with more tools and resources than ever before to protect their populations. According to this announcement, the COVID-19 vaccine will remain available, and COVID-19 home testing may or may not be covered by private insurance, but treatment will remain available, and monitoring the impact of COVID-19 and the effectiveness of prevention and control strategies will remain a public health priority for CDC. Accordingly, health informatics, which played a significant role in managing patients and populations during the pandemic (Dixon & Holmes, 2021), will continue operating, but the frequency, source, or availability of some metrics will change; however, the CDC will continue to be a trusted source of sustainable, accurate, and timely information to inform decision-making (CDC, September 12, 2023).

Although the COVID-19 pandemic posed challenges to individuals and governments, many lessons were learned that can empower humanity and healthcare systems to face similar future pandemics.

This chapter will discuss how the COVID-19 pandemic impacted healthcare informatics integration in healthcare systems and how to optimize this integration in the future. Additionally, the chapter will explore the challenges and solutions for maintaining data security and present strategies that were utilized in enhancing patient privacy in healthcare informatics systems, telehealth, and remote patient monitoring during the pandemic and discuss how to incorporate these strategies into future healthcare informatics models. Besides, this chapter will review how data analysis shaped COVID-19 response strategies and what improvements and adjustments are needed in healthcare informatics to deal with future pandemics, explain how to achieve interoperability in healthcare information systems, and overcome challenges to ensure seamless data exchange during pandemics.

This chapter will assess the resilience of healthcare information technology infrastructure during the COVID-19 pandemic, describe strategies for building a robust and adaptable healthcare informatics system, and outline lessons on adapting and improving user experiences and engagement in healthcare informatics. Moreover, this chapter will discuss the impact of COVID-19 on digital health literacy, outline strategies for enhancing health literacy in the future of healthcare informatics, review the successful implementation of healthcare informatics during the COVID-19 pandemic, describe the lessons learned from the pandemic that can be built upon in the future, explore international collaboration in managing informatics during pandemics, and outline recommendations for fostering international partnerships in healthcare informatics to deal with any pandemics similar to COVID-19 in the future.

This chapter is based on published articles in peer-reviewed journals from the last 5 years, governmental and nongovernmental formal reports, gray literature, and other resources such as media and reports by stakeholders and policymakers.

2.2 COVID-19 AND HEALTHCARE INFORMATICS: INTEGRATION AND THE FUTURE OF DATA EXCHANGE

The COVID-19 pandemic underlined the critical role of healthcare informatics in global health crisis management. The pandemic not only highlighted the growing necessity for digital health solutions but also focused on assessing the resilience of IT infrastructure to understand human factors and enhance digital health literacy.

The healthcare industry faces unprecedented challenges of global collaboration and partnerships created beyond borders that are focused on human health. Integrating health informatics during COVID-19 was an urgent and effective solution that allowed the optimization of public health and supported field data collection, contact tracing, and the prompt generation of epidemiological information for decision-makers (Ahmed et al., 2020).

Developing and implementing healthcare informatics undoubtedly enables local and federal health departments to meet the health needs of a population, implement routine surveillance, and rapidly manage disease outbreaks. Studies found that using and implementing health informatics during the pandemic enhanced the speed of the reporting system, enabled fast case processing, provided accurate data with low follow-up, and minimized the number of employees needed to do data entry (Walker et al., 2021).

During the COVID-19 pandemic, health informatics provided different data elements at various levels (national, state, regional/local agencies, hospitals/healthcare enterprises, and patients/individuals). Examples of these data include the number of new infections/new positive tests, types of tests performed, personal protective equipment availability/burn rate, hospital bed availability/occupancy, current number of admitted patients, number of previously admitted or COVID-positive patients, immunizations, mobility and disease protection, non-pharmaceutical interventions (mask mandates, social distancing, mandatory closures, etc.), social media campaigns, and crowdfunding (Basit et al., 2021). However, it became evident that the resilience of health information technology (HIT) infrastructure was more crucial than ever. In the following subsection, we will discuss the importance of building robust and adaptable HIT systems that can withstand and rapidly recover from crises. Additionally, we will explore various strategies that healthcare organizations can implement to enhance the resilience of their HIT infrastructure and ensure reliable data exchange.

2.3 RESILIENCE OF HIT INFRASTRUCTURE AND STRATEGIES FOR ROBUST AND ADAPTABLE HIT SYSTEMS

Dixon and Holmes (2021) reported that during the period of the COVID-19 pandemic, academics made considerable efforts to find the best methods of utilizing healthcare informatics to respond to COVID-19 and contribute to the recovery and preparedness phases. These efforts resulted in a large corpus of peer-reviewed publications. Furthermore, according to Dixon and Holmes (2021), the following four manuscripts were selected as the best papers for managing pandemics using health informatics in the Yearbook of Medical Informatics 2021 (Ahmed et al., 2020; Garcia et al., 2020; Gong et al., 2020; and Reeves et al., 2020).

Ahmed et al.'s (2020) paper describes how health informatics played a role in the WHO response to the COVID-19 pandemic in low- and middle-income countries in the African region. The authors designed, developed, and implemented a surveillance tool called the COVID-19 Data Visualization and Summarization (DVS) tool. The DVS tool was used to collect and report data through various available information systems and open standards from each WHO member state in Africa. DVS successfully and flexibly reported WHO and Ministry of Health requirements in each country. The authors recommended improving future public health informatics initiatives in pandemics similar to COVID-19 in low- and middle-income countries.

Garcia et al.'s (2020) paper discusses how the free online COVID-19 Information Management Resources Repository developed by the US-CDC provided excellent information and rapid reporting that helped manage the pandemic. This system was efficient and effectively made data standards accessible to public healthcare organizations and the healthcare system, facilitating healthcare providers in documenting and sharing data related to the disease, diagnoses, symptoms, interventions, and other clinical information when they used an electronic health record (EHR).

A third example of how healthcare informatics served humanity in responding to and managing the COVID-19 pandemic was discussed by Gong et al. (2020). The authors developed a cloud-based system for conducting effective surveillance and controlling COVID-19 in one Chinese city. This healthcare informatics model was developed and deployed over 72 hours and was designed to collect various types of data that helped detect COVID-19 and diagnose and manage patients. The data were then integrated with laboratory test results and the hospital EHR system data using a cloud-based platform to infer population trends at the community level.

Reeves et al. (2020) developed and deployed healthcare informatics to manage and control the pandemic. Their model is based on a case report documenting various activities from many hospitals and health systems, influencing EHRs and other information systems to manage their response to COVID-19.

In addition to the four aforementioned informatics models, a remote patient monitoring (RPM) technologies model was successfully used during the pandemic to facilitate data sharing and interaction between patients and their healthcare providers. This type of digital health platform had already been used before the pandemic, but during the outbreak, the platform could control infection and prevent the spread of the virus (Mantena & Keshavjee, 2021). These are a few other examples of HIT utilized during COVID-19 (to read about them, see Eappen, 2022).

In conclusion, the COVID-19 pandemic was a test for healthcare systems, enabling preparation for future pandemics that are a threat in the twenty-first century (Peek et al., 2020). This pandemic exposed vulnerabilities in many healthcare systems worldwide and outlined the need to develop a resilient global healthcare informatics system (Sundararaman et al., 2021). Assessing the resilience of healthcare IT infrastructure involves crafting strategies for building a robust system, including investing in cloud-based solutions for collecting global data in a common platform, enhancing cybersecurity protocols to prevent any tampering with data at any level, and adopting interoperable standards that are compatible with various governments globally (Pai, 2020).

We recommend the continued use of RPM technologies after the pandemic because they have the potential to enhance healthcare delivery by offering support to symptomatic individuals before hospitalization and ensuring continuity of care for discharged patients. Recent research on RPM technology has shown its effectiveness in enhancing patient satisfaction, lowering readmission rates, and streamlining healthcare system operations. There is an urgent necessity to broaden the adoption of evidence-backed RPM technologies in the future (Mantena & Keshavjee, 2021).

Peek et al. (2020) concluded that the rapid changes in the use of health informatics and telehealth technologies during the pandemic instilled trust in these technologies, supporting their continued use in healthcare systems even after the pandemic. Additionally, they emphasized the importance of continuing digital consultations to contribute to the future of healthcare informatics. However, they were unsure how healthcare systems could continue sharing health data without destroying public trust. Based on the world's short experience with artificial intelligence (AI) during the pandemic, the authors were optimistic about the future role of AI in enhancing healthcare informatics. However, they still have concerns about AI technology: "data quality, transferability of results across settings and health systems, the performance of algorithms when actually used in clinical systems, and about access to data and protection of privacy" (p. 2).

2.4   DATA SECURITY AND PATIENTS' INFORMATION PRIVACY IN HEALTHCARE INFORMATICS

The COVID-19 pandemic era has engendered an unprecedented surge in data collection from populations worldwide. The data are subsequently subjected to comprehensive analysis and dissemination among healthcare providers, policymakers, and the general public. While discussions about data security and patients' privacy have long been prominent among healthcare providers, researchers, and policymakers, the exigencies of the pandemic elevated these concerns to the forefront of discourse. Consequently, developing robust policies to safeguard data integrity and preserve patients' privacy has become crucial in the post-pandemic landscape (Combi et al., 2023).

During the COVID-19 pandemic, many new healthcare informatics tools were devised, and applications were developed and deployed to collect and analyze data and manage and control the pandemic, such as new health and illness applications, AI, smart devices, and wearable devices. Notably, these healthcare technologies promoted the health of populations besides saving and analyzing massive amounts of data and easing accessibility to patients' information. Unfortunately, much of these data were not protected by the Health Insurance Portability and Accountability Act (HIPAA), which was passed nearly three decades ago in the United States Senate (United States Senate, 2023).

Three decades ago, data security and patients' information privacy rules were formulated to protect data traditionally collected by healthcare institutions. However, the new revolution in technology and the expansion of AI technology adoption and applications, which were designed to collect, analyze, and share sensitive health data for different medical and nonmedical agencies, created a pressing need to revise these rules (IAAP, 2024). Therefore, in the context of COVID-19 and the period after the pandemic, new legislation, policies, and acts by healthcare policymakers have begun to be revised to address data security and patient privacy related to healthcare informatics (Combi et al., 2023).

Although HIT aided in controlling the COVID-19 pandemic and promoting population health, there are reports about the negative effects of this technology. For instance, it is well known that during the COVID-19 pandemic, most face-to-face healthcare services were moved online, and different platforms were utilized to provide healthcare or updated information related to COVID-19. Substantial data were released and shared through various platforms and applications during the pandemic, which increased cyberattack incidents that breached data security and violated patients' information privacy (Moulaei et al., 2023). These cyberattack incidents have pushed governments to find effective solutions to increase cybersecurity and protect individual and organizational data security and privacy. Potential risks that necessitate consideration include patient privacy breaches, premature decision-making based on preliminary or inaccurate data, and the potential misuse or misinterpretation of shared data.

Major stakeholders, such as EHR companies and healthcare providers, have cited privacy concerns as a key deterrent to data-sharing agreements (O'Reilly-Shah et al., 2020). Surprisingly, in some cases, during the COVID-19 pandemic, the governments of some countries such as South Korea and Singapore breached data security and patient privacy by disclosing to the public information such as the identities of infected individuals, their demographics, workplace, social contact, places they had visited, travel histories, and health information (Moulaei et al., 2023; Undale & Kulkarni, 2020; Wen et al., 2020; Yang & Tsai, 2020).

Although it is acknowledged that heightened interoperability may increase the risk of data breaches, interoperability does not inherently render these risks more probable. A robust implementation of safeguards, including encryption, authentication mechanisms, and stringent data usage protocols, can effectively mitigate these risks. It is important to underscore that the risk of EHR data exposure does not surpass that of financial data compromise. Consequently, these risks necessitate careful consideration vis-à-vis the potential benefits to individual patients and public health (O'Reilly-Shah et al., 2020). Furthermore, Moulaei et al. (2023) reported that COVID-19-infected individuals were worried about the release of their personal or health information through social media and websites. Unfortunately, many people share information on social media or unreliable websites without knowing that this information reflects their health or personal information. Therefore, Moulaei et al. (2023) urged people to become empowered, to know what information they can share, and to know which reliable websites, platforms, applications, or social media sites they can use.

The vast technological revolution that has occurred and the ubiquitous presence of AI applications in all aspects of life mean that healthcare providers, patients, and organizations have to constantly use social networks to share and analyze health information. This situation creates challenges in maintaining data security and privacy, especially when patients are unaware of the security risks of sharing their confidential health information through different telemedicine systems, social networks, and mHealth applications (Zhou et al., 2018).

Moulaei et al. (2023) reported about the vulnerability of all technology and social media to security threats and cyberattacks from within or without an organization. Notably, Babbs (2020) found that the majority (53%) of cyberattacks are reported as involving insiders or members of the workforce. The study also described the primary type of cyberattack as a "phishing scam" using email as the primary data vector to breach data security. Babbs (2020) identified some solutions, namely, email safety checks, website domain verification, and two-step verification for sensitive emails. Although the study identified some risks and solutions to challenges associated with data security, the author adopted a general business perspective—not a healthcare perspective. However, because the main risk factor for data breaches is human error, it is reasonable to compare Babbs' (2020) study to a healthcare setting based on the same vector of cyberattack: email usage.

Crafting security and privacy policies, facilitating ease of use, committing to ethical and transparency principles and practices, improving the quality of information, and complying with

HIPAA security rules are recommended ways to gain users' trust and protect their data and privacy (Armitage et al., 2020; Gerke et al., 2020). Moreover, Moulaei et al. (2023) emphasized the enhancement of people's trust in social media and technology by inviting governments and health policymakers worldwide to revise data usage regulations and policies and to understand people's concerns regarding their data security and privacy in social media and technology applications.

A qualitative assessment study was conducted in conjunction with Swiss hospitals and research institutions concerning patient data sharing in hospitals and research institutions (Scheibner et al., 2022). The assessment identified two possible data safety strategies: homomorphic encryption and distributed ledger technology (Scheibner et al., 2022). Homomorphic encryption is the ability to manipulate/compute data without moving them from an encrypted state to a decrypted state. Data in a decrypted state can be vulnerable to data leaks. In distributed ledger technology, data can be accessed through multiple agents, but all access, modification, and transfer are time-stamped and immutable (Scheibner et al., 2022). Having access to real-time immutable patient data can make conducting a privacy audit easy and fast.

Gerke et al. (2020) concluded that "the motto 'ethics by design, even in a pandemic' should guide makers in the development of home monitoring products to combat this public health emergency [and beyond]" (p. 1181), meaning that healthcare providers, technology companies, and public health officials should apply the highest standards of ethics, especially if privacy regulations for technologies do not exist. These ethical standards include not using patients' data without their consent, mandatory anonymization of data to maintain privacy and keep safeguards in place to reidentify risks, giving patients a choice to stop sharing data at any time they wish without being penalized, and adopting transparent principles with individuals. Individuals must be clearly informed about how their data are collected, used, and potentially shared with third parties, including for commercial purposes (Gerke et al., 2020).

In conclusion, COVID-19 has highlighted a pressing need to develop strategies for building a robust system, including investing in cloud-based solutions for collecting global data in a common platform, enhancing cybersecurity protocols to prevent any tampering with data at any level, and adopting interoperable standards that are in agreement with various governments across the globe (Gong et al., 2020; Pai, 2020). It is recommended that safe technology should be used to provide the highest level of patient data protection and safeguard patient privacy, considering the risks and benefits of using any new technology or application.

2.5   REMOTE PATIENT MONITORING DURING THE PANDEMIC AND HOW TO INCORPORATE IT INTO FUTURE HEALTHCARE INFORMATICS MODELS

Converting traditional healthcare to telehealth and the adoption of technology applications have become widespread in recent years because of the continuous development of new technologies and applications related to healthcare (Hood et al., 2023). The Internet, EHRs, and accessibility to medical devices are just a few factors that have accelerated the conversion process to telehealth and enabled healthcare providers to practice healthcare remotely. Telehealth acceleration adoption rates are multifactorial, but a particularly significant and recent factor has been the COVID-19 pandemic.

A study in Australia compared historically controlled cohorts of outpatient telehealth test requests and completion rates in March–May 2019 and 2020 (Liaw et al., 2021). The study showed that the participants in the March–May 2020 group had high test requests but low rates of completing the requested test (Liaw et al., 2021). The authors concluded that many people adopted telehealth-based services once the pandemic started, but the low completion rates require further investigation. The aforementioned study is also limited to comparing one set of time frames within the context of the beginning stages of the pandemic.

Chang et al. (2020) explored telehealth adoption rates among primary care providers during the COVID-19 outbreak in different socioeconomic settings. Their study found that all primary care providers significantly increased the use of telehealth options. The authors of the study used the

CDC Social Vulnerability Index (CDC-SVI) to compare adoption rates between high SVI areas and low SVI areas. They found that healthcare providers with high SVI used telephone telehealth modalities more than they used video. Conversely, in low SVI areas, healthcare providers used video more than they used telephones. The authors concluded that conversion to telehealth did not unfold similarly across communities. To guarantee additional telehealth equity, policy changes must consider barriers faced overwhelmingly by marginalized patients and those who serve them.

When telehealth was implemented during the pandemic, there was a sudden and rapid shift in the type of care provided. For example, Puspitasari et al.'s (2020) study created a series of guidelines to help with the transition of teletherapy to treat mental illness rapidly. The barriers to the transition included access to hardware, the scope of roles and responsibilities, technical problems, coordination and communication, and interventions implemented for each barrier. The study developed an implementation framework for teletherapy regarding the transfer of care from in-person to a telehealth model, along with a series of interventions for each piece of the framework. The study had 90 patient participants in total, with 81 patients completing the program. After their telehealth discharge from therapy, 86 patients had at least one appointment booked, and a majority (55 patients) had two appointments booked. Even with only two weeks of preparation time, the transition of the therapy programs to a telehealth-based model was achievable.

RPM is one type of telehealth that allows healthcare providers to assess and follow up with their patients remotely. Healthcare providers can use digital devices to conduct physiological tests, such as blood pressure monitors, blood glucose meters, body weight scales, and pulse oximeters. The data collected by these devices are transmitted electronically to healthcare providers for further planning and interventions. Literature reports the many advantages of using telehealth over traditional healthcare. For example, telehealth provides some opportunities for patients to become engaged in their medical plans, increases their compliance with their treatment protocols, expands healthcare providers' reach, and provides care to patients remotely (Hood et al., 2023), which is cost-effective and helps in controlling the spread of infectious diseases such as COVID-19 because there is no need for patients to travel and interact personally with healthcare providers.

RPM played a significant role during the COVID-19 pandemic in monitoring and managing COVID-19 patients, following up on new cases, and the continued remote management of other patients with chronic diseases to minimize the spread of the virus. There is no doubt that the COVID-19 pandemic and measures instituted to control it, namely, physical distancing, lockdowns, and quarantines, forced healthcare systems to convert their services to a remote format using technology as a solution to control the spread of the virus, minimize congestion in healthcare service facilities, protect patients and their healthcare providers, and provide an optimum level of safe and competent healthcare services (Bouabida et al., 2022).

During the pandemic, RPM was an effective solution that had positive outcomes such as enhancing accessibility to healthcare services; minimizing the feelings of isolation, anxiety, and depression in patients and their families; providing patients with practical and timely care; and enhancing communication between patients and their healthcare providers. Furthermore, healthcare providers indicated that RPM could guarantee continuity of care and support the administrators and healthcare system.

During the pandemic, the workload of clinicians greatly increased, but new technologies such as RPM can decrease their workload. Shah and Schulman's (2021) study examined the utilization of app-based remote patient monitoring by comparing a clinician's workload between a telephone-only group and an app-based group. The study found that clinicians had fewer working hours when working with the app-based remote monitoring group compared to the number of hours they had with the telephone-based group.

Remote monitoring of the poorly understood long-term effects of COVID-19 is necessary. Consequently, Izmailova and Reiss (2021) studied the remote monitoring of the pulmonary symptoms of symptomatic COVID-19 survivors and identified three sets of remote data, namely, remote spirometry, remote pulse oximetry, and at-home exercise stress tests. For remote spirometry and pulse oximetry, the authors noted that both sets of data were comparable based on clinical assessment; however, spirometry could have variable results, and the pulse oximeters provided to patients had to meet specific regulatory standards.

Bouabida et al. (2022) evaluated two remote monitoring platforms and concluded that the RPM platforms were functional, user-friendly, and well-received by users. For the future use of RPM platforms, the authors emphasized the importance of training healthcare providers, patients, and families to collaborate with health system leaders, decision-makers, and RPM platform providers. In this context, Muller et al. (2022) concluded that

> One lesson from the COVID-19 pandemic is the need to optimize healthcare provision outside of traditional settings and potentially over longer periods of time. An important strategy is remote patient monitoring (RPM), allowing patients to remain at home while they transmit health data and receive follow-up services.
>
> **(p. 2)**

Remote monitoring can significantly benefit the current healthcare system in many ways. However, there have been major challenges in adopting large-scale remote monitoring. One study reviewed the challenges that remote monitoring faces on a large scale. The first challenge is known as the signal-to-noise ratio, which is explained as follows: if every person with a cardiac implantable electronic device in the United States were to use remote monitoring, then over 10 million transmissions would be generated annually (Vandenberk & Raj, 2023). Consequently, future informatics would require increased staffing, optimized alert programming, and streamlined workloads to address these levels of transmissions. Another challenge is that the data gathered could vary with different manufacturers of remote monitoring technologies. This challenge should be addressed through enhanced manufacturer interoperability and standardization. Reimbursement is another challenge clinicians face. A European Heart Rhythm Association survey found that reimbursement was the greatest barrier to implementing remote monitoring. Due to the different laws/structures of healthcare economics worldwide, solutions should be examined based on each country's policy (Vandenberk & Raj, 2023).

2.6 DATA ANALYTICS FOR PANDEMIC RESPONSE: ADAPTING AND IMPROVING USER EXPERIENCE

As mentioned earlier, the data were collected and shared during the pandemic to enable the best measures to be taken to control the virus. By using COVID-19 testing data and tracking the data accordingly, healthcare policymakers could calculate the spread of the virus and make an appropriate response (Konchak et al., 2021).

Data analytics plays a role in epidemiology in pandemic response. Data were used during the COVID-19 pandemic to track the number of COVID-19 patients in local hospitals and triage them, ensuring resources were distributed based on patient needs (Konchak et al., 2021). However, collecting and analyzing accurate and timely data, identifying patients quickly, and making accurate decisions were not always feasible during the pandemic. Basit et al. (2021) discussed four failures or challenges and four successes in accurately collecting and analyzing data. These challenges or failures are outlined below.

First, strategy and data collection harmonization were lacking. In large countries such as the United States and Canada, where health systems are not centralized and there is no standard for data collection, accurate COVID-19 data were not consistently reported, leading to inaccurate responses to the data analysis results. Second, there was a deficiency in a skilled workforce that could combine a specialty in infectious diseases and healthcare informatics. This deficiency led to misinterpretation of data and a lack of understanding of the data required to be reported to the government at different levels (federal, state, and local levels) and for what reason the reporting was to be done, ultimately leading to inaccurate decision-making. Third, healthcare providers face a failure in the information system when collecting accurate data. COVID-19 data had to be reported using various formats over different periods and deadlines through various public healthcare informatics systems, which created a challenge and burden for healthcare organizations. Fourth was a challenge related to reporting errors, delays, and misrepresentations of the collected and analyzed data because there was a lack of unified collecting, analyzing, and reporting systems.

In addition to technical challenges, some ethical difficulties related to using health informatics in collecting and analyzing data were experienced during the pandemic (Basit et al., 2021; Bruneau et al., 2020; Garett & Young, 2022; Kilgallon et al., 2022). These ethical challenges concerned the following aspects:

1. Rationing resources (i.e., suggested utilizing scoring tools in EHRs for outcome prediction rather than for resource allocation or triaging patients in the context of deciding on scarce resource allocations).
2. Advanced directives (i.e., there was a lack of advanced directives and code status in the EHRs).
3. Testing and tracing (e.g., collecting data through technology that could put patients at risk of discrimination, bias, denial of employment or insurance, or collecting data that could be abused, sold, and used for unintended purposes).
4. Unintended consequences of using telehealth (i.e., telehealth created some ethical challenges related to creating a psychological burden and drain caused by overuse of virtual platforms and frustration because of a delay in audio/visual transmission, screen fatigue, decreased attention, and miscommunication; Basit et al., 2021).
5. Other ethical challenges concerning data privacy, surveillance, transparency, accountability, and robustness of data analyses in the context of fairness, equality, and power (Bruneau et al., 2020). The pandemic revealed power asymmetries, discrimination, and disparity in using technology in marginalized societies.
6. Additionally, patients and their families had ethical challenges in providing and signing consent forms. Furthermore, the ownership of the collected and analyzed data was unclear (i.e., there was no consensus on how best to address passive data storage aside from ownership problems).

In summary, the pandemic was eye-opening and revealed the need to study the challenges above, find evidence-based solutions, and plan and prepare for similar future pandemics.

Despite the foregoing challenges and failures, Basit et al. (2021) identified four successes in data collection and analysis as a result of using healthcare informatics during the pandemic. First, there was an improvement and transformational shift in clinical care because of the rapid development of health informatics infrastructure, the furnishing of healthcare providers with new technological skills, and the practice of virtual health assessment and interventions. Second, many healthcare systems successfully used technology and healthcare informatics for contact tracing to identify and inform persons potentially contacted by individuals infected with COVID-19. Third, forecasting COVID-19 data using traditional and innovative technological methods helped healthcare policymakers make decisions and craft health policies and measures. Fourth, COVID-19 enhanced scientific discovery and innovation by fostering the development and use of AI for data collection and analysis.

AI has saved money and effort because it is an accurate and cost-effective tool, contributing to the pharmaceutical industry and drug repurposing (Basit et al., 2021). Ma et al. (2021) reported that one relatively new informatics area is the use of AI for informatics. Furthermore, deep neural network AI can efficiently screen potential drugs to treat COVID-19 through different learning databases (Ma et al., 2021). With consistent improvement to AI and its data processing speed alongside bioinformatic genome sequencing, there are major potential applications of AI in combating future pandemics on a vast scale and at a fast speed.

The COVID-19 pandemic has provided many lessons regarding how healthcare data should be analyzed and utilized to meet the challenges posed by the next pandemic. Bioinformatic developments during the COVID-19 pandemic include third-generation gene sequencing, public databases with genome/protein structure, interactive models, and variants related to the COVID-19 virus (Ma et al., 2021). If these types of informatics can be improved over time before the next pandemic occurs, researchers can be greatly aided when analyzing a new pathogen.

Adapting to informatics tools, including RPM after the COVID-19 pandemic, requires careful consideration of human factors. Healthcare professionals play a pivotal role in this adaptation, and it is crucial to provide them with adequate training and support and to teach the basics of informatics during new healthcare professional orientations (Marquard, 2021). The addition of healthcare informatics does not end with training healthcare professionals but also includes user-friendly customization according to the language and culture of a place, which enhances performance by displaying customized clinical data, having measures in place to improve user safety, and diversifying health informatics designs according to the scope of the healthcare provider accessing it (Marquard, 2021). Other strategies for healthcare professionals include creating awareness campaigns and integrating digital literacy into healthcare curricula.

2.7 FUTURE OF HEALTHCARE INFORMATICS: LESSONS LEARNED FROM COVID-19

In this chapter, based on the global challenges faced during the COVID-19 pandemic regarding the utilization of healthcare informatics, many recommendations, suggestions, and possible solutions to enhance healthcare informatics in the future are presented in different sections. This section is an in-depth discussion of how the lessons learned from the COVID-19 pandemic will contribute to significantly improving the future outlook for healthcare informatics and enhancing preparedness for any similar pandemics in the future.

One of the lessons learned from the pandemic is that to implement healthcare informatics in the future, healthcare providers must be digitally literate and capable of using digital technologies. This literacy and capability can be imparted to these providers by enrolling them in training programs. They must be flexible and able to adapt to new digital clinical care models and be ready to integrate them into their practice. Moreover, healthcare organizations need to renovate their digital infrastructure to adopt the latest digital care model by enhancing telecommunication services and data management systems and improving accessibility to digital tools for healthcare providers. However, implementing healthcare informatics needs transformational leadership and management that will adopt digital technologies, provide necessary support and training for technology use and AI applications, and foster a culture of innovation to keep healthcare providers updated and prepared to face any new development in healthcare informatics (Clarke-Darrington et al., 2023; Powell et al., 2022).

Sadasivaiah et al. (2021) recommended adopting the following enabling measures to effectively enhance the capacity of the safety net healthcare and public health system capacity for adopting healthcare informatics in the future:

> (1) inviting different members of IT [sic] and informatics specialists as members of the incident management team; (2) creating governance [sic] about the approval process for EHRs to support the response; (3) close alignment with operational leaders to gain comprehensive insight of the key objectives; (4) keeping agility [sic] to adjust to changing conditions and priorities; and (5) upholding commitments to bolstering the care of vulnerable populations and mitigating disparities in healthcare accessibility.
>
> **(p. 7)**

In a paper entitled "Primary Care Informatics Response to Covid-19 Pandemic: Adaptation, Progress, and Lessons from Four Countries with High ICT Development," Liaw et al. (2021) discussed how primary care informatics in four countries (the United States, the United Kingdom, Canada, and Australia) responded to the COVID-19 pandemic and the lessons learned. The authors reported that there is a need to upgrade the digital health capacity infrastructure of primary care in Australia, creating standards for virtual health competencies, applying electronic referrals, and computerized physician order entry.

Canada has learned the following lessons regarding taking the next steps and future planning: There is a need to enhance primary care and public integration and improve equity and healthcare accessibility conditions for vulnerable populations. Furthermore, standards should be created for virtual care to protect privacy and security, and enhanced training and education should be offered to optimize workforce competency to effectively implement virtual healthcare.

Regarding the next steps and future planning, the United Kingdom has learned to accelerate the use of digital systems in healthcare, enhance partnerships with research and surveillance centers to improve data sharing and collaboration, and found satisfactory solutions for data sharing and linking data among agencies across its provinces.

The USA has learned the importance of

1. crafting federal rather than local strategies, regulations, and policies regarding health informatics;
2. enhancing the accessibility and coverage areas of high-speed Internet for telehealth use to encompass remote areas of the United States; and
3. providing enough resources for continuity and sustainability in the use of telehealth.

Dixon and Holmes (2021) recommended utilizing health informatics to manage COVID-19 survivors over the long term and address other physical and mental impacts of the pandemic. Therefore, Ambalavanan et al. (2023) developed a concept map of clinical pathways for long COVID-19 and recommended the use of the map. This innovative and highly standard digital framework could reduce the management gaps of long-term COVID-19 impacts and offer insights into the data required for health informatics for controlling the long-term effects of COVID-19 or other similar future pandemics. However, clear policies and legislation are needed to enhance healthcare informatics.

Telehealth utilization patterns during the COVID-19 period were investigated by Hamadi et al. (2022), and the authors recommended that policymakers must

1) ascertain which elements of the new telehealth landscape will be retained, 2) modernize the regulatory, accreditation and reimbursement framework to maintain pace with care model innovation, and 3) address disparities in access to broadband connectivity with a particular focus on rural and underserved communities.

(p. 43)

It is recommended that stakeholders in each country evaluate healthcare informatics applications used in their countries during the pandemic and make proper recommendations for reusability or further enhancements. The effectiveness and usefulness of official healthcare informatics applications in addressing COVID-19 in some countries were evaluated. For example, Alassaf et al. (2021) reviewed three applications that were developed and used in Saudi Arabia. One application was used to track individuals when visiting stores and institutions, the second one was aimed at providing people with their test results and checking their symptoms, and the third was developed and used to notify users if they were exposed to the virus. The authors recommended using these applications not only during the COVID-19 pandemic but also during similar future pandemics.

A study conducted in North India recommended incorporating healthcare informatics such as telehealth in a future healthcare system to serve as a supplementary measure rather than a replacement for traditional in-person outpatient clinic visits to lower the burden of outpatient clinic services in hospitals (Guleria et al., 2021).

During the pandemic, Payne et al. (2022) found an alignment between biomedical informatics and HIT; therefore, they recommended a potential synergy between the two models in modern biomedical research and healthcare delivery. This synergy will enhance healthcare outcomes by improving healthcare service value, quality, and safety through collaboration, shared respect, transformational leadership support, and knowledge-sharing. However, understanding how both models can synergize is necessary to create a "rapid learning" healthcare system in the future that includes healthcare providers and policymakers.

Technology and ethics must go hand-in-hand in developing and using future healthcare informatics. Therefore, to protect individual privacy in future applications, Informatics Europe (2020) recommended that policymakers and technical experts consider the following ethical principles when using healthcare informatics to collect data from the population:

1-Track individuals with their consent and under their direct control, allowing them to freely and easily switch tracking on and off even during the same day. To achieve this goal, we recommend that technical experts develop software that is not only [General Data Protection Regulation] GDPR-ready but also dynamically reconfigurable by the end users within the limits defined by the current jurisdiction. 2-Track only aggregated data that cannot be traced back to particular individuals if they have not given their explicit consent. 3-Keep the tracking process transparent and open to the scrutiny of public opinion from the beginning of its use and rely on the evaluation by independent scientific advisors to assess the impact of security measures taken. 4-Make any software and hardware used open to examination by civil society. 5-Specify the time limit for tracking without allowing for any extension in the absence of an independent evaluation of the motivations.

(Para. 7)

The pandemic was a major blow and is a stark wake-up call for countries to invest in public health and work cooperatively to become empowered and find the most evidence-based and cost-effective solution to similar pandemics in the future. Consequently, the healthcare system must be reformed, and healthcare informatics should be integrated with traditional healthcare practices.

2.8 CONCLUSION

The COVID-19 pandemic served as an unprecedented stress test, underscoring the critical importance of resilient, adaptable, and data-driven healthcare informatics systems. Throughout this global crisis, the rapid development and deployment of digital health tools and technologies played a pivotal role in pandemic response and management. Healthcare informatics enabled fast case processing, accurate data collection, and enhanced population-level insights to inform real-time decision-making by policymakers and healthcare providers.

Innovative solutions such as cloud-based surveillance platforms, remote patient monitoring systems, and AI-powered predictive models helped health systems overcome challenges posed by decentralized data, interoperability problems, and the need for timely information sharing. These informatics-powered capabilities proved invaluable in supporting clinical care delivery, resource allocation, and public health interventions during the pandemic. However, the COVID-19 experience also exposed underlying vulnerabilities in many healthcare IT infrastructures, underscoring the urgent need for secure, interoperable, and scalable informatics capabilities at the global level. Key priorities for the future of healthcare informatics include investing in robust cybersecurity protocols, adopting common data standards across jurisdictions, and leveraging emerging technologies such as AI to enhance predictive modeling and decision support.

The ethical considerations surrounding patient data privacy and consent are crucial. As the use of digital health applications surged during the pandemic, policymakers had to act swiftly to revise outdated privacy regulations and entrench principles of transparency to maintain public trust. Upholding the highest standards of data stewardship will be essential in realizing the full potential of healthcare informatics.

Ultimately, the COVID-19 pandemic has underscored the indispensable role of healthcare informatics in navigating public health crises. The lessons learned will be instrumental in shaping a resilient, data-driven, and patient-centric future for healthcare systems globally. By embedding informatics capabilities and digital literacy across all levels of care, health providers and policy-makers can prepare to respond well to the challenges of today and tomorrow. Through sustained investment, cross-sector collaboration, and a commitment to ethical principles, the healthcare sector can harness the transformative power of informatics to deliver equitable, efficient, and effective care for all.

REFERENCES

Afrin, S. Z., Islam, M. T., Paul, S. K., Kobayashi, N., & Parvin, R. (2022). Dynamics of SARS-CoV-2 variants of concern (VOC) in Bangladesh during the first half of 2021. *Virology, 565*, 29–37. https://doi.org/10.1016/j.virol.2021.10.005

Ahmed, K., Bukhari, M. A., Mlanda, T., Kimenyi, J. P., Wallace, P., Okot Lukoya, C., Hamblion, E. L., & Impouma, B. (2020). Novel approach to support rapid data collection, management, and visualization during the COVID-19 outbreak response in the World Health Organization African region: development of a data summarization and visualization tool. *JMIR Public Health and Surveillance, 6*(4), e20355. https://doi.org/10.2196/20355

Alassaf, N., Bah, S., Almulhim, F., AlDossary, N., & Alqahtani, M. (2021). Evaluation of official healthcare informatics applications in Saudi Arabia and their role in addressing COVID-19 pandemic. *Healthcare Informatics Research, 27*(3), 255–263. https://doi.org/10.4258/hir.2021.27.3.255

Aldiabat, K. M., Alsrayheen, E., Prabha Valsaraj, B., Abu Baker, R., Al-Harthi, I., Qutishat, M. G., & Aldamery, K. (2022). The lived experiences of COVID-19 quarantined Omani adults: a phenomenological study. *American Journal of Qualitative Research, 6*(3).

Ambalavanan, R., Snead, R. S., Marczika, J., Kozinsky, K., & Aman, E. (2023). Advancing the management of long COVID by integrating into health informatics domain: current and future perspectives. *International Journal of Environmental Research and Public Health, 20*(19), 6836. https://doi.org/10.3390/ijerph20196836

Armitage, L., Lawson, B. K., Whelan, M. E., & Newhouse, N. (2020). Paying SPECIAL consideration to the digital sharing of information during the COVID-19 pandemic and beyond. *BJGP open, 4*(2), bjgpopen20X101072. https://doi.org/10.3399/bjgpopen20X101072

Babbs A. (2020). How to leverage data security in a post-Covid world. *Computer Fraud & Security, 2020*(10), 8–11. https://doi.org/10.1016/S1361-3723(20)30107-X

Basit, M. A., Lehmann, C. U., & Medford, R. J. (2021). Managing pandemics with health informatics: successes and challenges. *Yearbook of Medical Informatics, 30*(1), 17–25. https://doi.org/10.1055/s-0041-1726478

BBC. (December 8, 2020). BBC Covid-19 vaccine: first person receives Pfizer jab in UK. https://www.bbc.com/news/uk-55227325

Bouabida, K., Malas, K., Talbot, A., Desrosiers, M. È., Lavoie, F., Lebouché, B., Taghizadeh, N., Normandin, L., Vialaron, C., Fortin, O., Lessard, D., & Pomey, M. P. (2022). Healthcare professional perspectives on the use of remote patient-monitoring platforms during the COVID-19 pandemic: a cross-sectional study. *Journal of Personalized Medicine, 12*(4), 529. https://doi.org/10.3390/jpm12040529

Bruneau, Gabriela Arriagada, Müller, Vincent, C., & Gilthorpe, Mark S. (2020). The ethical imperatives of the COVID-19 pandemic: a review from data ethics. *Veritas: Revista de Filosofía y Teología, 46*, 13–35.

Centers for Disease Control and Prevention (CDC). (September 12, 2023). *End of the Federal COVID-19 Public Health Emergency (PHE) Declaration.* Retrieved from https://archive.cdc.gov/#/details?url=https://www.cdc.gov/coronavirus/2019-ncov/your-health/end-of-phe.html

Chang, S., Pierson, E., Koh, P. W., Gerardin, J., Redbird, B., & Grusky, D. (2020). Mobility network models of COVID-19 explain inequities and inform reopening. *Nature, 589*, 82–87. https://doi.org/10.1038/s41586-020-2923-3

Clarke-Darrington, J., McDonald, T., & Ali, P. (2023). Digital capability: an essential nursing skill for proficiency in a post-COVID-19 world. *International Nursing Review, 70*(3), 291–296. https://doi.org/10.1111/inr.12839

Combi, C., Facelli, J. C., Haddawy, P., Holmes, J. H., Koch, S., Liu, H., Meyer, J., Peleg, M., Pozzi, G., Stiglic, G., Veltri, P., & Yang, C. C. (2023). The IHI Rochester report 2022 on healthcare informatics research: resuming after the CoViD-19. *Journal of Healthcare Informatics Research, 7*(2), 169–202. https://doi.org/10.1007/s41666-023-00126-5

Dixon, B. E., & Holmes, J. H. (2021). Section editors for the IMIA yearbook section on managing pandemics with health informatics. Managing pandemics with health informatics. *Yearbook of Medical Informatics, 30*(1), 69–74. https://doi.org/10.1055/s-0041-1726504

Eappen, Philip. (2022). Healthcare informatics during the COVID-19 pandemic. In *Global Risk and Contingency Management Research in Times of Crisis*. https://doi.org/10.4018/978-1-6684-5279–0.ch010

Flahault, A. (2020). COVID-19 cacophony: is there any orchestra conductor? *Lancet (London, England), 395*(10229), 1037. https://doi.org/10.1016/S0140–6736(20)30491–8

Ganjali, R., Eslami, S., Samimi, T., Sargolzaei, M., Firouraghi, N., Mohammad Ebrahimi, S., Khoshrounejad, F., & Kheirdoust, A. (2022). Clinical informatics solutions in COVID-19 pandemic: scoping literature review. *Informatics in Medicine Unlocked, 30*, 100929. https://doi.org/10.1016/j.imu.2022.100929

Garcia, M., Lipskiy, N., Tyson, J., Watkins, R., Esser, E. S., & Kinley, T. (2020). Centers for disease control and prevention 2019 novel coronavirus disease (COVID-19) information 8: management: addressing national health-care and public health needs for standardized data definitions and codified vocabulary for data exchange. *Journal of the American Medical Informatics Association, 27*(9), 1476–1487.

Garett, R., & Young, S. D. (2022). Ethical views on sharing digital data for public health surveillance: analysis of survey data among patients. *Frontiers in Big Data, 5*, 871236. https://doi.org/10.3389/fdata.2022.871236

Gerke, S., Shachar, C., Chai, P. R., & Cohen, I. G. (2020). Regulatory, safety, and privacy concerns of home monitoring technologies during COVID–19. *Nature Medicine, 26*(8), 1176–1182. https://doi.org/10.1038/s41591-020-0994-1

Gong, K., Xu, Z., Cai, Z., Chen, Y., & Wang, Z. (2020). Internet hospitals help prevent and control the epidemic of COVID-19 in China: multicenter user profiling study. *Journal of Medical Internet Research, 22*(4), e18908. https://doi.org/10.2196/18908

Guleria, K., Patiyal, N., Negi, A., Kanwar, V., & Kansal, D. (2021). Utilization of outpatient eSanjeevani National Teleconsultation Service during the COVID-19 pandemic in a public healthcare institution in North India. *Indian Journal of Pharmacy and Pharmacology, 7*, 265–269. https://doi.org/10.18231/j.ijpp.2020.045

Hamadi, H. Y., Zhao, M., Haley, D. R., Dunn, A., Paryani, S., & Spaulding, A. (2022). Medicare and telehealth: the impact of COVID-19 pandemic. *Journal of Evaluation in Clinical Practice, 28*(1), 43–48. https://doi.org/10.1111/jep.13634

Hood, C., Sikka, N., Van, C. M., & Mossburg, S. E. (2023, March 15). Remote Patient Monitoring. *PSNet: Patient Safety Network*. Retrieved from https://psnet.ahrq.gov/perspective/remote-patient-monitoring

IAAP. (2024, April 3–4). *Global Privacy Summit*. Washington-DC. Retrieved from https://iapp.org/conference/global-privacy-summit/

Informatics Europe. (2020, April 3). Recommendation on the Use of IT for COVID-19 Infection Mitigation. *Informatics Europe News*. https://www.informatics-europe.org/news/541-policy-recommendation-covid19.html

Izmailova, E. S., & Reiss, T. F. (2021). Being closer to the patient means better decisions, such as wearable remote monitoring of patients with COVID-19 lung disease. *Clinical and Translational Science, 14*(6), 2091–2094. https://doi.org/10.1111/cts.13085

Jassim, G., Jameel, M., Brennan, E., Yusuf, M., Hasan, N., & Alwatani, Y. (2021). Psychological impact of COVID-19, isolation, and quarantine: a cross-sectional study. *Neuropsychiatric Disease and Treatment, 17*, 1413–1421. https://doi.org/10.2147/NDT.S311018

Kilgallon, J. L., Tewarie, I. A., Broekman, M. L. D., Rana, A., & Smith, T. R. (2022). Passive data use for ethical digital public health surveillance in a postpandemic world. *Journal of Medical Internet Research, 24*(2), e30524. https://doi.org/10.2196/30524

Konchak, C. W., et al. (2021). From testing to decision-making: a data-driven analytics COVID-19 response. *Academic Pathology, 8*. https://doi.org/10.1177/23742895211010257

Liaw, S. T., Kuziemsky, C., Schreiber, R., Jonnagaddala, J., Liyanage, H., Chittalia, A., Bahniwal, R., He, J. W., Ryan, B. L., Lizotte, D. J., Kueper, J. K., Terry, A. L., & de Lusignan, S. (2021). Primary care informatics response to Covid-19 pandemic: adaptation, progress, and lessons from four countries with high ICT development. *Yearbook of Medical Informatics, 30*(1), 44–55. https://doi.org/10.1055/s-0041–1726489

Ma, A., Ba, Z., Zhao, Y., Mao, J., & Li, G. (2021). Understanding and predicting the dissemination of scientific papers on social media: a two-step simultaneous equation modelling–artificial neural network approach. *Scientometrics, 126*(8), 7051–7085. https://doi.org/10.1007/s11192-021-04051-5

Mantena, S., & Keshavjee, S. (2021). Strengthening healthcare delivery with remote patient monitoring in the time of COVID–19. *BMJ Health & Care Informatics, 28*(1), e100302. https://doi.org/10.1136/bmjhci-2020–100302

Marquard, J. (2021). Human factors and organizational issues in health informatics: innovations and opportunities. *Yearbook of Medical Informatics, 30*(1), 91–99. https://doi.org/10.1055/s-0041–1726511

Moulaei, K., Iranmanesh, E., Amiri, P., & Ahmadian, L. (2023). Attitudes of COVID-19 patients toward sharing their health data: a survey-based study to understand security and privacy concerns. *Health Science Reports, 6*(3), e1132. https://doi.org/10.1002/hsr2.1132

Muller, A. E., Berg, R. C., Jardim, P. S. J., Johansen, T. B., & Ormstad, S. S. (2022). Can remote patient monitoring be the new standard in primary care of chronic diseases, post-COVID-19? *Telemedicine Journal and e-Health: The Official Journal of the American Telemedicine Association, 28*(7), 942–969. https://doi.org/10.1089/tmj.2021.0399

O'Reilly-Shah, V. N., Gentry, K. R., Van Cleve, W., Kendale, S. M., Jabaley, C. S., & Long, D. R. (2020). The COVID-19 pandemic highlights shortcomings in US health care informatics infrastructure: a call to action. *Anesthesia and Analgesia, 131*(2), 340–344. https://doi.org/10.1213/ANE.0000000000004945

Pai, M. (2020, April 6). *Can we Reimagine Global Health in the Post-Pandemic World?* Forbes. https://www.forbes.com/sites/madhukarpai/2020/04/06/can-we-reimagine-global-health-in-the-post-pandemic-world/

Payne, P. R. O., Wilcox, A. B., Embi, P. J., & Longhurst, C. A. (2022). Better together: integrating biomedical informatics and healthcare IT operations to create a learning health system during the COVID-19 pandemic. *Learning Health Systems, 6*(2), e10309. https://doi.org/10.1002/lrh2.10309

Peek, N., Sujan, M., & Scott, P. (2020). Digital health and care in pandemic times: impact of COVID–19. *BMJ Health & Care Informatics, 27*, e100166. https://doi.org/10.1136/bmjhci-2020–100166

Powell, K. R., Winkler, A. E., Liu, J., & Alexander, G. L. (2022). A mixed-methods analysis of telehealth implementation in nursing homes amidst the COVID-19 pandemic. *Journal of the American Geriatrics Society, 70*(12), 3493–3502. https://doi.org/10.1111/jgs.18020

Puspitasari, I. M., Garnisa, I. T., Sinuraya, R. K., & Witriani, W. (2020). Perceptions, knowledge, and attitude toward mental health disorders and their treatment among students in an Indonesian University. *Psychology Research and Behavior Management, 13*, 845–854. https://doi.org/10.2147/PRBM.S274337

Reeves, J. J., Hollandsworth, H. M., Torriani, F. J., Taplitz, R., Abeles, S., Tai-Seale, M., Millen, M., Clay, B. J., & Longhurst, C. A. (2020). Rapid response to COVID-19: health informatics support for outbreak management in academic health system. *Journal of the American Medical Informatics Association (JAMIA).* https://academic.oup.com/jamia/advance-article/doi/10.1093/jamia/ocaa037/5811358

Sadasivaiah, S., Shaffer, E., Enanoria, W., Su, G., Goldman, S., Scarafia, J., Lee, T., Yu, A., Goldman, L. E., & Ratanawongsa, N. (2021). Informatics response to address the COVID-19 pandemic in a safety net healthcare system. *JAMIA Open, 4*(3), ooaa057. https://doi.org/10.1093/jamiaopen/ooaa057

Scheibner, J., Nielsen, J., & Nicol, D. (2022). An ethical-legal assessment of intellectual property rights and their effect on COVID-19 vaccine distribution: an Australian case study. *Journal of Law and the Biosciences, 9.* https://doi.org/10.1093/jlb/lsac020.

Shah, B. R., & Schulman, K. (2021). Do not let a good crisis go to waste: health care's path forward with virtual care. *NEJM Catal, 19*, 1–14. https://doi.org/10.1056/CAT.20.0693

Sundararaman, T., Muraleedharan, V. R., & Ranjan, A. (2021). Pandemic resilience and health systems preparedness: lessons from COVID-19 for the twenty-first century. *Journal of Social and Economic Development, 23*(Suppl 2), 290–300. https://doi.org/10.1007/s40847-020-00133-x

Undale, S., & Kulkarni, A. (2020). Perceived eWallet security: impact of COVID-19 pandemic. *Vilakshan, XIMB Journal of Management.* ahead-of-print. https://doi.org/10.1108/xjm-07-2020-0022

United States Senate. (2023). *A Request by US Senator Bill Cassidy, MD (R-LA), Ranking Member of the Senate Health, Education, Labor, and Pensions (HELP) Committee, for Information from Stakeholders on Ways to Improve the Privacy Protections of Health Data to Safeguard Sensitive Information.* https://www.help.senate.gov/ranking/newsroom/press/ranking-member-cassidy-seeks-information-from-stakeholders-on-improving-Americans-health-data-privacy

Vandenberk, B., & Raj, S. (2023). Remote patient monitoring: what have we learned and where are we going? *Current Cardiovascular Risk Reports, 17*, 1–13. https://doi.org/10.1007/s12170-023-00720-7

Walker, D. M., Yeager, V. A., Lawrence, J., & McAlearney, A. S. (2021). Identifying opportunities to strengthen the public health informatics infrastructure: exploring hospitals' challenges with data exchange. *The Milbank Quarterly, 99*(2), 393–425. https://doi.org/10.1111/1468-0009.12511

Wen, H., Zhao, Q., Lin, Z., Xuan, D., & Shroff, N. (2020, October 21–23). A study of the privacy of COVID-19 contact tracing apps. In *Security and Privacy in Communication Networks: 16th EAI International Conference, SecureComm, Proceedings, Part I* (pp. 297–317). Springer. (2024, April 2). Coronavirus cases, deaths, recovered. Retrieved from https://www.worldometers.info/coronavirus/

Yang, W.-Y., & Tsai, C.-H. (2020). Democratic values, collective security, and privacy: Taiwan people's response to COVID–19. *Asian Journal for Public Opinion Research, 8.* 222–245. https://doi.org/10.15206/ajpor.2020.8.3.222

Zhou, L., Parmanto, B., & Joshi, J. (2018). Development and evaluation of a new security and privacy track in a health informatics graduate program: multidisciplinary collaboration in education. *JMIR Medical Education. 4*(2), e19.

3 Telehealth Revolution
Bridging the Digital Divide

Ruiling Guo, Christopher Thompson, and Myllissa Reyes

3.1 INTRODUCTION

The coronavirus disease 2019 (COVID-19) pandemic is a substantial public health crisis of the 21st century. This infectious disease is caused by the severe acute respiratory syndrome corona-virus 2 (SARS-COV-2). The COVID-19 pandemic had profound impacts on many healthcare systems worldwide. For instance, the pandemic exposed vulnerabilities in international healthcare delivery systems while simultaneously stressing and overwhelming hospital emergency department capacity as well as intensive care bed availability (Ahmed et al., 2024). In many countries such as Canada, Germany, the United Kingdom and the United States, surgical procedures were severely restricted and reduced due to the uncertain potential for virus spread within the public. COVID-19's impact on the worldwide economy simultaneously had a devastating impact on the medical supply chain. Pharmaceutical and other resource management became as equally challenging as containing the contagion (Verschuur et al., 2021). To reduce the risks of COVID-19 transmission and protect lives, the US healthcare system, like those in other countries, had to adopt alternative models to continue meeting the health needs of patients and the population seeking medical services (Centers for Medicare and Medicaid Services [CMS], 2021). The pandemic has not only presented unprecedented challenges to many countries' healthcare systems but also significantly changed the ways of delivering patient care. As a noncontact and non-travel modality tool, telehealth became the most promising solution to these challenges that transformed the provision of medical and health services in many international healthcare systems such as in the United States, Canada, China, India, Italy, the United Kingdom, and Spain during this difficult time (Hincapié et al., 2020).

The objective of this chapter is to investigate the use of telehealth as a means to bridge the digital divide by rapidly adopting telehealth services in healthcare systems in the United States and some other countries in the world during the COVID-19 pandemic. Through a review of existing research and analysis of relevant data, this chapter aims to examine the trends in telehealth utilization, advantages, challenges, barriers, and lessons learned from the pandemic. Furthermore, this chapter attempts to generate evidence-based recommendations and explore new opportunities for future improvement in reducing health disparities, and promoting equitable access and quality of care in the healthcare systems.

3.2 LITERATURE REVIEW

To achieve the objective of this chapter, a literature review was conducted to identify telehealth utilization before and during the COVID-19 pandemic, the advantages of the rapid adoption of telehealth, and disparities, challenges, and barriers in the existing research. The literature searches were performed in electronic databases such as PubMed, CINAHL, Academic Search Complete, Web of Sciences, and Google Scholar. Search terms such as "telehealth," "telemedicine," "COVID-19 pandemic," "information technology," "health disparities," "digital literacy," and "quality of care" were used to identify the relevant studies and data sources. The inclusion criteria for selecting

DOI: 10.1201/9781003485629-3

evidence included publications in peer-reviewed journals and higher-level studies such as systematic reviews, meta-analysis, randomized clinical trials, and retrospective studies. In addition, the literature review included government reports, reputable web resources, and white papers from the US Centers for Disease Control and Prevention (CDC), the Centers for Medicare & Medicaid Services (CMS), National Center for Health Statistics (NCHS), World Health Organization (WHO), and professional associations such as the American Medical Association (AMA) and the Healthcare Information and Management Systems Society (HIMSS). Data were compiled and analyzed following the literature searches. The analysis and review results are presented in the following sections of this chapter.

3.3 DEFINITION OF TELEHEALTH AND ITS CLASSIFICATIONS

Telehealth is broadly defined as the remote delivery of healthcare services via telecommunications technology, and encompasses various modalities such as video visits, telephone consultations, remote monitoring, and secure messaging. Various healthcare organizations give several definitions for telehealth. For instance, the WHO defines telehealth as the "delivery of health care services, where patients and providers are separated by distance. Telehealth uses Information and Communication Technologies (ICT) for the exchange of information for the diagnosis and treatment of diseases and injuries, research and evaluation, and for the continuing education of health professionals" (World Health Organization [WHO], 2022). The US CMS defines telehealth as "two-way, real-time interactive communication between a patient and a physician or practitioner at a distant site through telecommunications equipment that includes, at a minimum, audio and visual equipment" (American Medical Association [AMA], 2024). The US Health Resources and Services Administration (HRSA) gives a similar definition: "Telehealth is defined as the use of electronic information and telecommunication technologies to support long-distance clinical health care, patient and professional health-related education, health administration, and public health" (Health Resources and Services Administration [HRSA], 2022).

Telehealth and telemedicine are often used interchangeably. For instance, the US National Library of Medicine defines both telehealth and telemedicine as "providing clinical services (either in real time or asynchronously) between patient and clinician and/or between clinician and clinician when the two parties are physically remote from one another using some form of information-communication technology. The term telehealth is a larger umbrella term encompassing other remote health-related services, such as administration, continuing medical education, and/or provider training" (Shaver, 2022). However, the American Academy of Family Physicians gives a different explanation. It says that "Telehealth is different from telemedicine in that it refers to a broader scope of remote healthcare services than telemedicine. While telemedicine refers specifically to remote clinical services, telehealth can refer to remote non-clinical services such as provider training, continuing medical education or public health education, administrative meetings, and electronic information sharing to facilitate and support assessment, diagnosis, consultation, treatment, education, and care management" (American Academy of Family Physician [AAFP], 2022). In this chapter, telehealth refers to a broader scope of remote healthcare services, including telemedicine.

Telehealth services can be divided into two categories: synchronous and asynchronous. Synchronous refers to either real-time, audio-video communication or real-time audio and telephone communications that connect physicians and patients in different locations. Asynchronous refers to store-and-forward technologies that collect images and data to be transmitted and interpreted later; online digital visits and brief check-in services furnished using communication technology (via patient portal and smartphone); and interprofessional online consultations between physicians and/or other qualified healthcare professionals for patients by sharing verbal or written reports for further assessment or care management (AMA, 2024).

3.4 HISTORY OF TELEHEALTH AND ITS EVOLUTION

The early stages of telehealth can be traced as far back as the 1950s. The development of telecommunication technologies made it possible for healthcare providers in urban hospitals to connect people in remote clinics. In the United States, one of the early uses of telemedicine was in an experiment conducted by the National Aeronautics and Space Association (NASA) in 1960, for monitoring astronauts in flight by physicians and medical teams during their mission Project Mercury (Link, 1965). In 1966, the US National Library of Medicine designated $42 million for multiple telemedicine projects spanning over 19 years to help medically isolated areas (Li, 1999). The University of Nebraska's telepsychiatry services began the first major telehealth project in 1959 by connecting a hospital and a state mental hospital to provide telepsychiatry services to patients; and in 1969 Massachusetts General Hospital (MGH) provided psychiatric consultations for adults and children at a Logan International Airport health clinic (Von Hafften, 2024).

In the 1980s and 1990s, with the development of new technologies, more telehealth projects were carried out using satellite communication and videoconferencing. People began to use the Internet for communication, and telehealth networks were formed to provide opportunities that allowed healthcare providers to collaborate and offer distance consultations. For instance, radiologists could analyze medical images remotely through the use of telehealth (Hyder & Razzak, 2020). During this period, telehealth was adopted by various countries such as the United States, Canada, Australia, China, Norway, and the United Kingdom, primarily to address the challenges of providing healthcare to remote and underserved populations. The development and implementation of telehealth laid the foundation for the more widespread use of telemedicine seen in later years. The United States was one of the pioneers in telehealth, with early projects focused on providing healthcare to remote and rural areas of the country.

From 2000 to 2019, the rapid advances in telecommunications technology opened a new door that allowed telehealth to grow faster in both scope and scale. For instance, broadband Internet and wireless technologies made it feasible to reach patients in their homes or remote locations with ease of use. Government and insurance companies began to discuss telehealth regulations and reimbursements for healthcare providers who use telehealth. With the rapid evolution of information technology, most people in many countries have at least one digital device that can provide a means for communication between a patient and a healthcare provider (World Health Organization [WHO], 2022). Telehealth is a promising tool with many advantages in healthcare delivery systems. It has the potential to significantly increase access to healthcare and cost-effective health services for patients no matter where people live (De Oliveira et al., 2023). In particular, it is valuable for medically underserved populations who live in remote areas. Overall, telehealth has evolved along with advanced technological development. The utilization of telehealth has transformed the landscape of the healthcare systems in the United States and many other countries around the world.

The researchers of this chapter conducted literature searches in PubMed, a premier database in the field of medicine and health sciences in the world. This medical database, developed by the US National Library of Medicine, can be openly accessed worldwide. PubMed collects more than 37 million citations in biomedical and health sciences from peer-reviewed journals around the world (National Library of Medicine [NLM], 2024). Literature review results showed a total of 76,592 publications (as of May 17, 2024) in the use of telehealth and telemedicine from 1962 to 2024 around the world. Figure 3.1 illustrates the trends in practicing telehealth and telemedicine, showing significant increases, particularly in the periods 1995–2000, 2010–2019, and 2020–2023 during the pandemic. The results demonstrate the evolution of telehealth and the trends in telehealth use with the advanced development of technologies over the past six decades around the world.

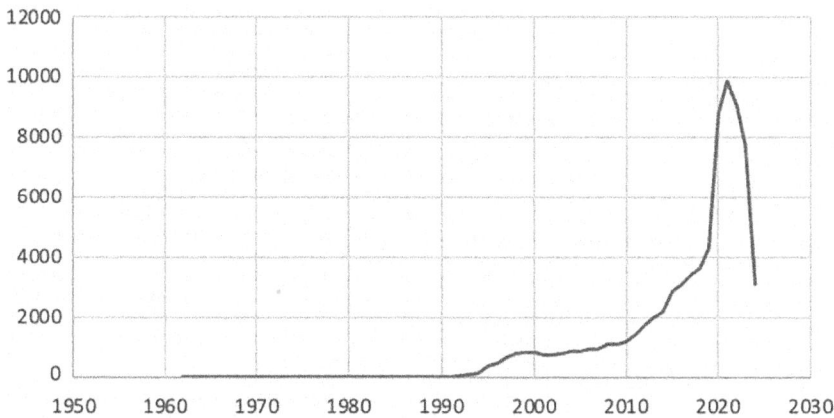

FIGURE 3.1 Trends in Practicing Telehealth and Telemedicine from 1962 to 2024 in the World.

3.5 BRIDGING THE DIGITAL DIVIDE DURING THE COVID-19 PANDEMIC

Telehealth has been implemented over the past six decades around the world as outlined above. Research evidence in Figure 3.1 showed that telehealth has gained recognition as a viable and convenient healthcare delivery model since 2010. The level of utilizing telehealth varied from country to country. However, the COVID-19 pandemic has promoted and accelerated the implementation of telehealth in many countries' healthcare systems around the world (Webster, 2020). This chapter presents three countries as examples to demonstrate the implementation of telehealth during the pandemic.

3.5.1 TELEHEALTH IN THE UNITED STATES

The utilization of telehealth in the United States was relatively low and was not as widespread or deeply integrated into mainstream healthcare practices prior to the COVID-19 pandemic. Telehealth primarily served as a supplemental option for certain consultations, follow-ups, and specialized services, with limited adoption in some urban medical centers and healthcare sectors (Shaver, 2022). It is noted that the utilization of telehealth was influenced by factors such as geographic accessibility, patient preferences, limited reimbursement, regulatory barriers, provider resistance, and limited Internet access. Additionally, the landscape was marked by mixed enthusiasm for the potential benefits of using telehealth, which resulted in the cautious exploration of the technology's capabilities prior to the pandemic.

The outbreak of the COVID-19 pandemic first occurred in Wuhan, Hubei Province, in China in December 2019. The WHO declared the COVID-19 pandemic on March 11, 2020 (WHO, 2020). As the virus spread rapidly in the United States, public health measures were implemented such as social distancing and lockdown. Hospitals and healthcare facilities faced unprecedented challenges. Traditional care delivery models became increasingly difficult to sustain. Healthcare providers had to find alternative ways to deliver patient care. In response to the increasing need to extend the reach of healthcare without physically changing the location of either the provider or the patient, telehealth medical practice emerged as a critical tool for ensuring continuity of care while minimizing viral transmission, which was otherwise a risk with face-to-face consultation (Chang et al., 2021).

The COVID-19 pandemic dramatically accelerated the widespread adoption of telehealth in the US healthcare system. Literature review results revealed that telehealth utilization experienced significant growth during the pandemic, as compared to before the pandemic. For instance, the AMA indicated that telehealth utilization surged to 70% in 2020, even though the healthcare system in the United States was not adequately prepared to manage the significant influx of patients during the pandemic (Chang). The statistical data from the CDC indicated that during the first quarter of 2020, the number of telehealth visits increased by 50%, compared with that in the same period in 2019. In addition, there was a 154% increase in visits noted in surveillance week 13 in 2020, compared with the same period in 2019 (Centers for Disease Control and Prevention [CDC], 2020). This rapid expansion of telehealth services enabled healthcare providers to maintain continuity of care for patients with chronic conditions while simultaneously expanding access to medical consultation for acute illnesses and preventive care needs (Davila et al., 2023).

White-Williams et al. (2023) conducted a retrospective study by examining the electronic health records of privately insured patients in the COVID-19 Research Database. The researchers examined 17.98 million unique visit records of 2.93 million patients from March through December 2019 and 22.17 million records of 3.55 million patients from March through December 2020. The purpose of White-Williams' study was to identify whether there was any difference in the use of telehealth services among the non-Hispanic White, non-Hispanic Black, and Hispanic racial and ethnic groups. The research results indicate that from March through December 2020, the overall mean percentage of telehealth visits per month was 11.1%, and the monthly percentage peaked at 15.5% in April 2020. In 2019, the overall mean percentage of telehealth visits per month among non-Hispanic Black patients was 10.4%, and the monthly percentage peaked at 19.6% in November.

Another study on telemedicine use among adults in the United States was conducted by Lucas and Villarroel (2022). The researchers observed the differences in telemedicine use by sex, age, race and Hispanic origin, family income, education level, region, and urbanicity. The data were collected from the US National Health Interview Survey. The results showed that in 2021, 37.0% of adults used telemedicine in the past 12 months. Telemedicine use increased with age and was higher among women (42.0%) compared with men (31.7%). Non-Hispanic White (39.2%) and non-Hispanic American Indian or Alaska Native (40.6%) adults were more likely to use telemedicine compared with Hispanic (32.8%), non-Hispanic Black (33.1%), and non-Hispanic Asian (33.0%) adults.

Another important factor of a rapid adoption of telehealth services was that the US government expanded reimbursement policies and coverage (Rinkle, 2020). During the pandemic, the Department of Health and Human Services changed its policy to reimburse healthcare providers for the use of telehealth for patient care (Department of Health and Human Services [HHS], 2023, 2024). The reimbursement policy change included relaxed licensing requirements and broader insurance coverage for telehealth services. The AMA stated these changes were intended to "aggressively expand telehealth policy, research, and resources to ensure physician practice sustainability and fair payment" (AMA, 2023a).

3.6   TELEHEALTH IN THE UNITED KINGDOM

The adoption of telehealth in the United Kingdom has been driven by the National Health Service (NHS). As the central governing body for healthcare in the United Kingdom, the NHS has been advocating for further investment in and inclusion of telehealth as a primary delivery vehicle of their 21st-century healthcare system. In 2019, the NHS published its "Long Term Plan," which includes and explicitly delineates how telehealth is central to its strategy to modernize healthcare delivery via the expansion of digital healthcare services (National Health Service [NHS], 2019). Utilization of telehealth was already on the rise since the early 2010s, but the COVID-19 pandemic catapulted it to become the primary method of primary care delivery by mid-2020. Nearly one year after the discovery of the novel coronavirus that sparked the COVID-19 pandemic, 99% of primary care practices in the United Kingdom were offering video consultations. Pre-pandemic, telehealth was only offered in just over 10% of primary care offices (NHS, n.d.).

In 2018, the NHS created and implemented the "NHS App." This app helped usher in a "soft launch" of how digital resources can be used in the delivery of healthcare. As with most medical apps nowadays, the "NHS App" allows patients to chat with their healthcare provider, review their medical records, and even create appointments to discuss their health concerns in more depth. Citizens of the United Kingdom have recognized the NHS's push toward a more digital healthcare system and have largely embraced the change. With strong support from the government and widespread buy-in from citizens across the country, the integration of telehealth into the NHS framework has been crucial in achieving the "Long Term Plan."

Even with these challenges, patients and providers have provided largely positive reviews of telehealth. In 2021, Peters and colleagues reported that "80% of patients found video consultations to be as effective as face-to-face appointments, and 75% of healthcare providers felt that telehealth had improved access to care" (Peters et al., 2021). When evaluated as a whole, the successful integration of telehealth in the United Kingdom has been dependent on prioritizing patient-centered care and supporting providers in healthcare delivery.

3.7   TELEHEALTH IN CANADA

Canada is known for its immense geography and heavily dispersed population among many of its various territories in provinces. Because of this, telehealth is an attractive solution to expanding healthcare in Canada and has been since prior to the pandemic. One of the primary aims of implementing telehealth within the various provincial healthcare systems is to reach rural and remote areas where access to healthcare has traditionally been extremely limited. The implementation of telehealth in Canada was rapidly set ablaze as the accelerant that was the COVID-19 pandemic unfolded. In fact, according to the Canadian Institute for Health Information (CIHI), virtual care accounted for 39% of primary care visits in Canada during the height of the pandemic in 2020, a dramatic increase from just 4% in 2019 (Canadian Institute for Health Information [CIHI], 2022).

The CIHI also conducted an analysis of the physician billing data in five provinces (Ontario, Manitoba, Saskatchewan, Alberta, and British Columbia). The results showed that during the first year of the pandemic in 2020, up to twice as many physicians provided care virtually compared to 2019. At the same time, the rate at which patients received virtual services quadrupled (Husak et al., 2022).

Like the United States, Canada has also struggled with establishing a reliable digital infrastructure to aid in the permanent implementation of telehealth. However, bolstered by a centralized governing healthcare body, the success of telehealth can be attributed to Canada's federal government's investment in furthering the digital infrastructure and rapid development of virtual care platforms.

3.8   ADVANTAGES OF UTILIZING TELEHEALTH

The results of a comprehensive literature review and data analysis demonstrated that the utilization of telehealth presents advantages such as patient and provider satisfaction, improved access to care, convenience, slowing spread of infection, and potential cost-saving (De Oliveira et al., 2023; Gajarawala & Pelkowski, 2021).

3.8.1   PATIENT AND PROVIDER SATISFACTION WITH TELEHEALTH

As telehealth revolutionizes the healthcare landscape, understanding its impact on patient satisfaction and potential cost-saving is crucial for healthcare providers and policymakers. While quantitative data provide a broad overview of telehealth usage and outcomes, qualitative data such as patient testimonials and survey responses offer a more nuanced and personal perspective on the efficacy and challenges of telehealth services.

Telehealth, depending on the specific service, offers a preferable alternative for patients, enhancing healthcare accessibility, especially for those in remote or underserved areas. It reduces travel time and costs, decreases wait times, and provides scheduling flexibility. This convenience allows patients to receive care without the disruptions associated with traditional healthcare visits. Telehealth has proven effective in facilitating continuity of care, particularly for follow-up consultations, chronic condition management, and mental health services. The ability for patients to access care from the comfort of their homes also minimizes the risk of exposure to contagious illnesses. This benefit has become increasingly important considering recent global health challenges.

Some specialty services, however, such as orthopedic medicine, may present challenges when delivered through telehealth, or so we would assume. Tilmon et al. (2023) conducted a survey of 175 patients in a cross-sectional study, in which 82 patients were seen via telehealth services and 93 were in person. The study indicated that "most patients presenting to an orthopedic sports medicine clinic are open to telehealth, recognize its utility, and believe it to be just as comparable with in-person clinical visits" (Tilmon et al., 2023). The study showed that the two groups' patient satisfaction scores did not differ, suggesting that telehealth and in-person consultations provided comparable satisfaction levels. This finding highlights the potential for telehealth to be as effective as traditional in-person visits in meeting patient needs and preferences.

In the wake of the COVID-19 pandemic, a compelling study led by Buchalter and colleagues (2020) has shed light on the high levels of satisfaction associated with telehealth. Patients rated their telehealth experiences an impressive 4.25 out of 5, with 37% favoring telehealth for future consultations. The study shows that patient satisfaction was particularly high among those who found scheduling telehealth visits easy (odds ratio [OR] = 3.058; 95% confidence interval [CI] = $1.621 - 5.768$; $p < 0.001$) and felt their communication during these sessions was effective $\left(OR = 20.268; 95\% \; CI = 5.033 - 81.631; p < 0.001\right)$ (Buchalter et al., 2020).

Surgeons also reported a high level of satisfaction with telehealth, scoring an average of 3.94 out of 5. Even though they rated the effectiveness of physical examinations via telehealth as moderate, with a score of 2.64 out of 5, they were quite confident in their diagnoses, scoring 4.03 out of 5. Interestingly, 36.7% of surgeons felt that some telehealth patients still required in-person visits. However, an overwhelming 93.9% of surgeons planned to continue utilizing telehealth in the future, as noted by Buchalter et al. (2020).

A survey conducted by Canada Health Infoway in 2021 found that 91% of patients were satisfied with their virtual care experience (Canada Health Infoway, 2021a), and 80% of healthcare providers reported that telehealth had improved the efficiency of care delivery (Canada Health Infoway, 2021b). Thus, despite the challenges of a geographically diverse nation such as Canada, patient and provider satisfaction with telehealth has been immensely positive. Moving forward, targeted approaches to address the shortcomings of the current digital infrastructure and digital divide will result in an even more positive opinion of telehealth among Canadian citizens. Telehealth remains a significant mode of delivery and has important implications for the future of patient care and the relationships between patients and providers in Canada (Husak et al., 2022).

Despite reservations about its limitations in conducting thorough physical examinations, surgeons were still enthusiastic about telehealth's potential benefits. They valued its convenience and effectiveness, demonstrated by their confidence in making accurate diagnoses and their commitment to integrating telehealth into their practice. This reflects a broader trend of acceptance and adaptation to telehealth in the medical community.

Based on the studies presented, telehealth holds significant promise as a viable alternative to traditional in-person healthcare delivery. The satisfaction levels among both patients and healthcare providers indicate that telehealth effectively meets the needs of various populations, particularly those in remote or underserved areas. Despite certain limitations in specialties, the ability of telehealth to provide continuity of care, reduce exposure to infectious diseases, and enhance communication and convenience for patients cannot be understated.

3.8.2 FINANCIAL COST-SAVING

While telehealth is not a universal solution for all healthcare challenges, it has demonstrated significant potential to reduce medical costs in various areas such as reduced hospital readmissions, fewer emergency room visits, and decreased travel expenses during the COVID-19 pandemic. For instance, the Stanford hospital addiction consult service (ACS) adapted to the pandemic by transforming an in-person ACS to a telehealth ACS (Deng et al., 2023). Deng et al. compared 30-day readmission rates in patients with and without an addiction medicine consult pre-pandemic (in-person ACS) and during the pandemic (telehealth ACS). Their study results showed that patients seen by telehealth ACS had decreased 30-day readmission rates consistent with those seen before COVID-19. Another study showed the decrease in emergency department visits ranged from 41.5% in Colorado to 63.5% in New York.

Vosburg and Robinson (2022) compared studies by 23 primary care providers and 1,692 patients in Massachusetts, wherein US patients and providers reported high levels of satisfaction with telemedicine visits in a primary care setting. Providers felt that telemedicine visits usually take the same amount or less time than in-person visits. Patients who saved more than 30 min of travel time found it easy to connect. The rapid expansion of telehealth not only highlighted its resilience in times of crisis but also prompted a broader recognition of its potential to reduce health costs, increase healthcare accessibility, improve patient outcomes, and enhance the overall efficiency of healthcare delivery ((De Oliveira et al., 2023; Koonin et al., 2020). Additionally, the rapid and widespread utilization of telehealth and changes to reimbursement policies are considered a revolution in bridging the digital divide in the US healthcare system.

As telehealth continues to evolve, its role in cost reduction is likely to expand, particularly as technology improves and adoption increases. In the future, it is crucial for healthcare providers and policymakers to recognize and address the challenges posed by certain medical specialties to optimize telehealth services further. By doing so, telehealth can continue to expand its reach and efficacy, ensuring that it remains a cornerstone of modern healthcare delivery, especially in a world increasingly aware of the importance of reducing contagion risk and enhancing patient accessibility. Overall, the widespread adoption of telehealth was a direct response driven by the urgent need for remote access to healthcare services while satisfying the necessity of minimizing the risk of viral transmission, reducing travel costs and time, and saving lives. Many healthcare providers used telehealth during the pandemic to provide patients with virtual consultations, remote monitoring, patient education, and teletherapy around the world.

3.9 CHALLENGES AND BARRIERS TO TELEHEALTH UTILIZATION

The widespread use of telehealth during the pandemic saved many lives and protected numerous individuals from virus infection. However, not all people were able to have access to this technology. Literature review results showed that disparities, challenges, and barriers to telehealth do exist (Gajarawala & Pelkowski, 2021). Similar to in-person healthcare, access to telehealth services was not equitable across all populations (Ahmed et al., 2024). Ensuring equitable access to digital healthcare services is the main obstacle for telehealth implementation in the United Kingdom. In Canada, even with this staunch support, struggles in some regions without adequate Internet connectivity have voiced concerns about equitable access, particularly among the Indigenous communities in Canada (CIHI, 2022). These communities are typically located in rural areas, separated by great geographic distances and difficult-to-traverse terrains.

The ever-increasing population of older adults with limited digital literacy has throttled the widespread success of telehealth. The challenges of digital literacy extend far beyond the screen as older adults are among the heaviest utilizers of healthcare resources in many modern countries. Efforts to target interventions to support this specific population as they navigate the challenges of telehealth are ongoing, but there is no immediate solution at hand. Notable disparities were observed in rural areas, in low-income communities, and among racial and ethnic minorities (Park et al., 2023). The relative scarcity of access to the appropriate technological infrastructure impeded the expansion of this modality, as technological limitations, such as lack of broadband Internet access and digital literacy, cast a stark light on the absence of fully accessible Internet services in many regions of the United States (Zhu et al., 2024).

The use of telehealth services among racial and ethnic minority groups before and during the COVID-19 pandemic was investigated by White-Willliams et al. (2023). The study results showed that the likelihood of using telehealth was lower among Hispanic patients than among non-Hispanic White and non-Hispanic Black patients during the pandemic. It is suggested that culturally sensitive measures are needed to support telehealth use among the Hispanic population.

Lucas and Villarroel (2022) conducted research that closely examined the disparities of telemedicine use among ethnic groups and their education level, family income, and geographic locations. The research results indicated that the percentage of adults who used telemedicine increased with education level, revealing a correlation between higher education and increased usage, as well as variations based on income.

Additionally, the geographical landscape played a defining role, as telemedicine usage demonstrated regional discrepancies and diminishes with decreasing urbanization levels. Telemedicine use was highest among those living in the Northeast and West regions, and use increased with age, education level, and family incomes at or above 200% of the federal poverty level (FPL). Telemedicine use was highest in large metropolitan areas and decreased with lower urbanization levels. This compilation of insights underscores the multifaceted nature of telemedicine adoption, intricately woven with demographic, socioeconomic, and geographic factors, offering a comprehensive understanding of its diverse patterns in the year 2021 (Lucas & Villarroel, 2022).

Zhang et al. (2024) investigated the prevalence and factors associated with telehealth utilization among US adults during the COVID-19 pandemic using a nationally representative survey in the United States. The results indicated that 43% of the sample reported having used telehealth, representing 114.5 million adults in the nation. East and Southeast Asians used telehealth less than non-Hispanic Whites (OR = 0.5; 95% CI: 0.3–0.8). Being uninsured (compared with private insurance: OR = 0.4; 95% CI: 0.2–0.8) and those with limited broadband coverage in the community (OR = 0.5; 95% CI: 0.3–0.8) were less likely to use telehealth (Zhang et al., 2024).

Despite the seemingly overwhelming potential for public benefit, progress was also hindered by government regulatory barriers, which included variations in telehealth reimbursement policies across payers and state licensing requirements for healthcare providers. Work to overcome these challenges to telehealth implementation and sustainability is ongoing. Telehealth further demonstrated its applicability to even broader medical interactions between patients and their care providers in practically all service lines worldwide.

There are some concerns about the utilization of telehealth. For instance, several crucial elements of comprehensive medical care can only be delivered in face-to-face encounters, especially for particularly complex or sensitive medical cases and conditions. Telehealth performs well in managing nonurgent medical conditions and questions but lacks the ability for providers to physically evaluate a patient. Another big concern is about privacy and security related to telehealth visits during the COVID-19 pandemic (Jalali et al., 2021; Ftouni et al., 2022). Data breaches in healthcare have risen in the past 5 years, increasing a massive 42% in 2020 when the pandemic occurred. Of the total amount of ransomware attacks reported in 2020, 60% specifically targeted the healthcare sector (Witts, 2024). Houser et al. (2023) conducted a systematic review and identified the three risk factors related to privacy and security in telehealth practice during the COVID-19 pandemic. These three factors included environmental factors (e.g., lack of private space for vulnerable populations, and difficulty sharing sensitive health information remotely); technology factors (e.g., data security issues, limited access to the Internet, and technology); and operational factors (e.g., reimbursement, payer denials, technology accessibility, training, and education).

3.10   RECOMMENDATIONS

Telehealth has become an essential medical service, especially in the post-pandemic world. It is believed that telehealth will continue to transform today's landscape of healthcare systems in the

United States and around the world. With the new technologies such as artificial intelligence (AI), machine learning, and patient remote monitoring, telehealth will continue to play an important role in improving access to healthcare and the health and well-being of people. Despite its impressive growth, the rapid and widespread adoption of telehealth has made many health leaders ask questions about the implementation process and how it might affect workflows, staffing resources, and data security and patient privacy and confidentiality. Based on the research evidence, the following recommendations are proposed with the hope to improve telehealth utilization in international healthcare systems in the future.

3.10.1 EXPAND BROADBAND INFRASTRUCTURE

Much progress in telehealth utilization has been made in recent years, especially with a rapid adoption during the COVID-19 pandemic, but a digital gap still exists in many countries of the world. Internet service providers still primarily rely on "wired" connectivity to optimize speed and reliability of digital communication (Sheets et al., 2021; Ftouni et al., 2022). Wireless technology in many ways is more practical to deploy to remote locations. However, there is often diminished speed and reliability compared to the wired standard. Addressing the digital divide is crucial for ensuring equitable access to telehealth services (Park et al., 2023). The hardware and software development needed to close this gap and enhance the delivery of reliable Internet access, even in remote and underserved areas, is crucial to enabling equitable healthcare access and expansion (Carretier et al., 2023). The research evidence revealed that telehealth use was highest in large metropolitan areas and lowest with decreasing urbanization levels in the United States during the COVID-19 pandemic (Lucas & Villarroel, 2022). The United Kingdom also saw higher telemedicine usage in cities like London, Birmingham, and Manchester. In Canada, telehealth use was particularly high in major cities like Toronto, Vancouver, and Montreal. The CIHI (CIHI, 2022) reported that urban areas saw a much higher uptake of virtual care compared to rural and remote regions, where challenges like Internet access and technological resources were more pronounced. Urban areas had more robust healthcare systems capable of quickly integrating telemedicine, while rural areas lagged behind due to technological and logistical barriers.

Therefore, expanding broadband infrastructure is critical to the success of telehealth, particularly in rural and underserved areas. It is recommended to develop government funding, public–private partnerships, community engagement, and strategic investments in technology to create a robust infrastructure that supports widespread telehealth adoption. For instance, the Rural Digital Opportunity Fund (RDOF) in the United States provides $20.4 billion in funding over 10 years to support broadband expansion in rural areas. This funding has been crucial in improving access to telehealth services in remote regions (Universal Service Administrative Co., n.d.). In Australia, National Broadband Network (NBN) is a government initiative aimed at providing high-speed broadband to all Australians. The NBN has been instrumental in enabling telehealth services, particularly in rural and remote areas (Australian Government, 2020a).

Another suggestion for expanding broadband infrastructure is to engage local communities in the planning and deployment process to ensure that infrastructure meets local needs. This can include community consultations, local government involvement, and collaboration with regional health networks. For instance, in Scotland, UK, the Scottish Futures Trust worked with local councils to develop community broadband solutions, particularly in the Highlands and Islands (Scottish Futures Trust, 2024).

3.10.2 ENHANCE USER DIGITAL LITERACY

There must be increased efforts on digital literacy and competency for the public and healthcare providers. The literature review revealed a correlation between education level and telehealth use in American adults (Lucas & Villarroel, 2022). Some underserved populations that face challenges of decreased education levels or inadequate financial resources to purchase appropriate hardware will continue to lag in their access to healthcare even as telemedicine continues to expand (Chu et al., 2022). Populations such as the elderly or individuals with language barriers may still struggle with interacting via telehealth despite its increased availability (Wong et al., 2023). Education and training programs to improve digital literacy can help bridge the gap in access to telehealth services, but only as education in general is able to extend its reach into this population base. Ftouni et al. (2022) in their study pointed out that telehealth training for both healthcare providers and patients was deficient. Therefore, not only is it in the best interest of the public to increase digital literacy and understand how to use technology for communication with healthcare providers, but there is a need to develop comprehensive training and support programs to train healthcare providers with the necessary skills and knowledge to effectively deliver care via telehealth.

Therefore, to enhance user digital literacy, it is recommended to create education and training programs that teach patients how to use telehealth platforms, including navigating software, understanding privacy settings, and troubleshooting common issues. For instance, Telehealth Education for Seniors in Ontario, Canada, was developed by the Ontario Telemedicine Network (OTN) to help seniors use telehealth services effectively (Ontario Telemedicine Network, n.d.). This program includes workshops, one-on-one training sessions, and instructional videos. As a result, many elderly patients who were previously unfamiliar with digital technologies are now actively using telehealth services for their healthcare needs. Additionally, a Digital Health Literacy Project supported by the Australian government partnered with local libraries and senior centers to deliver digital health literacy workshops. The workshops provided were tailored to different levels of digital literacy and included hands-on practice with telehealth platforms (Australian Digital Health Agency, 2022).

Another recommendation for enhancing user digital literacy is to incorporate digital literacy in school curriculums. For instance, Digital Health in Schools in Finland incorporated digital health literacy into its national curriculum. Students learn how to use telehealth platforms as part of their health and technology education, preparing them for future healthcare interactions (International Literacy Association, 2015).

With regard to training for healthcare providers, it is recommended that healthcare providers need to have a fundamental understanding of the working of Internet communications and electronic health records to properly make use of these tools (CMS, 2021). Healthcare providers possibly may even be called upon to help educate their patient base regarding this technology to enhance the uptake of this model of care in the place of, or in conjunction with, traditional in-person office visits (Wong et al., 2023). Telehealth Advocate Training by the AMA provides training for healthcare providers on how to assist their patients with telehealth. The training includes how to explain the process, demonstrate the technology, and provide follow-up support. As a result, providers can effectively guide their patients in using telehealth services, particularly those who are less tech-savvy. The enthusiasm that healthcare providers demonstrate in promoting telehealth as being equally beneficial to the patient will certainly stimulate the interest and willingness of the public to accept this as yet another tool that the provider can employ to manage healthcare conditions in both acute and chronic diseases (Chen et al., 2023). Such expanded healthcare provider training should emphasize telehealth technologies, communication techniques, and cultural competency to ensure high-quality, patient-centered care.

3.10.3 PROTECT PATIENT INFORMATION PRIVACY AND SECURITY

Protecting patient data privacy and security is very critical when using telehealth services. With the increased adoption of telehealth and massive 42% of data breaches in healthcare when the pandemic hit in 2020, healthcare providers must ensure that patient information is safeguarded against breaches and unauthorized access (Witts, 2024). Privacy and security threats are likely to be encountered post-pandemic. Without adequate security and privacy protections for underlying telehealth data and systems, healthcare providers and patients will lack trust in the use of telehealth solutions.

To protect patients' privacy and improve the quality of telehealth for patient safety, it is necessary for health leaders, policymakers, healthcare providers, and IT experts to comprehensively analyze potential risks and security threats in remote healthcare and institute appropriate countermeasures. It is recommended that federal and state guidelines, protocols, and policies for telehealth security and privacy be updated and that sufficient resources be allocated toward improving telehealth capabilities to ensure patient safety, privacy, and security when implementing telehealth. For instance, Kaiser Permanente in the United States has developed detailed data privacy policies that govern the use of patient data within its telehealth services (Kaiser Permanente, n.d.). These policies are regularly reviewed and updated to ensure compliance with the latest regulations. One of the effective strategies for protecting patient data privacy and security is to implement strong encryption protocols recommended by the Health Sector Coordinating Council Cybersecurity Working Group (2023).

Another important recommendation is to adopt secure telehealth platforms that are compliant with legal and regulatory standards and healthcare regulations such as the Health Insurance Portability and Accountability Act (HIPAA) in the United States or the General Data Protection Regulation (GDPR) in Europe. These platforms should have built-in security features, including user authentication, audit trails, and secure data storage.

For protecting patient data privacy and security, another effective strategy is to develop clear consent procedures for telehealth services, ensuring that patients understand how their data will be used and have the opportunity to opt-in or opt-out of specific services. Document consent digitally to maintain accurate records. The good example is that the Ontario Telemedicine Network (OTN) has implemented a robust informed consent process that clearly explains to patients how their data will be used, stored, and shared when using telehealth services. Patients are required to provide digital consent before any telehealth session begins (Ontario Telemedicine Network, n.d.).

Finally, it is important to set up monitoring systems to detect and respond to security incidents in real time. Have a response and preparedness plan in place for breaches, including notification procedures, mitigation strategies, and communication with affected patients. A good example is that International Business Machines Corporation (IBM) Security in the United States provides incident response services to healthcare organizations, including those offering telehealth. Their services include 24/7 monitoring, rapid response to breaches, and post-incident analysis to prevent future occurrences (International Business Machines Corporation [IBM], n.d.). Overall, by implementing strong encryption, adopting secure platforms, conducting regular audits, educating users, and staying compliant with regulations, healthcare providers can safeguard patient information effectively.

3.10.4 Promote Telehealth Equity and Accessibility

In the previous section, the researchers identified some access disparities in the utilization of telehealth. Therefore, promoting telehealth equity and accessibility is very important to ensure that all populations, including those in medically underserved communities and areas, have equal access to healthcare services. Strategies to promote telehealth equity should be integrated into broader initiatives aimed at addressing social determinants of health such as housing, transportation, and food insecurity. The challenge of establishing reliable and stable technology in older, more remotely established communities remains (Davila et al., 2023). However, given the success already realized with the delivery of healthcare via telehealth, current and future community and city planners must also make dedicated efforts to include technology access as the new "standard of living" in developing and newly planned living communities. Providing this foundational infrastructure in communities will lead to enhanced acceptance in surrounding municipalities and vastly accelerate the potential for further future expansion and enhancements as it pertains to healthcare equity and accessibility. It is recommended that community-based partnerships and outreach programs can help raise awareness of telehealth services and facilitate access for vulnerable populations by working in conjunction with city and county government planners. Some programs are successfully implemented to reduce disparities. A good example is that the California Telehealth Network (CTN) was established to bridge the digital divide and expand telehealth services in rural and low-income communities across California. The CTN provides the necessary infrastructure, training, and support to healthcare providers in underserved areas, enabling them to offer telehealth services to their patients (California Telehealth Network [CTN], n.d.). The CTN has successfully expanded telehealth services to over 1,000 healthcare sites across California, many of which are located in rural or underserved areas. This program has increased access to care, particularly for populations that previously faced significant barriers to healthcare services.

Another good example is that the Indigenous Telehealth Project was launched to improve healthcare access for Indigenous communities in remote parts of Australia (Australian Government, 2020b). The program leverages telehealth technology to connect Indigenous patients with healthcare providers, including specialists, who are often located in urban centers. The project also includes cultural competency training for healthcare providers to ensure that telehealth services are delivered in a culturally sensitive manner. The Indigenous Telehealth Project has successfully reduced healthcare disparities in indigenous communities by increasing access to care, improving the management of chronic conditions, and reducing the need for patients to travel long distances for medical appointments.

3.10.5 Monitor the Impacts of Emerging Technologies and Innovations on Telehealth

Emerging technologies like AI, wearable monitoring devices, and other innovations are revolutionizing the way healthcare is delivered, making it more accessible, efficient, and personalized. Therefore, it is important to monitor some key emerging technologies and their potential impact on the future of telehealth. For instance, with technological advancements, we are able to remotely monitor patients' health in real time, leverage AI for accurate diagnostics and predictive analytics, provide high-quality virtual consultations, and utilize wearable devices to track vital signs and ensure adherence to treatment plans. These innovations not only enhance the quality of care but also empower patients to take a more active role in managing their health, ultimately leading to better outcomes and a more sustainable healthcare system.

In just a few short years, AI has made a significant impact on various industries by improving efficiency, enabling advanced data analysis, and transforming patient experiences. For example, AI-powered diagnostics uses algorithms that analyze medical images, pathology slides, and other diagnostic data with high accuracy. This technology aids in the early detection of diseases such as cancer, diabetic retinopathy, and cardiovascular conditions (AMA, 2023b).

The primary benefit of AI-powered diagnostics is its ability to process data quickly, transforming the healthcare field. Advanced algorithms, supported by machine learning and neural networks, drive these AI systems, allowing them to analyze vast amounts of data in seconds. This remarkable speed in diagnostics not only accelerates the detection of diseases but also equips healthcare professionals to delve deeper into complex medical conditions, ultimately improving patient outcomes and enabling more personalized treatment plans (The Healthcare Daily, 2023).

In addition to AI-powered diagnostics, wearable monitoring devices have also revolutionized healthcare by providing real-time data on patients' vital signs and activities. This continuous stream of information allows for early detection of potential health issues, more proactive management of chronic conditions, and personalized treatment adjustments. These wearable devices enhance patient engagement and adherence to treatment plans by offering insights into their health metrics and encouraging healthier lifestyle choices.

In the future, AI will have a greater impact on healthcare as it continues to advance and integrate into various aspects of patient care and medical research. AI's capabilities in analyzing vast amounts of data will enhance diagnostic accuracy, personalize treatment plans, and streamline administrative processes within healthcare organizations. With improved predictive analytics, AI will aid in early detection of diseases and more effective management of chronic conditions. Additionally,

AI-driven tools will support medical professionals by providing real-time insights and decision support, ultimately leading to more efficient and effective healthcare delivery (Healthcare Daily, 2023).

3.11 CONCLUSION

Telehealth is revolutionizing the delivery of healthcare services in the United States and the world. The COVID-19 pandemic has accelerated the widespread adoption of telehealth in many healthcare systems worldwide. Research evidence revealed that telehealth utilization was found to improve access to health services and decrease the risks of the virus transmission among people during the pandemic. However, widespread use of telehealth is still hampered by barriers and challenges. There is limited evidence available about specific cost-effectiveness of telehealth utilization except saving travel costs. Further research is required to improve the credibility of evidence on telehealth outcomes. In addition, patient privacy and security have to be addressed to ensure the success of telehealth use and patient safety in the long-term.

The future of telehealth holds tremendous promise and potential for continuing to transform the landscape of healthcare delivery systems in the post-pandemic era. However, the analysis findings showed some challenges and disparities in the use of telehealth during the pandemic. As healthcare systems move on to the post-pandemic era, information technology and medicine continue advancing to strengthen healthcare delivery systems for the future. AI and machine learning will be able to help analyze electronic patient records, support clinical decision-making, and enhance the efficiency of telehealth services. Telehealth's ongoing evolution will be driven by the need for accessible, efficient, and patient-centered healthcare services. Hopefully, the recommendations, including some samples and successful programs presented in this chapter, will help governments, policymakers, and health leaders create better health policies to continuously promote widespread telehealth utilization and implementation and reduce disparities, especially in medically underserved populations and areas. AI and digital health technological advancements will encourage healthcare providers to embrace new changes to improve telehealth and virtual care. All the improvements will allow healthcare professionals and healthcare systems to build a more resilient, accessible, cost-effective, and equitable telehealth infrastructure that is better prepared to respond to future health crises while reducing disparities and improving quality care and health outcomes for all.

3.12 CONFLICT OF INTEREST STATEMENT

The authors declare no conflict of interests.

3.13 FUNDING

None

REFERENCES

Ahmed, A., Mutahar, M., Daghrery, A. A., AlbarPark, N. H., Alhadidi, I. Q. I., Asiri, A. M., Boreak, N., Alshahrani, A. A. S., Shariff, M., Shubayr, M. A., & Al Moaleem, M. M. (2024). A systematic review of publications on perceptions and management of chronic medical conditions using telemedicine remote consultations by primary healthcare professionals April 2020 to December 2021 during the COVID-19 pandemic. *Medical Science Monitor: International Medical Journal of Experimental and Clinical Research, 30*, e943383. https://doi.org/10.12659/MSM.943383

American Academy of Family Physician. (2022, January). *Telehealth and Telemedicine.* https://www.aafp.org/about/policies/all/telehealth-telemedicine.html#:~:text=While%20telemedicine%20refers%20specifically%20to,facilitate%20and%20support%20assessment%2C%20diagnosis%2C

American Medical Association (AMA). (2023a, January 9). *What to Expect in Telehealth in 2023? Here Are 5 Predictions.* https://www.ama-assn.org/practice-management/digital/what-expect-telehealth-2023-here-are-5-predictions

American Medical Association (AMA). (2023b, September 1). *How the AMA's Working to Improve Access to Telemedicine.* https://www.ama-assn.org/practice-management/digital/how-ama-s-working-improve-access-telemedicine

American Medical Association. (2024, May 15). *Telehealth Resource Center: Definitions.* https://www.ama-assn.org/practice-management/digital/telehealth-resource-center-definitions#:~:text=Telehealth%2C%20 telemedicine%20and%20related%20terms,to%20another%20through%20electronic%20communication

Australian Digital Health Agency. (2022). *Digital Health Literacy: Final Program Report.* Retrieved August 12, 2024, from https://library.alia.org.au/sites/default/files/documents/digital_health_literacy_final_report_feb_2022.pdf

Australian Government. (2020a). *National Broadband Network.* Retrieved August 15, 2024, from https://www.infrastructure.gov.au/media-communications-arts/internet/national-broadband-network

Australian Government. (2020b). *Indigenous Telehealth Initiative: Improving Healthcare Access in Remote Australia.* Retrieved August 15, 2024, from https://www.health.gov.au

Buchalter, D. B., Moses, M. J., Azad, A., Kirby, D. J., Huang, S., Bosco, J. A., III, & Yang, S. S. (2020). Patient and surgeon satisfaction with telehealth during the COVID-19 pandemic. *Bulletin of the Hospital for Joint Disease (2013), 78*(4), 227–235.

California Telehealth Network. (n.d.). *California Telehealth Network: Expanding Telehealth Services across California.* Retrieved August 10, 2024, from https://www.caltelehealth.org

Canada Health Infoway. (2021a). *Canadian Digital Health Survey 2021: What Canadians Think.* Retrieved on August 11, 2024, from https://www.infoway-inforoute.ca/en/component/edocman/resources/reports/benefits-evaluation/4011-canadian-digital-health-survey-2021-what-canadians-think

Canada Health Infoway. (2021b). *2021 National Survey of Canadian Physicians.* Retrieved August 12, 2024, from https://www.infoway-inforoute.ca/en/component/edocman/resources/reports/benefits-evaluation/3935–2021-national-survey-of-canadian-physicians

Canadian Institute for Health Information. (2022). *Virtual Care: A Major Shift for Canadians Receiving Physician Services.* Retrieved on August 11, 2024, from https://cihi.ca/en

Carretier, E., Bastide, M., Lachal, J., & Moro, M. R. (2023). Evaluation of the rapid implementation of telehealth during the COVID-19 pandemic: a qualitative study among adolescents and their parents. *European Child & Adolescent Psychiatry, 32*(6), 963–973. https://doi.org.libpublic3.library.isu.edu/10.1007/s00787-022-02108-1

Centers for Disease Control and Prevention. (2020, October 30). *Trends in the Use of Telehealth during the Emergence of the COVID-19 Pandemic—United States, January–March 2020.* https://www.cdc.gov/mmwr/volumes/69/wr/mm6943a3.htm

Centers for Medicare and Medicaid Services. (2021, December 3). *Medicare Telehealth Trends.* Retrieved August 10, 2024, from https://data.cms.gov/summary-statistics-on-use-and-payments/medicare-service-type-reports/medicare-telehealth-trends

Chang, J. E., Lai, A. Y., Gupta, A., Nguyen, A. M., Berry, C. A., & Shelley, D. R. (2021). Rapid transition to telehealth and the digital divide: implications for primary care access and equity in a post-COVID era. *Milbank Quarterly, 99*(2), 340–368. https://doi.org.libpublic3.library.isu.edu/10.1111/1468–0009.12509

Chen, K., Zhang, C., & Jackson, H. B. (2023). Relative billing complexity of in-person versus telehealth outpatient encounters. *Journal of Evaluation in Clinical Practice, 29*(6), 887–892. https://doi.org.libpublic3.library.isu.edu/10.1111/jep.13905

Chu, C., Brual, J., Fang, J., Fleury, C., Stamenova, V., Bhattacharyya, O., & Tadrous, M. (2022). The use of telemedicine in older-adults during the COVID-19 pandemic: a weekly cross-sectional analysis in Ontario, Canada. *Canadian Geriatrics Journal, 25*(4), 380–389. https://doi.org.libpublic3.library.isu.edu/10.5770/cgj.25.610

Davila, J., House, M., Brockman, M., Dayama, N., & Shaver, C. (2023). Telehealth utilization to reduce hospital admissions in high-risk patient populations. *Journal of Business & Behavioral Sciences, 35*(3), 123–135.

De Oliveira, C. R. A., da Silva Etges, A. P. B., Marcolino, M. S., Paixão, M. C., Mendes, M. S., Ribeiro, L. B., Alkmim, M. B. M., Polanczyk, C. A., & Ribeiro, A. L. P. (2023). COVID-19 telehealth service can increase access to the health care system and become a cost-saving strategy. *Telemedicine Journal and E-health, 29*(7), 1043–1050. https://doi.org/10.1089/tmj.2022.0240

Deng, H., Raheemullah, A., Fenno, L. E., & Lembke, A. (2023). A telehealth inpatient addiction consult service is both feasible and effective in reducing readmission rates. *Journal of Addictive Diseases, 41*(3), 225–232. https://doi.org/10.1080/10550887.2022.2090822

Department of Health and Human Services. (2023). *Telehealth Policy Changes after the COVID-19 Public Health Emergency.* https://telehealth.hhs.gov/providers/telehealth-policy/policy-changes-after-the-covid-19-public-health-emergency

Department of Health and Human Services. (2024). *Billing for Telehealth.* https://telehealth.hhs.gov/providers/billing-and-reimbursement

Ftouni, R., AlJardali, B., Hamdanieh, M., Ftouni, L., & Salem, N. (2022). Challenges of telemedicine during the COVID-19 pandemic: a systematic review. *BMC Medical Informatics and Decision Making*, *22*(1), 207. https://doi.org/10.1186/s12911-022-01952-0

Gajarawala, S. N., & Pelkowski, J. N. (2021). Telehealth benefits and barriers. *Journal for Nurse Practitioners: JNP*, *17*(2), 218–221. https://doi.org/10.1016/j.nurpra.2020.09.013

Health Resources and Services Administration. (2022, March). *What Is Telehealth?* https://www.hrsa.gov/telehealth/what-is-telehealth#:~:text=Telehealth%20is%20defined%20as%20the,health%20administration%2C%20and%20public%20health.HRSA

Health Sector Coordinating Council Cybersecurity Working Group. (2023). *Health Industry Cybersecurity—Securing Telehealth and Telemedicine.* Retrieved August 15, 2024, from https://healthsectorcouncil.org/wp-content/uploads/2023/10/HIC-STAT_2023.pdf

The Healthcare Daily. (2023). *AI-Powered Diagnostics: Revolutionizing Healthcare with Speed and Precision.* Retrieved August 12, 2024, from https://thehealthcaredaily.com/ai-powered-diagnostics/

Hincapié, M. A., Gallego, J. C., Gempeler, A., Piñeros, J. A., Nasner, D., & Escobar, M. F. (2020). Implementation and usefulness of telemedicine during the COVID-19 pandemic: a scoping review. *Journal of Primary Care & Community Health*, *11*, 2150132720980612. https://doi.org/10.1177/2150132720980612

Houser, S. H., Flite, C. A., & Foster, S. L. (2023). Privacy and security risk factors related to telehealth services—a systematic review. *Perspectives in Health Information Management*, *20*(1), 1f.

Husak, L., Sovran, V., Ytsma, A., & Comeau, M. (2022). Impact of the COVID-19 pandemic on virtual care: a major shift for physicians and patients. *Healthcare Quarterly (Toronto, Ont.)*, *25*(3), 11–13. https://doi.org/10.12927/hcq.2022.26948

Hyder, M. A., & Razzak, J. (2020). Telemedicine in the United States: an introduction for students and residents. *Journal of Medical Internet Research*, *22*(11), e20839. https://doi.org/10.2196/20839

International Business Machines Corporation. (n.d.). *Incident Response Cybersecurity Services.* Retrieved from https://www.ibm.com/security/services/incident-response

International Literacy Association. (2015). *Digital Literacies in the New Finnish National Core Curriculum.* Retrieved August 15, 2024 from https://www.literacyworldwide.org/blog/literacy-now/2015/08/28/digital-literacies-in-the-new-finnish-national-core-curriculum

Jalali, M. S., Landman, A., & Gordon, W. J. (2021). Telemedicine, privacy, and information security in the age of COVID–19. *Journal of the American Medical Informatics Association: JAMIA*, *28*(3), 671–672. https://doi.org/10.1093/jamia/ocaa310

Kaiser Permanente. (n.d.). *Health Data Privacy.* Retrieved August 12, 2024 from https://about.kaiserpermanente.org/commitments-and-impact/public-policy/our-key-issues/health-data-privacy

Koonin, L. M., Hoots, B., Tsang, C. A., Leroy, Z., Farris, K., Jolly, T., Antall, P., McCabe, B., Zelis, C. B. R., Tong, I., & Harris, A. M. (2020). Trends in the use of telehealth during the emergence of the COVID-19 pandemic—United States, January-March 2020. *Morbidity and Mortality Weekly Report (MMWR)*, *69*(43), 1595–1599. https://doi.org/10.15585/mmwr.mm6943a3

Li, H. K. (1999). Telemedicine and ophthalmology. *Survey of Ophthalmology*, *44*(1), 61–72. https://doi.org/10.1016/s0039–6257(99)00059–4

Link, M. M. (1965). *Space Medicine in Project Mercury. NASA SP–4003. NASA Special Publication.* Washington, DC: Office of Manned Space Flight, National Aeronautics and Space Administration.

Lucas, J. W., & Villarroel, M. A. (2022). Telemedicine use among adults: United States, 2021. *NCHS Data Brief*, (445), 1–8.

National Health Service. (2019). *The Implementation Framework.* Retrieved on August 11, 2024, from https://www.longtermplan.nhs.uk/publication/implementation-framework/

National Health Service. (n.d.). *Video Conferencing Technology in Primary and Secondary Care.* Retrieved August 11, 2024, from https://transform.england.nhs.uk/covid-19-response/technology-nhs/web-based-platform-which-offers-video-calls-services/

National Library of Medicine. (2024, May 17). *PubMed.* https://pubmed.ncbi.nlm.nih.gov/

Ontario Telemedicine Network. (n.d.). *Training and Help Resources.* Retrieved August 10, 2024, from https://otn.ca/support/

Park, J.-H., Lee, M. J., Tsai, M.-H., Shih, H.-J., & Chang, J. (2023). Rural, regional, racial disparities in telemedicine use during the COVID-19 pandemic among US adults: 2021 National Health Interview Survey (NHIS). *Patient Preference & Adherence*, *17*, 3477–3487. https://doi.org.libpublic3.library.isu.edu/10.2147/PPA.S439437

Peters, G. M., Kooij, L., Lenferink, A., van Harten, W. H., & Doggen, C. J. M. (2021). The effect of telehealth on hospital services use: systematic review and meta-analysis. *Journal of Medical Internet Research*, *23*(9), e25195. https://doi.org/10.2196/25195

Rinkle, V. A. (2020). CMS updates COVID-19 policies and guidance on testing, vaccination, and telehealth reimbursement. *Briefings on APCs*, *21*(11), 1–4.

Scottish Futures Trust. (2024). *A Guide to Smart Infrastructure—Scotland's Learning Estate*. Retrieved August 12, 2024, from https://www.scottishfuturestrust.org.uk/

Shaver, J. (2022). The state of telehealth before and after the COVID-19 pandemic. *Primary Care*, *49*(4), 517–530. https://doi.org/10.1016/j.pop.2022.04.002

Sheets, L. R., Wallach, E., Khairat, S., Mutrux, R., Edison, K., & Becevic, M. (2021). Similarities and differences between rural and urban telemedicine utilization. *Perspectives in Health Information Management*, 1–14.

Tilmon, J. C., Farooq, H., Metzger, C. M., Schlecht, S. H., & Klitzman, R. G. (2023). Telehealth in orthopedic sports medicine: a survey study on patient satisfaction and experience. *Telemedicine Journal and E-health*, *29*(6), 943–946. https://doi.org/10.1089/tmj.2022.0193

Universal Service Administrative Co. (n.d.). *Rural Digital Opportunity Fund*. Retried August 12, 2024 from https://www.usac.org/high-cost/funds/rural-digital-opportunity-fund/

Verschuur, J., Koks, E. E., & Hall, J. W. (2021). Global economic impacts of COVID-19 lockdown measures stand out in high-frequency shipping data. *PLoS ONE*, *16*(4), 1–16. https://doi.org.libpublic3.library.isu.edu/10.1371/journal.pone.0248818

Von Hafften, A. (2024, May 18). *The History of Telepsychiatry*. https://www.psychiatry.org/psychiatrists/practice/telepsychiatry/toolkit/history-of-telepsychiatry

Vosburg, R. W., & Robinson, K. A. (2022). Telemedicine in primary care during the COVID-19 pandemic: provider and patient satisfaction examined. *Telemedicine Journal and E-health: The Official Journal of the American Telemedicine Association*, *28*(2), 167–175. https://doi.org/10.1089/tmj.2021.0174

Webster P. (2020). Virtual health care in the era of COVID–19. *Lancet (London, England)*, *395*(10231), 1180–1181. https://doi.org/10.1016/S0140–6736(20)30818–7

White-Williams, C., Liu, X., Shang, D., & Santiago, J. (2023). Use of telehealth among racial and ethnic minority groups in the United States before and during the COVID-19 pandemic. *Public Health Reports (Washington, D.C.: 1974)*, *138*(1), 149–156. https://doi.org/10.1177/00333549221123575

Witts, J. (2024, February 9). *Healthcare Cyber Attack Statistics 2022: 25 Alarming Data Breaches You Should Know*. https://expertinsights.com/insights/healthcare-cyber-attack-statistics/

Wong, H., Razvi, Y., Hamid, M. A., Mistry, N., & Filler, G. (2023). Age and sex-related comparison of referral-based telemedicine service utilization during the COVID-19 pandemic in Ontario: a retrospective analysis. *BMC Health Services Research*, *23*(1), 1374. https://doi.org.libpublic3.library.isu.edu/10.1186/s12913-023-10373-2

World Health Organization. (2020, March 10). *WHO Director-General's Opening Remarks at the Media Briefing on COVID-19—11 March 2020*. https://www.who.int/director-general/speeches/detail/who-director-general-s-opening-remarks-at-the-media-briefing-on-covid-19-11-march-2020

World Health Organization. (2022, January 1). *WHO-ITU Global Standard for Accessibility of Telehealth Services*. https://www.who.int/publications/i/item/9789240050464

Zhang, D., Shi, L., Han, X., Li, Y., Jalajel, N. A., Patel, S., Chen, Z., Chen, L., Wen, M., Li, H., Chen, B., Li, J., & Su, D. (2024). Disparities in telehealth utilization during the COVID-19 pandemic: findings from a nationally representative survey in the United States. *Journal of Telemedicine and Telecare*, *30*(1), 90–97. https://doi.org/10.1177/1357633X211051677

Zhu, D., Paige, S. R., Slone, H., Gutierrez, A., Lutzky, C., Hedriana, H., Barrera, J. F., Ong, T., & Bunnell, B. E. (2024). Exploring telemental health practice before, during, and after the COVID-19 pandemic. *Journal of Telemedicine and Telecare*, 72–78. https://doi.org.libpublic3.library.isu.edu/10.1177/135763
33X211025943

4 Artificial Intelligence in Post-Pandemic Healthcare

Sarad Pawar Naik Bukke, Venkatesh Chandrakala, Anupam Maity, Chandrashekar Thalluri, Narayana Goruntla, Tadele Mekuriya Yadesa, and Soosamma John

4.1 INTRODUCTION

Coronaviruses come from a family of Coronaviridae. These are single-stranded RNA viruses with positive sense; their genomes are roughly 26–32 kilobases in size. The coronavirus commonly causes infections to the upper respiratory tract. Most of the virus of this family is noninfectious for humans (Jain & Barhate, 2020). Only a small number of the coronavirus family's viruses—229E, NL63, OC43, HKU1, SARS-CoV, and MERS-CoV—are known to infect humans (Lone & Ahmad, 2020). Coronaviruses are of round shape and approximately 80–120 nm in diameter. They have characteristic club-shaped spike-like projections on their outer structure, and for this reason, they are named as coronavirus. There are four main structural proteins in the coronavirus: spike proteins (S), envelop protein (E), membrane-bound protein (M), and nucleocapsid proteins (N) (Khadse NA et al., 2020).

Numerous instances of pneumonia with no identifiable cause were reported from Wuhan Province in China in December 2019. By January 2020, the causative organism was identified and named as severe acute respiratory syndrome coronavirus 2 (SARS-CoV-2; Cevik et al., 2020). Over the course of one month, the virus spread across the globe, and on January 30, 2020, WHO declared SARS-CoV-2 as pandemic (Cevik et al., 2020). Many methods were encountered to detect the infections in the communities during the pandemic; the mostly used methods were RT-PCR test, rapid antigen test, and serology-based antibody test (Mercer & Salit, 2021).

According to the World Health Organization (WHO) database, nearly 0.77 billion cases and 7 million deaths are reported till mid-January 2024 (*Coronavirus Disease [COVID-19]*, 2023). The COVID-19 pandemic highlights the most vulnerable components of the global healthcare infrastructure. Lack of healthcare facilities, shortage of infrastructure in existing facilities, insufficient healthcare providers, etc., were somehow responsible for such a deadly outbreak (Filip et al., 2022).

Artificial intelligence (AI) is often called an intelligent agent. It aims to mimic human cognitive functions in machines (Das et al., 2015). AI refers to simulate human minds in learning and analysis and can work to solve problems. In a clinical perspective, AI can have the potential to revolutionize the healthcare settings globally and can be a worthy tool to assist the healthcare practitioners (Jiang et al., 2017). Healthcare systems faced various challenges, including inefficiencies and diagnostic delays, which AI has partially alleviated by improving accuracy and streamlining processes.

4.2 CHALLENGES FACED BY HEALTHCARE SYSTEM DURING PANDEMIC

The pandemic exposed challenges in global healthcare, these are as follows.

4.2.1 IN-HOUSE CHALLENGES

The in-house challenges involve the challenges faced by hospitals and other healthcare facilities. The healthcare system has two major pillars: public healthcare services (government hospitals) and private healthcare services. The healthcare services had the major burden at the time of the out-break. Some of the key challenges are as follows:

A. Lack of materials support for the frontline workers
The sudden outbreak of COVID-19 has hampered the global supply of essential com-modities like personal protective equipment (PPE) kits, surgical gloves, and sanitizers. Factors contributing to delays include shortages of raw materials, machines, labor, over-dependence on China, border closures, and export bans (Asian Development Bank et al., 2020; Torrentira, 2020).

According to Ahmed et al., in the United States, 15% of doctors reported not having access to N95 respirators; moreover, 20% did not have gloves, roughly 12% lacked face shields, and roughly 50% lacked access to full robes or coveralls. Furthermore, roughly 7% of physicians said they had to treat COVID-19 patients without the proper PPE, and over 80% said they had to reuse some PPE (Ahmed et al., 2020).

B. Shortage of healthcare workers
Healthcare worker shortages during the pandemic led to inexperienced professionals step-ping in to meet the surge in cases (Filip et al., 2022).

Limited human resource in the healthcare facilities puts extra burden and workload on the existing workers during the outbreak. Moreover, due to infections significant numbers of healthcare professionals died and caused more burden to existing workers (Razu et al., 2021).

C. Disruption of non-COVID healthcare service
The global outbreak of COVID-19 has had a dramatic effect on healthcare systems across the globe, leading to a notable disturbance in non-COVID healthcare services. Consequently, the delivery of routine medical services, including screenings, elective surgeries, and ongoing treatments for chronic conditions, has been severely affected. The prioritization of COVID-19 response measures, such as lockdowns, resource reallocation, and infection control protocols, has led to delays, cancellations, and reductions in access to essential non-COVID healthcare services (Mahendradhata et al., 2021; Sengupta et al., 2021).

Lockdowns have reduced psychiatric emergency admissions, with anxiety disorders being the most common diagnosis in Spain and Switzerland, and intellectual disability, and neurotic, stress-related, somatoform and affective disorders in Germany (Tuczyńska et al., 2021). A study in Nigeria found worsening chronic diseases during COVID-19 due to limited medication access and rising treatment costs (Tuczyńska et al., 2021). Furthermore, projections of the COVID-19 pandemic's indirect effects on maternal and newborn health in Nigeria, Pakistan, India, and Indonesia over a one-year period have resulted in a further 31,980 maternal fatalities, 395,440 infant deaths, and 338,760 still-births (Mahendradhata et al., 2021).

D. Supply chain disruption
The COVID-19 pandemic has disrupted global supply chains, particularly in developing nations. Raj et al. identified major challenges, including demand uncertainty, supply vola-tility, material scarcity, delivery delays, and labor scarcity. They used the gray decision-making trial and evaluation laboratory approach to analyze these issues, emphasizing the impact of supply inconsistency. The article offers practical advice for navigating the post-pandemic supply chain (Raj et al., 2022).

E. Challenges in disease testing, screening, and tracing
Effective disease testing, screening, and tracing during the COVID-19 pandemic have encountered multifaceted challenges. While timely and accurate diagnosis is pivotal for clinical management, conventional methods like biochemical assays, ELISA, and RT-PCR have been hindered by their time-consuming nature and high costs. Moreover, these meth-ods often fail to identify past infections crucial for community-wide surveillance and

mitigation efforts. Particularly challenging is the identification of asymptomatic carriers. In this context, rapid antibody-based tests have emerged as frontline tools for mass testing, offering a more practical approach to initial diagnosis amidst the evolving landscape of a viral pandemic (Augustine et al., 2020).

4.2.2 SOCIAL/COMMUNITY CHALLENGES

The onset of the pandemic unleashed a wave of unprecedented challenges within our social and community landscapes. As communities grapple with the complexities of public health measures, economic instability, and social isolation, issues such as inequity, access to healthcare, and systemic disparities have been magnified. The pandemic has not only tested the resilience of our social fabric but also underscored the urgent need for collaborative solutions that address the multifaceted challenges faced by individuals, families, and communities worldwide. Some of the key social challenges are listed below:

A. **Misinformation and Infodemic**

The COVID-19 pandemic has exacerbated misinformation, with social media posts originating from unreliable sources and bots. Despite efforts by social media companies and public awareness, the problem persists (Greenspan & Loftus, 2021).

Misinformation during the COVID-19 pandemic has significantly impacted public perception, behavior, and memory, leading to an "infodemic." Cognitive science research shows that misinformation distorts memory and influences beliefs. To combat this, social media companies must implement measures, while users must discern information reliability. Strategies integrating cognitive science research can enhance media literacy and promote accurate information dissemination (Datta & Litt, 2020).

B. **Health inequities and vulnerable populations**

The COVID-19 pandemic worsened health disparities, especially among vulnerable populations. Lower income, education, and ethnic minorities face higher risks. Targeted strategies and research are needed to ensure equitable resource access (Häfliger et al., 2023).

Moreover, vulnerable populations of psychiatric patients have been disproportionately affected by the COVID-19 pandemic, compounding existing global health disparities. Pregnant women, children with impairments, ethnic minorities, and residents in rural and urban areas encounter particular difficulties that aggravate mental health consequences. To address these disparities, social programs aimed at reducing discrimination, enhancing community resilience, and overcoming systemic barriers to care are essential (Diaz et al., 2021).

C. **Patient and population mental health impact**

The COVID-19 pandemic has significantly impacted mental health, leading to conditions like depression, anxiety, and traumatic stress. To address this, researchers need to identify risk factors, anticipate outcomes, and develop intervention strategies. Innovative approaches, including nontraditional models and tailored preventive interventions, have the potential to effectively address mental health needs during and beyond the pandemic (Boden et al., 2021).

D. **Long-term health effects and post-COVID syndrome**

During the COVID-19 pandemic, post-COVID syndrome emerged, affecting 10%–35% of individuals and 85% of hospitalized patients. Common symptoms include fatigue, breathing difficulties, mental health issues, chest pain, and changes in taste and smell. Many patients have preexisting health conditions, increasing the burden on primary healthcare (Del Rio et al., 2020).

The post-pandemic era saw a significant surge in AI adoption and innovation in AI, driven largely by the challenges faced by the healthcare sector.

4.3 INNOVATIONS IN AI DURING THE PANDEMIC

The applications and innovations of AI were observed at the time of pandemic. Some of the innovations involved machine learning (ML), deep learning (DL), Artificial Neural Network (ANN), and Internet of Things (IoT).

The field of ML is concerned with two interconnected questions: How can computer systems be designed so that they automatically get better with time? And what basic laws of statistical computation and information theory control all learning systems, including those in computers, people, and organizations? ML is the preferred approach in AI for tasks like speech recognition, computer vision, natural language processing, and robot control, as it simplifies training systems by providing desired input–output behavior (Alpaydin, 2021; González García et al., 2019). One of the most significant applications of AI was seen during the pandemic, where the AI helped in various purposes like outbreak detection, contact tracing, and disease forecasting.

ML is termed as a specific branch of AI. It is a field within computer science that focuses on empowering computers to improve their performance at tasks without being explicitly programmed for each task. Instead, computers "learn" by gaining experience, typically through analyzing and fitting to data. This process blurs the distinction between ML and statistical approaches, as both rely on leveraging data to enable computers to make decisions or predictions autonomously (Bi et al., 2019; González García et al., 2019).

DL is also a part of AI and more specifically an upgradation of ML that uses multiple arrays of neural networks to solve complex problems. DL enhances classical ML methodologies by intricately augmenting model complexity and reshaping data through a multitude of functions, fostering hierarchical data representation across multiple abstraction levels. This approach leverages automatic feature extraction from raw data, where higher-level features are amalgamations of lower-level counterparts (González García et al., 2019; Schmidhuber, 2015).

ANNs are systems of artificial neurons organized in layers to uncover patterns in data. Typically consisting of input, hidden, and output layers, ANNs process external data through hidden layers to generate meaningful outputs. Their adaptability allows modeling of complex natural systems with numerous inputs, improving accuracy and usability. By mimicking brain neuron interconnections, ANNs excel in tasks resembling human cognition, showcasing their potential as versatile computational tools for complex problem-solving (Dongare et al., 2012; González García et al., 2019; Krenker et al., 2011).

The IoT encapsulates the interconnected network of physical objects, known as "things," integrated with sensors, software, and various technologies to enable communication and data exchange with other devices and systems via the Internet. By embedding objects with smart capabilities, IoT enhances efficiency, automation, and decision-making processes across various sectors, heralding a new era of interconnectedness and technological advancement (Ghosh et al., 2018).

Amidst the challenges posed by the pandemic, there has been a notable surge in innovations within the realm of AI. With the persistent threat of new variants and the ongoing need for proactive measures, healthcare providers and organizations have turned to AI technologies to enhance their response strategies. These innovations span a broad spectrum, encompassing advancements in areas such as IoT, cloud computing, DL, and blockchain. Particularly, the convergence of AI and IoT technologies has revolutionized healthcare, offering solutions like fog computing, DL algorithms, and blockchain integration to bolster efficiency, privacy, and security in patient care and management (Khan et al., 2022). With the rapid advancements in AI, it played a pivotal role during the pandemic.

These innovations in AI had a major role in pandemic and post-pandemic healthcare. AI enhances pandemic response through predictive analytics, diagnostics, and drug discovery, while revolutionizing post-pandemic healthcare with improved coding and risk assessment.

4.4 ROLE OF AI DURING PANDEMIC

Amidst the COVID-19 pandemic, AI stands as a crucial ally in various fronts. AI aids in outbreak detection and contact tracing through advanced data analysis, predicts disease trends, and identifies vulnerable populations. In medical imaging, AI assists in detecting COVID-19-related abnormalities, improving diagnostics. AI streamlines treatment monitoring, optimizes resource allocation, accelerates drug discovery and vaccine development, and helps curb misinformation. It plays a crucial role in mitigating pandemic impacts, offering innovative solutions across healthcare and public health.

4.4.1 Outbreak Detection and Contact Tracing

AI plays a pivotal role in outbreak detection and contact tracing during the pandemic, leveraging advanced technologies to enhance surveillance and prevention efforts. Natural language processing (NLP) is an AI subfield that interprets and extracts meaning from human languages, enabling automated analysis of unstructured data like social media posts and health records to identify potential outbreaks and trends (Arora et al., 2020; Shamman et al., 2023). For example, popular social media app Twitter was used along with supervised and semi-supervised AI algorithms to detect the regions of the outbreaks such as Wuhan, China (early 2020; Shamman et al., 2023).

Digital contact tracing, using AI-powered mobile apps with Bluetooth and GPS, tracks movements and interactions to identify potential exposures. This enables health authorities to quickly intervene, facilitating self-isolation or testing, offering an efficient, scalable solution to curb virus transmission (Agbehadji et al., 2020).

AI-powered outbreak detection systems improve disease surveillance, enabling early identification and proactive interventions by analyzing healthcare data, demographics, and environmental factors, helping contain outbreaks and allocate resources effectively (Agbehadji et al., 2020; Arora et al., 2020; Shamman et al., 2023).

4.4.2 Disease Forecasting

AI-based approaches can forecast the quantity of fatalities and positive cases in any given area. AI can assist in identifying the most susceptible nations, areas, and individuals so that appropriate action can be taken (Vaishya et al., 2020).

For example, ML regression and statistical models helped predict cumulative patient counts in Brazil at the early stages of the pandemic (Shamman et al., 2023).

Advanced AI models and techniques like NRANN, ANFIS, HFFA, BNN, LSTM, VAE, and SSA can improve surveillance and response strategies in healthcare. These models analyze complex datasets, identify patterns, and provide a mathematical framework for interpreting data, enabling timely interventions (Elsheikh et al., 2021).

4.4.3 Detection of COVID-19 by Medical Imaging

AI plays a critical role in the detection of COVID-19 on medical imaging during the pandemic, particularly in cases where clinical features of SAR-CoV-2 infection overlap with those of other viral illnesses. Chest X-rays (CXRs) and CT scans, while often revealing nonspecific bilateral infiltrates and ground-glass opacities, respectively, pose challenges in accurate diagnosis. However, efforts to leverage DL, specifically convolutional neural networks (CNNs), for COVID-19 detection from chest imaging have shown promise. By pretraining CNNs on broader datasets and fine-tuning them with limited medical data, researchers enhance AI models' performance, demonstrating their potential to outperform fully trained networks in specific scenarios (Khemasuwan & Colt, 2021).

4.4.4 Treatment Monitoring of the Infected Patients

AI has significantly aided in monitoring COVID-19 treatment, including quarantine and self-isolation protocols, using smartphone apps, algorithms, cameras, and GPS. Despite concerns about civil liberties, supply restrictions, and detection challenges, AI-driven monitoring systems have proven instrumental in managing and mitigating the pandemic's impact on public health (Shamman et al., 2023).

AI has transformed COVID-19 patient management by enhancing diagnostics, treatment monitoring, and telemedicine. It improves diagnostic accuracy and efficiency but raises concerns about medical privacy, patient evaluation, and potential AI system failures (Shamman et al., 2023).

4.4.5 Workload Reduction of Healthcare Workers

AI is assisting healthcare workers during the COVID-19 pandemic by facilitating early diagnosis, treatment, and training initiatives. It aids in managing cases, providing comprehensive training modules, automating processes like training dissemination, and treatment determination. AI-powered telemedicine solutions reduce hospital visits and infection transmission, while medical chatbots provide remote consultations, enhancing accessibility and efficiency in critical care services (Arora et al., 2020; Vaishya et al., 2020).

4.4.6 Drug and Vaccine Development

AI revolutionized COVID-19 drug discovery with algorithms like AOPEDF and DL-based models, expediting drug–target interaction prediction and repurposing existing compounds for potential treatments. Additionally, Zhang et al. proposed a dense fully connected neural network (DFCNN) pipeline where AI algorithms enable the quick screening of millions of chemicals against targets. These AI-driven strategies not only hold promise for COVID-19 drug discovery but also pave the way for developing novel treatments against other infectious diseases, underscoring the transformative potential of AI in advancing global healthcare initiatives (Arora et al., 2021). Hu et al. found eight SARS-CoV-2 proteins as potential drug targets using a DL model. They identified abacavir and darunavir as compounds with high binding affinity, with darunavir being the focus of a clinical trial in China. This highlights the potential of AI in drug discovery (Hu et al., 2022).

AI facilitates the development of therapies and vaccinations far more quickly than is typically possible. It also helps with clinical trials that are conducted while a vaccine is being developed (Arora et al., 2020; Vaishya et al., 2020). Ong et al. used AI to analyze SARS-CoV-2 protein sequences and human coronavirus strains. They used Vaxign-ML, a ML algorithm, to predict protegenicity scores. They identified six proteins, including the spike protein, as potential vaccine targets. The study highlights the importance of AI in vaccine development (Ong et al., 2020).

4.4.7 Protein Structure Prediction

AI has emerged as a transformative force in drug discovery efforts during the COVID-19 pandemic, particularly in predicting the structures of key proteins essential for virus entry and replication. By harnessing advanced algorithms such as AlphaFold and DeepTracer, researchers can accurately predict the structural configurations of crucial viral proteins, including membrane proteins and RNA polymerases. These predictions not only offer valuable insights into the molecular mechanisms underlying viral infection but also provide a foundation for the development of targeted therapeutics. Overall, AI-driven approaches hold immense promise in accelerating the discovery and development of novel antiviral agents to combat the COVID-19 pandemic (Arora et al., 2020; Swayamsiddha et al., 2021).

4.4.8 Curbing the Spread of Misinformation

The COVID-19 pandemic caused an infodemic. Analyzing social media data with ML helps track public sentiment, debunk misinformation, and provide updates on recovery rates and healthcare, aiding clinicians and reducing public fear and panic (Arora et al., 2020).

4.5 ROLE OF AI IN POST-PANDEMIC HEALTHCARE INFRASTRUCTURE

4.5.1 CLINICAL DECISION-MAKING FOR PATIENTS IN HEALTHCARE ORGANIZATION

AI aids healthcare by improving surgical risk stratification, identifying high-risk patients, optimizing resources, and enhancing preoperative support (Giordano et al., 2021).

AI is revolutionizing patient outcome optimization by providing data-driven insights for clinical decision-making. ML methods optimize patient care, from medication dosing to surgical interventions, analyzing complex patient data from electronic health records (EHRs; Giordano et al., 2021).

Furthermore, AI can be used in early warning systems for acute patient decompensation, detecting physiological trends in EHRs. These systems offer a proactive approach to patient monitoring, enabling timely interventions to mitigate adverse outcomes. Despite challenges, ongoing research is advancing AI capabilities (Giordano et al., 2021).

4.5.2 HEALTH INFORMATION MANAGEMENT IN HEALTHCARE ORGANIZATIONS

In the post-pandemic era, AI's integration into health information management (HIM) promises to enhance patient care and efficiency. Automated medical coding, diagnosis specificity, and early detection are key areas. While natural language processing (NLP) aids in coding, successful AI implementation requires workflow adjustments and HIM oversight. Effective integration also needs interdisciplinary collaboration to update coding guidelines and navigate complexities. (Stanfill & Marc, 2019).

4.5.3 PRECISION MEDICINE

AI plays a crucial role in precision medicine post-pandemic by personalizing treatments through genomic analysis, optimizing therapy for diseases like medulloblastoma, enhancing cancer imaging via radio genomics, and integrating environmental factors and clinical data. This ensures equitable, tailored, and effective interventions while minimizing adverse effects (Alowais et al., 2023; Johnson et al., 2021).

4.5.4 PREDICTION OF POPULATION HEALTH

Predictive analytics, utilizing AI, ML, and data mining, is increasingly vital in population health management, analyzing past and recent data to forecast trends and guide targeted health interventions (Schwalbe & Wahl, 2020).

During the post-pandemic era, the application of AI can be extensively used for mortality and morbidity risk assessment for the sake of public healthcare. For example, in order to evaluate the probability of dengue fever severity, Phakhounthong et al. applied ML algorithms on administrative records from a large tertiary care hospital in Thailand (Phakhounthong et al., 2018).

AI enhances disease outbreak prediction by analyzing data, enabling early detection, proactive containment, and stronger global health crisis response (D. Jiang et al., 2018).

4.5.5 CONTACTLESS HEALTHCARE SERVICE

The COVID-19 pandemic has accelerated the adoption of contactless services, facilitated by advanced technologies like AI, IoT, augmented reality, and virtual reality. These services, which offer non-face-to-face interactions, have gained prominence in sectors like distribution. The pandemic has accelerated digital transformation, positioning information and communication technologies (ICT) at the forefront of the post-pandemic era (Alowais et al., 2023; Lee & Lee, 2021).

The global telemedicine market, driven by the COVID-19 pandemic, is projected to reach $175.5 billion by 2026. Growth is fueled by chronic disease prevalence, smartphone adoption, and cost-effective care. Advanced ICT integration and regulatory changes are needed to unlock its full potential, with AI and big data playing vital roles post-pandemic (Alowais et al., 2023; Fikry et al., 2023; Lee & Lee, 2021).

4.5.6 MENTAL HEALTH SUPPORT

AI chatbots are transforming mental health services by providing empathetic interactions and resources. With digital government policies, platforms like Woebot, Emma, Sermo, and Tess offer accessible and cost-effective solutions for anxiety and depression. The COVID-19 pandemic has increased the demand for digital mental health interventions, prompting increased investment in chatbot technologies. These chatbots address loneliness and uncertainty, promoting mental resilience and personalized support worldwide (Damij & Bhattacharya, 2022).

4.5.7 INFECTIOUS DISEASE TESTING

AI and ML are revolutionizing infectious disease testing post-pandemic, improving accuracy, speed, and early detection of diseases like Lyme disease and meningitis, leading to better patient outcomes (Alowais et al., 2023; Tran et al., 2023).

Furthermore, AI/ML-driven approaches can improve infectious disease diagnostics, particularly in early recognition of life-threatening conditions like sepsis. By leveraging electronic medical record (EMR) data and integrating clinical parameters, AI/ML models can enhance diagnostic accuracy and specificity, particularly for special sepsis populations. This technology holds promise for improved patient care and public health outcomes (Kaur et al., 2021; Tran et al., 2023).

4.6 BENEFITS AND LIMITATIONS OF AI IN POST-PANDEMIC HEALTHCARE

A. Benefits of AI

- *Enhanced Diagnostic Accuracy:* Large amounts of medical data, such as imaging scans, lab findings, and patient records, can be analyzed by AI algorithms to help medical personnel diagnose patients more accurately, particularly in cases of complex or uncommon illnesses.

  Khalifa et al. highlight AI's potential in diagnostic imaging, suggesting funding, moral standards, and patient-focused research. They recommend teamwork for effective integration and healthcare inequities (Khalifa & Albadawy, 2024).
- *Streamlined Workflow:* AI-powered solutions can reduce administrative costs and free up time for healthcare providers to concentrate more on patient care by automating repetitive administrative chores like monitoring electronic health records, making appointment schedules, and processing paperwork (Johnson et al., 2021).
- *Personalized Treatment Plans:* AI can assist in customizing treatment plans and interventions to each patient's distinct traits, including genetics, lifestyle factors, and medical history, by analyzing individual patient data. This will result in more efficient and individualized care (Alowais et al., 2023; Johnson et al., 2021).
- *Predictive Analytics:* AI-driven predictive modeling can forecast healthcare demands, identify at-risk populations, and predict disease outbreaks, enabling proactive interventions and resource allocation to mitigate the spread of infectious diseases and improve population health (Alowais et al., 2023; Jiang et al., 2018; Phakhounthong et al., 2018).
- *Remote Monitoring and Telemedicine:* AI-powered telemedicine systems and remote monitoring equipment can improve access to healthcare services, especially in underserved or

distant locations, and allow continuous monitoring of patients' health state. They can also make virtual consultations easier (Fikry et al., 2023; Lee & Lee, 2021).

- *Drug Discovery and Development:* By evaluating enormous volumes of biological and chemical data to find promising drug candidates, anticipate medication interactions, and improve treatment regimens, AI algorithms might hasten the drug discovery process and hasten the development of new treatments (Hu et al., 2022; Ong et al., 2020).
- *Continuous Learning and Improvement:* Healthcare practitioners may stay updated on medical knowledge and best practices by using AI systems, which can learn continuously from fresh data and feedback. This improves patient care and results over time.

B. Limitations of AI

- *Data Bias and Quality:* AI algorithms rely heavily on the quality and representativeness of the data they are trained on. Biases in healthcare data, such as underrepresentation of certain demographics or populations, can lead to biased AI predictions and recommendations, potentially exacerbating healthcare disparities and inequities (Daneshjou et al., 2021). It can be training data bias, algorithmic bias and cognitive bias. A study by IBM showed underrepresented data of women or minority groups in predictive AI algorithms. For example, computer-aided diagnosis (CAD) systems have been found to return lower accuracy results for Black patients than White patients.
- *Lack of Transparency:* A lot of AI algorithms function as "black boxes," which means that it is challenging to understand or comprehend how they make decisions. Healthcare practitioners may find it difficult to comprehend and trust AI-driven advice as a result of this lack of transparency, especially in situations where crucial decisions must be made (Daneshjou et al., 2021; Kiseleva et al., 2022). An AI system is deemed sufficiently transparent if it enables its users to interpret the AI's system output and apply it appropriately [EC Proposal for the AI Act, art 13(1)]. Yet, what interpretation exactly mean and what are the relevant measures that are acceptable by the legislator are still open questions.
- *Patient Privacy and Data Security:* For AI systems to work well, they frequently need access to a lot of private patient data. It is crucial to protect the privacy and security of these data since data breaches or improper use could have detrimental effects on patient confidentiality and public confidence in the healthcare system, among other things (Khan et al., 2023). A common example would include facing workplace discrimination if one's medical history is made public or facing inflated health insurance premiums as a result of additional information accessible due to a breach of privacy (Yadav et al., 2023).
- *Regulatory and Legal Challenges:* The rapid advancement of AI in healthcare poses challenges for regulatory bodies and legal frameworks to keep pace. Unclear regulations and liability issues surrounding AI-driven healthcare technologies may hinder their widespread adoption and integration into clinical practice (Ganapathy, 2021). Prof. Dr. Heinz-Uwe Dettling, Partner, Ernst & Young Law GmbHand EY GSA Life Sciences Law Lead, explains that healthcare AI and Software as a Medical Device require a rewrite of the regulatory rule book. He says this is because existing regulatory frameworks do not allow medical devices to change without first undergoing a drawn-out re-authorization process which threatens to stifle adoption and innovation. By its nature however, ML wants to learn from data and improve its performance over time (How the challenge of regulating AI in healthcare is escalating | EY—Global).
- *Interpretability and Accountability:* As AI algorithms become increasingly complex, understanding how they arrive at their conclusions can be challenging. Lack of interpretability makes it difficult for healthcare professionals to verify the accuracy and reliability of AI-generated insights, raising concerns about accountability in the event of errors or adverse outcomes.

- *Informed Consent and Autonomy:* Informed consent involves communication between patients and healthcare providers, including decision capacity, documentation, and ethical disclosure. Patients have the right to receive information and ask questions about procedures, and to know who is accountable if robotic medical devices fail or cause errors. This transparency is crucial for patient rights and the medical labor market. With the rise of AI in healthcare, concerns about autonomy have increased (Farhud & Zokaei, 2021).
- *Ethical Consideration in AI:* According to the Thomson Reuters report, one of the top five fears is that AI will "push ethics out of the window." Professionals should keep in mind that AI is most effective when used to initiate processes or streamline routine tasks such as research. It is not advisable to depend solely on AI for delivering precise answers or conclusions (Navigate ethical and regulatory issues of using AI [thomsonreuters.com]).

4.7 CONCLUSION

In the wake of the pandemic, it has become increasingly evident that the integration of AI in healthcare systems is not only advantageous but also imperative for building resilient and effective healthcare infrastructures. AI has demonstrated its potential to streamline processes, enhance diagnostic accuracy, optimize resource allocation, and facilitate remote patient monitoring, all of which are crucial in navigating the challenges presented by public health crises like pandemics. However, to fully leverage the benefits of AI in post-pandemic healthcare, it is essential to address pertinent issues such as data privacy, algorithm transparency, and ethical considerations. Interdisciplinary collaboration in AI blends diverse expertise to drive innovation, enhance design, and tackle ethical issues, resulting in more effective, comprehensive, and balanced solutions while accelerating development. Ongoing monitoring and adaptation of AI technologies are essential for ensuring they remain effective, secure, and aligned with ethical standards. This continuous process helps address

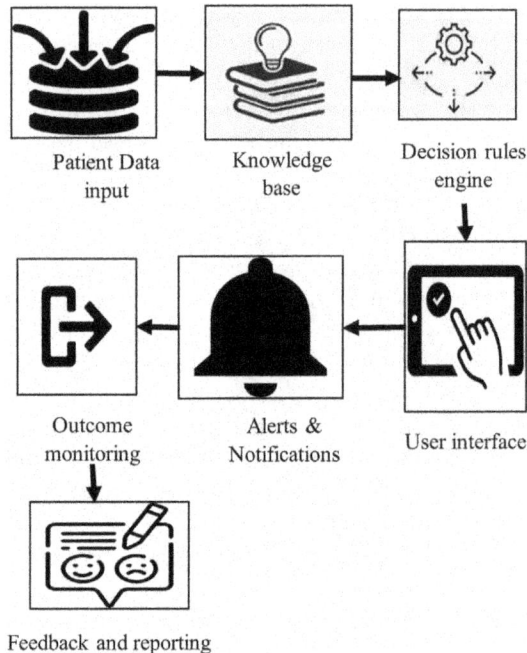

FIGURE 4.1 Artificial Intelligence in Post-Pandemic Healthcare.

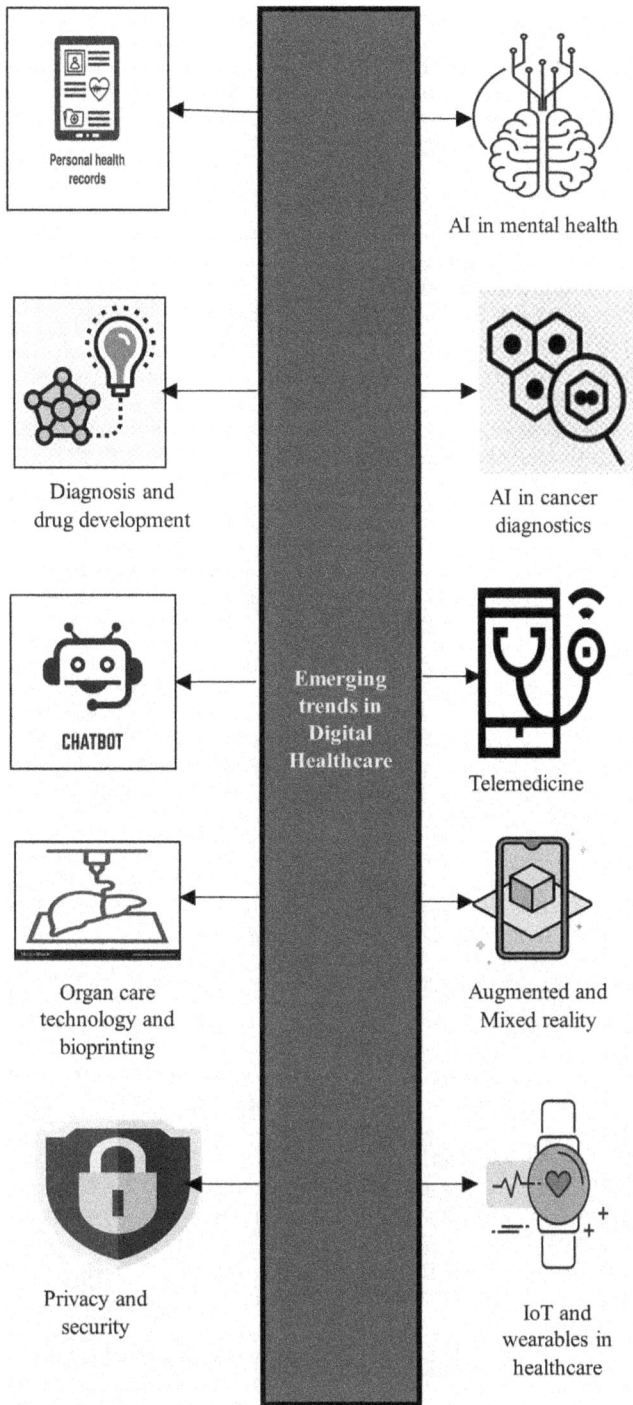

FIGURE 4.2 Emerging trends in Digital Healthcare.

emerging issues, refine performance, and adapt to new challenges. Future AI research will focus on ethical and bias mitigation, enhancing explainability, advancing toward general AI, ensuring safety and robustness, integrating with emerging technologies, optimizing human–AI collaboration, and developing regulatory frameworks.

REFERENCES

Agbehadji, I. E., Awuzie, B. O., Ngowi, A. B., & Millham, R. C. (2020). Review of big data analytics, artificial intelligence and nature-inspired computing models towards accurate detection of COVID-19 pandemic cases and contact tracing. *International Journal of Environmental Research and Public Health, 17*(15), 5330. https://doi.org/10.3390/ijerph17155330

Ahmed, J., Malik, F., Bin Arif, T., Majid, Z., Chaudhary, M. A., Ahmad, J., Malik, M., Khan, T. M., & Khalid, M. (2020). Availability of personal protective equipment (PPE) among US and Pakistani doctors in COVID-19 pandemic. *Cureus, 12*(6), e8550. https://doi.org/10.7759/cureus.8550

Alowais, S. A., Alghamdi, S. S., Alsuhebany, N., Alqahtani, T., Alshaya, A. I., Almohareb, S. N., Aldairem, A., Alrashed, M., Bin Saleh, K., Badreldin, H. A., Al Yami, M. S., Al Harbi, S., & Albekairy, A. M. (2023). Revolutionizing healthcare: the role of artificial intelligence in clinical practice. *BMC Medical Education, 23*(1), 689. https://doi.org/10.1186/s12909-023-04698-z

Alpaydin, E. (2021). *Machine Learning* (Revised and updated edition). The MIT Press.

Arora, G., Joshi, J., Mandal, R. S., Shrivastava, N., Virmani, R., & Sethi, T. (2021). Artificial intelligence in surveillance, diagnosis, drug discovery and vaccine development against COVID–19. *Pathogens (Basel, Switzerland), 10*(8), 1048. https://doi.org/10.3390/pathogens10081048

Arora, N., Banerjee, A. K., & Narasu, M. L. (2020). The role of artificial intelligence in tackling COVID–19. *Future Virology, 15*(11), 717–724. https://doi.org/10.2217/fvl-2020–0130

Asian Development Bank, Park, C.-Y., Kim, K., Asian Development Bank, Roth, S., Asian Development Bank, Beck, S., Asian Development Bank, Kang, J. W., Asian Development Bank, Tayag, M. C., Asian Development Bank, Grifin, M., & World Health Organization. (2020). *Global Shortage of Personal Protective Equipment amid COVID-19: Supply Chains, Bottlenecks, and Policy Implications*. Asian Development Bank. https://doi.org/10.22617/BRF200128–2

Augustine, R., Das, S., Hasan, A., S, A., Abdul Salam, S., Augustine, P., Dalvi, Y. B., Varghese, R., Primavera, R., Yassine, H. M., Thakor, A. S., & Kevadiya, B. D. (2020). Rapid antibody-based COVID-19 mass surveillance: relevance, challenges, and prospects in a pandemic and post-pandemic world. *Journal of Clinical Medicine, 9*(10), 3372. https://doi.org/10.3390/jcm9103372

Bi, Q., Goodman, K. E., Kaminsky, J., & Lessler, J. (2019). What is machine learning? A primer for the epidemiologist. *American Journal of Epidemiology, 188*(12), 2222–2239. https://doi.org/10.1093/aje/kwz189

Boden, M., Zimmerman, L., Azevedo, K. J., Ruzek, J. I., Gala, S., Abdel Magid, H. S., Cohen, N., Walser, R., Mahtani, N. D., Hoggatt, K. J., & McLean, C. P. (2021). Addressing the mental health impact of COVID-19 through population health. *Clinical Psychology Review, 85*, 102006. https://doi.org/10.1016/j.cpr.2021.102006

Cevik, M., Bamford, C. G. G., & Ho, A. (2020). COVID-19 pandemic-a focused review for clinicians. *Clinical Microbiology and Infection: The Official Publication of the European Society of Clinical Microbiology and Infectious Diseases, 26*(7), 842–847. https://doi.org/10.1016/j.cmi.2020.04.023

Damij, N., & Bhattacharya, S. (2022). The role of AI chatbots in mental health related public services in a (Post) pandemic world: a review and future research agenda. In *2022 IEEE Technology and Engineering Management Conference (TEMSCON EUROPE)*, 152–159. https://doi.org/10.1109/TEMSCONEUROPE54743.2022.9801962

Daneshjou, R., Smith, M. P., Sun, M. D., Rotemberg, V., & Zou, J. (2021). Lack of transparency and potential bias in artificial intelligence data sets and algorithms: a scoping review. *JAMA Dermatology, 157*(11), 1362–1369. https://doi.org/10.1001/jamadermatol.2021.3129

Das, S., Dey, A., Pal, A., & Roy, N. (2015). Applications of artificial intelligence in machine learning: review and prospect. *International Journal of Computer Applications, 115*(9), 31–41. https://doi.org/10.5120/20182–2402

Datta, R., & Litt, T. B. (2020). Infodemic with misinformation and disinformation in pandemic COVID-19 situation: a global case study. *International Journal of Advance Research and Innovative Ideas in Education, 6*(4), 1732–1743.

Del Rio, C., Collins, L. F., & Malani, P. (2020). Long-term health consequences of COVID–19. *JAMA, 324*(17), 1723–1724. https://doi.org/10.1001/jama.2020.19719

Diaz, A., Baweja, R., Bonatakis, J. K., & Baweja, R. (2021). Global health disparities in vulnerable populations of psychiatric patients during the COVID-19 pandemic. *World Journal of Psychiatry, 11*(4), 94–108. https://doi.org/10.5498/wjp.v11.i4.94

Dongare, A. D., Kharde, R. R., & Kachare, A. D. (2012). Introduction to artificial neural network. *International Journal of Engineering and Innovative Technology (IJEIT)., 2*(1), 189–194.

Elsheikh, A. H., Saba, A. I., Panchal, H., Shanmugan, S., Alsaleh, N. A., & Ahmadein, M. (2021). Artificial intelligence for forecasting the prevalence of COVID-19 pandemic: an overview. *Healthcare*, *9*(12), 1614. https://doi.org/10.3390/healthcare9121614

Farhud, D. D., & Zokaei, S. (2021, November). Ethical issues of artificial intelligence in medicine and healthcare. *Iran Journal of Public Health*, 50(11), i-v. https://doi.org/10.18502/ijph. v50i11.7600

Fikry, A., Shafie, I. S. M., Yusof, Y. L. M., Mahamood, S. F., & Jamil, N. (2023). When contactless service matters: the use of robotic services in the healthcare sector. *IEEE Engineering Management Review*, *51*(2), 26–34. https://doi.org/10.1109/EMR.2023.3266604

Filip, R., Gheorghita Puscaselu, R., Anchidin-Norocel, L., Dimian, M., & Savage, W. K. (2022). Global challenges to public health care systems during the COVID-19 pandemic: a review of pandemic measures and problems. *Journal of Personalized Medicine*, *12*(8), 1295. https://doi.org/10.3390/jpm12081295

Ganapathy, K. (2021). Artificial intelligence and healthcare regulatory and legal concerns. *Telehealth and Medicine Today*. https://doi.org/10.30953/tmt.v6.252

Ghosh, A., Chakraborty, D., & Law, A. (2018). Artificial intelligence in Internet of things. *CAAI Transactions on Intelligence Technology*, *3*(4), 208–218. https://doi.org/10.1049/trit.2018.1008

Giordano, C., Brennan, M., Mohamed, B., Rashidi, P., Modave, F., & Tighe, P. (2021). Accessing artificial intelligence for clinical decision-making. *Frontiers in Digital Health*, *3*, 645232. https://doi.org/10.3389/fdgth.2021.645232

González García, C., Núñez-Valdez, E., García-Díaz, V., Pelayo G-Bustelo, C., & Cueva-Lovelle, J. M. (2019). A review of artificial intelligence in the Internet of Things. *International Journal of Interactive Multimedia and Artificial Intelligence*, *5*(4), 9. https://doi.org/10.9781/ijimai.2018.03.004

Greenspan, R. L., & Loftus, E. F. (2021). Pandemics and infodemics: research on the effects of misinformation on memory. *Human Behavior and Emerging Technologies*, *3*(1), 8–12. https://doi.org/10.1002/hbe2.228

Häfliger, C., Diviani, N., & Rubinelli, S. (2023). Communication inequalities and health disparities among vulnerable groups during the COVID-19 pandemic—a scoping review of qualitative and quantitative evidence. *BMC Public Health*, *23*(1), 428. https://doi.org/10.1186/s12889-023-15295-6

Hu, F., Jiang, J., & Yin, P. (2022). Prediction of potential commercially available inhibitors against SARS-CoV-2 by multi-task deep learning model. *Biomolecules*, *12*(8), 1156. https://doi.org/10.3390/biom12081156

Jain, M. S., & Barhate, S. D. (2020). Corona viruses are a family of viruses that range from the common cold to MERS corona virus: a Review. *Asian Journal of Research in Pharmaceutical Science*, *10*(3), 204. https://doi.org/10.5958/2231–5659.2020.00039.9

Jiang, D., Hao, M., Ding, F., Fu, J., & Li, M. (2018). Mapping the transmission risk of Zika virus using machine learning models. *Acta Tropica*, *185*, 391–399. https://doi.org/10.1016/j.actatropica.2018.06.021

Jiang, F., Jiang, Y., Zhi, H., Dong, Y., Li, H., Ma, S., Wang, Y., Dong, Q., Shen, H., & Wang, Y. (2017). Artificial intelligence in healthcare: past, present and future. *Stroke and Vascular Neurology*, *2*(4), 230–243. https://doi.org/10.1136/svn-2017–000101

Johnson, K. B., Wei, W.-Q., Weeraratne, D., Frisse, M. E., Misulis, K., Rhee, K., Zhao, J., & Snowdon, J. L. (2021). Precision medicine, AI, and the future of personalized health care. *Clinical and Translational Science*, *14*(1), 86–93. https://doi.org/10.1111/cts.12884

Kaur, I., Behl, T., Aleya, L., Rahman, H., Kumar, A., Arora, S., & Bulbul, I. J. (2021). Artificial intelligence as a fundamental tool in management of infectious diseases and its current implementation in COVID-19 pandemic. *Environmental Science and Pollution Research International*, *28*(30), 40515–40532. https://doi.org/10.1007/s11356-021-13823-8

Khadse, N. A., Wankhade, A. M., Patil, S. R., & Kathale, S. V. (2020). A review on corona virus disease. *European Journal of Biomedical and Pharmaceutical Sciences*, *7*(4), 1–8.

Khalifa, M., & Albadawy, M. (2024). AI in diagnostic imaging: revolutionising accuracy and efficiency. *Computer Methods and Programs in Biomedicine Update*, *5*, 100146. https://doi.org/10.1016/j.cmpbup.2024.100146

Khan, B., Fatima, H., Qureshi, A., Kumar, S., Hanan, A., Hussain, J., & Abdullah, S. (2023). Drawbacks of artificial intelligence and their potential solutions in the healthcare sector. *Biomedical Materials & Devices (New York, N.Y.)*, 1–8. https://doi.org/10.1007/s44174-023-00063-2

Khan, J. I., Khan, J., Ali, F., Ullah, F., Bacha, J., & Lee, S. (2022). Artificial intelligence and Internet of Things (AI-IoT) technologies in response to COVID-19 pandemic: a systematic review. *IEEE Access*, *10*, 62613–62660. https://doi.org/10.1109/ACCESS.2022.3181605

Khemasuwan, D., & Colt, H. G. (2021). Applications and challenges of AI-based algorithms in the COVID-19 pandemic. *BMJ Innovations*, *7*(2), 387–398. https://doi.org/10.1136/bmjinnov-2020–000648

Kiseleva, A., Kotzinos, D., & De Hert, P. (2022). Transparency of AI in healthcare as a multilayered system of accountabilities: between legal requirements and technical limitations. *Frontiers in Artificial Intelligence*, *5*, 879603. https://doi.org/10.3389/frai.2022.879603

Krenker, A., Bester, J., & Kos, A. (2011). Introduction to the Artificial Neural Networks. In K. Suzuki (Ed.), *Artificial Neural Networks—Methodological Advances and Biomedical Applications*. InTech. https://doi. org/10.5772/15751

Lee, S. M., & Lee, D. (2021). Opportunities and challenges for contactless healthcare services in the post-COVID-19 Era. *Technological Forecasting and Social Change, 167*, 120712. https://doi.org/10.1016/j. techfore.2021.120712

Lone, S. A., & Ahmad, A. (2020). COVID-19 pandemic—an African perspective. *Emerging Microbes & Infections, 9*(1), 1300–1308. https://doi.org/10.1080/22221751.2020.1775132

Mahendradhata, Y., Andayani, N. L. P. E., Hasri, E. T., Arifi, M. D., Siahaan, R. G. M., Solikha, D. A., & Ali, P. B. (2021). The capacity of the Indonesian healthcare system to respond to COVID–19. *Frontiers in Public Health, 9*, 649819. https://doi.org/10.3389/fpubh.2021.649819

Mercer, T. R., & Salit, M. (2021). Testing at scale during the COVID-19 pandemic. *Nature Reviews. Genetics, 22*(7), 415–426. https://doi.org/10.1038/s41576-021-00360-w

Ong, E., Wong, M. U., Huffman, A., & He, Y. (2020). COVID-19 coronavirus vaccine design using reverse vaccinology and machine learning. *Frontiers in Immunology, 11*, 1581. https://doi.org/10.3389/fimmu.2020.01581

Phakhounthong, K., Chaovalit, P., Jittamala, P., Blacksell, S. D., Carter, M. J., Turner, P., Chheng, K., Sona, S., Kumar, V., Day, N. P. J., White, L. J., & Pan-Ngum, W. (2018). Predicting the severity of dengue fever in children on admission based on clinical features and laboratory indicators: application of classification tree analysis. *BMC Pediatrics, 18*(1), 109. https://doi.org/10.1186/s12887-018-1078-y

Raj, A., Mukherjee, A. A., de Sousa Jabbour, A. B. L., & Srivastava, S. K. (2022). Supply chain management during and post-COVID-19 pandemic: mitigation strategies and practical lessons learned. *Journal of Business Research, 142*, 1125–1139. https://doi.org/10.1016/j.jbusres.2022.01.037

Razu, S. R., Yasmin, T., Arif, T. B., Islam, M. S., Islam, S. M. S., Gesesew, H. A., & Ward, P. (2021). Challenges faced by healthcare professionals during the COVID-19 pandemic: a qualitative inquiry from Bangladesh. *Frontiers in Public Health, 9*, 647315. https://doi.org/10.3389/fpubh.2021.647315

Schmidhuber, J. (2015). Deep learning. *Scholarpedia, 10*(11), 32832. https://doi.org/10.4249/scholarpedia.32832

Schwalbe, N., & Wahl, B. (2020). Artificial intelligence and the future of global health. *Lancet (London, England), 395*(10236), 1579–1586. https://doi.org/10.1016/S0140–6736(20)30226–9

Sengupta, M., Roy, A., Ganguly, A., Baishya, K., Chakrabarti, S., & Mukhopadhyay, I. (2021). Challenges encountered by healthcare providers in COVID-19 times: an exploratory study. *Journal of Health Management, 23*(2), 339–356. https://doi.org/10.1177/09720634211011695

Shamman, A. H., Hadi, A. A., Ramul, A. R., Abdul Zahra, M. M., & Gheni, H. M. (2023). The artificial intelligence (AI) role for tackling against COVID-19 pandemic. *Materials Today. Proceedings, 80*, 3663–3667. https://doi.org/10.1016/j.matpr.2021.07.357

Stanfill, M. H., & Marc, D. T. (2019). Health information management: implications of artificial intelligence on healthcare data and information management. *Yearbook of Medical Informatics, 28*(1), 56–64. https://doi.org/10.1055/s-0039–1677913

Swayamsiddha, S., Prashant, K., Shaw, D., & Mohanty, C. (2021). The prospective of artificial intelligence in COVID-19 pandemic. *Health and Technology, 11*(6), 1311–1320. https://doi.org/10.1007/s12553-021-00601-2

Torrentira, M. (2020). Combating COVID-19 pandemic: the best management practices of a designated hospital in southern Philippines. *Journal of Business and Management Studies, 2*(2), 11–15. https://al-kindipublisher.com/index.php/jbms/article/view/462

Tran, N. K., Albahra, S., Rashidi, H., & May, L. (2023). Innovations in infectious disease testing: leveraging COVID-19 pandemic technologies for the future. *Clinical Biochemistry, 117*, 10–15. https://doi.org/10.1016/j.clinbiochem.2021.12.011

Tuczyńska, M., Matthews-Kozanecka, M., & Baum, E. (2021). Accessibility to non-COVID health services in the world during the COVID-19 pandemic: review. *Frontiers in Public Health, 9*, 760795. https://doi.org/10.3389/fpubh.2021.760795

Vaishya, R., Javaid, M., Khan, I. H., & Haleem, A. (2020). Artificial intelligence (AI) applications for COVID-19 pandemic. *Diabetes & Metabolic Syndrome: Clinical Research & Reviews, 14*(4), 337–339. https://doi.org/10.1016/j.dsx.2020.04.012

World Health Organization. (2023). *Advice for the Public: Coronavirus Disease (COVID-19)*. https://www.who.int/emergencies/diseases/novel-coronavirus-2019/advice-for-public

Yadav, N., Pandey, S., Gupta, A., Dudani, P., Gupta, S., & Rangarajan, K. (2023, October 27). Data privacy in healthcare: in the era of artificial intelligence. *Indian Dermatology Online Journal, 14*(6), 788–792. https://doi.org/10.4103/idoj.idoj_543_23

5 Navigating Post-Pandemic Mental Health Challenges
Unleashing the Potential of Artificial Intelligence

Abilash K, Sindhuja Manisha Kamini P, and Ruchi Joshi

5.1 INTRODUCTION

The COVID-19 virus has made mental health an even more important issue. Given the more than 150 million people living with mental health problems in the World Health Organization (WHO) European region, new approaches to mental health care are more important than ever (World Health Organization Europe, 2023). Artificial Intelligence's (AI's) ability to help improve mental health treatment, diagnose and monitor mental health problems, and expand our understanding of complex diseases is unparalleled in this field (World Health Organization Europe, 2023).

It is a very powerful tool that can easily discover subtle connections or patterns among large datasets by reading them (Bajwa et al., 2021). AI-based mental health apps and platforms offer users accessible and individualized assistance. These tools are able to evaluate the inputs from the users and suggest specific coping mechanisms, calming practices such as mindfulness exercises, and approaches to therapy that will assist people in dealing with their stress levels, anxiety attacks, or other depressive symptoms. For example, AI interventions provide constant support throughout the week, thus narrowing down geographical barriers of access especially in cases where nonconventional means of therapy may be limited.

Additionally, AI improves the efficacy of therapies through virtual therapy and chatbots. These AI-driven systems can provide on-demand therapy sessions at scale that can be used alongside traditional counseling methods. They enable individuals to share their worries openly in a safe environment, while also helping them practice therapeutic techniques including cognitive behavioral therapy (CBT) and receive CBT if they choose so, making mental healthcare more adaptable.

Furthermore, AI helps in mental health studies by making use of large datasets to reveal various insights into mental health issues and treatment results. This approach based on data helps in identifying the best approaches to treatment, understanding the intricacies of mental disorders, and creating new solutions. The integration of AI into the field of mental healthcare is expected to make support better in terms of quality and more accessible, and provide a basis for further research, enabling an informed and compassionate approach to mental wellness.

Finally, AI plays a significant role in predictive analytics and early intervention. Advanced algorithms can detect trends in wearable devices' data or analyze content from electronic medical records or social media that signify early symptoms of psychological problems. In this regard, an early intervention model is very relevant as it can prevent further escalation of a disease and help in early recovery. On the one hand, through mood or behavior change detection systems, these systems may alert individuals/users/healthcare providers to initiate preventive measures before severe symptoms occur.

The surging tide of mental health burdens worldwide is nothing less than a pandemic and accounts for about 16% of the global burden of disease (Arias et al., 2022). Preponderant mental

DOI: 10.1201/9781003485629-5

illnesses, such as major depression and anxiety disorders, already cost the global economy about $1 trillion annually in lost productivity, so the urgency for effective solutions is hard to overstate. Second to this, the stigma that permeates mental health only worsens the crisis, leaving many without the care they need—further feeding into a cycle of neglect and suffering. At the same time, AI in healthcare does open up a chink of light for some optimism. AI integrated into mental health services gives us a concrete opportunity not only to attenuate the consequences of this global pandemic but also to change the status quo in mental health treatment (Naik et al., 2022). The potential for AI to enhance early detection, provide personalized options for treatment, and then support these with new platforms holds the potential to revolutionize the very concept of mental wellness and accessibility of treatment with reduced associated stigma. That is where this narrative review comes in—at a critical juncture (Health, 2020). As the AI boom unfurls across the world, there comes a juncture for reflection on how far the field of AI and mental health has come and when to start speculating about challenges and opportunities lying ahead. In essence, this review seeks to further elucidate the ways in which AI can be fruitfully integrated into mental healthcare while charting its prospects, progress, and pitfalls.

In accordance with Minerva and Giubilini (2023) and Johnson et al. (2020), it can improve treatment outcomes, reduce stigma, and widen healthcare access. AI potentially is capable of transforming mental health entirely because it provides answers and insights where other methods have been inadequate. This is especially relevant to the field of mental health treatment (Nilsen et al., 2022a) because understanding human behavior and emotions is essential there (Langarizadeh et al., 2017). In fact, this innovative system combines online therapy, virtual reality technologies, and specialized counseling in a revolutionary way. Dynamic changes in integrated treatment for mental cases and cognitive behavioral treatments are changing too (Tai, 2020). However, even though this change has potential for universal accessibility, ease of early intervention, and individualized care, ethical concerns, managing technological issues or problems, and further research need to be done (Bouhouita-Guermech et al., 2023; Naik et al., 2022; Gerke et al., 2020). While our world is becoming increasingly connected, the integration of AI with human knowledge could open up newer vistas within the domain of mental healthcare; at the same time, blanket use and the impact of AI in this sphere are also under scanner. Digitization poses opportunities and threats to mental health. For example, social media platforms offer access to knowledge, support, and a sense of community, but they can foster unrealistic beauty standards, addictive behaviors, or glamorize mental health issues. Mental Health Europe underlines the need to factor in human rights within the use of digital platforms and calls for actions oriented to enhance digital literacy and commitments held in these platforms, and refrain from harmful or misleading practices (Stoumpos et al., 2023).

The COVID-19 pandemic has prompted a more rapid adoption of digital technology in mental health treatment, bringing with its wearables, AI, telemedicine, and mental health applications. These technologies provide never-before-seen opportunities for care, assistance, and assessment. But issues with profit-driven business strategies and the requirement for sufficient industry regulation surface. Risks associated with digital mental health therapies include those related to privacy and data security, as well as inequalities in access and abilities (Lee et al., 2022).

Mental Health Europe emphasizes the need for effective management to maximize potential while minimizing harm. The EU and national governments have recognized that the safety, effectiveness, fairness, and overall visibility of mental health are important considerations in the development of laws and regulations. It is recommended that the human approach, collaborative decision-making by all parties, and human rights be followed as a guide (Leka et al., 2014). Ensuring the safety and effectiveness of digital health technology requires important steps such as addressing ethical issues, cost evidence, and self-defense.

It is important not to look at digital technology as a solution to social psychological problems. Recognizing the complexity of mental health issues, policymakers should concentrate on community-based treatment while taking socioeconomic and environmental variables into account. True innovation is found in both our approach to mental health treatment and technical breakthroughs

(Berardi et al., 2024). According to Mental Health Europe, digitization should be viewed as a tool to help achieve the dual goals of improving access to mental healthcare services and creating a mentally healthy society. The focus should be shifted from technology itself to the people who stand to gain and may be impacted by these developments, making sure that actual needs are met and meaningful involvement occurs through the use of a psychosocial model and inclusive governance (*Digitalisation & Mental Health: Navigating the Future | MHE, 2024*).

The domain of AI applications in mental healthcare is quite fast-moving, and the key developments took place only in the very recent past. Research studies proved that AI works well in diagnosis, case planning, and monitoring patients. For example, AI algorithms were applied successfully to predict a possible eruption of mental health disorders in patients, including depression and anxiety, by analyzing data about patients and noticing the first signs of a disorder.

Moreover, AI-powered platforms, including virtual therapists and chatbots, have been deployed to provide mental health services to those with no access to traditional therapy. These tools also have the potential to provide CBT interventions and real-time support for their users.

Nevertheless, fast-tracking of the application of AI in mental healthcare has equally raised a number of ethical concerns over the technologies. Literature has voiced concerns on data privacy, algorithmic bias, and the ability of AI to worsen already existing disparities in healthcare. These concerns need to be attended to if AI-driven innovations in mental healthcare are to be appropriate and fair.

The COVID-19 pandemic accelerated this "digital revolution" across sectors; mental healthcare was no different. AI in mental healthcare presents a distinctive opportunity that can improve the service delivery, treatment efficiency, and, finally, patient outcomes. Despite the potential benefits, there are important gaps in our understanding of the ethical, practical, and clinical implications of AI-driven mental health solutions.

5.2   RESEARCH OBJECTIVES

The chapter will look to explore the following objectives:

1) Critically appraise the role of AI in responding to post-pandemic mental health challenges.
2) Identify main AI-driven innovations in mental healthcare and their potential impact on service delivery.
3) Appraise the ethical implications and challenges in the adoption of AI in mental health settings.
4) Recommend how AI technologies can be integrated into mental healthcare in the near future and ensure that innovations will contribute to a more fair and effective healthcare system in all aspects.

5.3   STUDY DESIGN

This will be a systematic review with a meta-analysis of available literature to determine the effectiveness of AI-based mental health interventions. In this study, an attempt will be made to pool and synthesize data to get a good understanding of AI's impact on mental health contexts amid the COVID-19 pandemic and its aftermath.

5.4   INCLUSION CRITERIA

1. Study Design: Randomized controlled trials, quasi-experimental studies, and cohort studies offering quantitative data on the effectiveness of AI-driven mental health interventions.
2. Population: Studies involving adult participants aged 18 years and above who have mental health challenges in which the effects of COVID-19 have been heightened, such as anxiety disorder, major depressive disorder, and stress-related disorder.

3. Intervention: Research into AI-driven mental health tools that are virtual assistants or AI-based chatbots, digital CBT, and other AI-supported solutions for mental health.
4. Outcome Measures: The studies must report at least one outcome of interest that has to do with some aspect of mental health, for example, anxiety or depression levels or changes in these levels. This could be measured, for example, by utilizing generalized anxiety disorder 7-item for anxiety, patient depression questionnaire-9 for depression, or five well-being index-5 for general well-being.
5. Publication Type: Peer-reviewed articles, theses, and dissertations available in English and published from January 2020 up to date.
6. Sample Size: Not below 20, just to ensure there is enough robustness in data.

5.5 EXCLUSION CRITERIA

1. Study Design: Nonexperimental studies, qualitative research, case reports, or editorials without quantitative outcome data.
2. Population: Studies involving populations other than adults (e.g., children or adolescents) or those not directly affected by COVID-19-related mental health issues.
3. Intervention: Studies focusing on non-AI interventions or interventions without an AI component (e.g., purely human-operated services).
4. Outcome Measures: Studies lacking specific numerical data on mental health outcomes or those without pre- and post-intervention measures.
5. Publication Type: Articles not published in peer-reviewed journals or those not available in English.
6. Sample Size: Studies with fewer than 20 participants, due to potential limitations in generalizability.

5.6 DATA EXTRACTION

Data will be systematically extracted using a standardized form to include details on study design, sample characteristics, AI intervention specifics, outcome measures, and effect sizes. This information will be utilized to calculate pooled effect sizes and assess the overall efficacy of AI-driven mental health interventions.

5.7 THE IMPACT OF COVID-19 ON MENTAL HEALTHCARE

Public mental health, COVID-19 patients, healthcare professionals, and those with preexisting mental health issues have all been significantly impacted by the epidemic. Preventive measures including lockdowns, social distance, and self-isolation have reduced face-to-face social interaction for the general population, which can raise the risk of depressive illnesses (Teo et al., 2015). While social connections can be facilitated by online platforms, in-person human touch remains essential. Because of the increased attention to hygiene and cleanliness, this condition may cause temporary mild to moderate depression symptoms and elevated anxiety. Drug misuse, loneliness, spousal violence, and child abuse are all expected to rise as a result of the epidemic. Substance misuse may be used as a coping mechanism by some, and lockdowns and isolation may increase the number of incidences of child abuse and domestic violence. Post-traumatic stress disorder (PTSD) or depression symptoms might manifest in patients with COVID-19 infection (Galea et al., 2020).

Government and organizational assistance, psychological fortitude, and social support would help reduce the mental health issues of healthcare professionals. In particular, those who already have mental health issues are at risk during the epidemic (Tam et al., 2004). The role of stress in the development, course, and severity of mental health problems has been determined for a long time. The general population has higher rates of anxiety and depression, although individuals with preexisting conditions are more susceptible and prone to symptoms. For example, the levels of stress and anxiety caused by the pandemic may intensify the condition of patients with schizophrenia, bipolar disorder, or obsessive-compulsive disorder. Due to COVID-19, the mental health of so many communities have declined, and identifying and addressing the problems is very essential to help people during and after the pandemic.

5.8   THE ROLE OF AI IN MENTAL HEALTH DIAGNOSIS AND TREATMENT

- **Predictive Modeling for Early Detection and Intervention**
  Predictive models will improve treatment outcomes and indicate patients at risk. AI can power models for the prediction of a patient's response to several treatments, including medication, psychotherapy, and lifestyle changes. This individualized strategy increases expectations and reduces the likelihood of adverse outcomes by ensuring everyone receives treatment. Predictive models also have the potential to anticipate how a disease will proceed, which helps medical professionals make educated decisions regarding therapy and resource allocation (Yang, 2022). Healthcare systems can better prepare to handle the need for mental health services and efficiently distribute resources by forecasting the likely trajectory of mental health diseases.

- **Sentiment Analysis: Understanding Patient Emotions and Behaviors**
  Sentiment analysis is the process of classifying a text block as good, negative, or neutral. The primary goal will be to analyze public interest in a way that supports corporate growth. It illustrates emotions (such as happiness, sadness, and anger) in addition to polarity (positive, negative, and neutral). It makes use of several algorithms for natural language processing (Marreddy & Mamidi, 2023). The social sentiment of a brand is revealed through the contextual mining of words. Determining if the product being manufactured will create demand in the market is also helpful to the firm. Sentiment analysis is based on rules to determine the text opinion: It employs polarity-labeled words and a set of rules. Sentences with dependent clauses, sarcasm, or negations usually require the addition of other powers to be understood in addition to sentiment value (Chakraborty & Das, 2023). Sentiment analysis powered by machine learning entails utilizing a sentiment-labeled training set to teach a machine learning model to comprehend the polarity based on word order.

- **Digitalized Psychometric Assessments: Enhancing Accuracy and Timeliness**
  Digital psychological assessment has the potential to enhance time and accuracy in psychological assessment. The tests are administered and graded by the use of technology and offer very valuable information about a person's intellectual ability, personality, and work habits. Among others, the benefits of digital psychological testing are content creation and result personalization in business-focused terminologies that improve results. This has led to the promotion of working with psychometric tools across the business, which helps back up the decisions of the HR team in talent decisions and provides a place for multiple behavioral testing products to be accessed. Digital psychometric testing platforms, such as Aptitude, simplify and upgrade the measurement procedure. As a result, this makes the recruitment process effective and helps quickly screen the best candidates. Digital psychological testing not only increases accuracy but also saves time. In this regard, the time that is consumed by online test administration and grading systems will be saved compared to traditional paper exams. This speed comes in handy, for instance, during recruitment at high levels, say, graduate program applications. Not to forget that the psychometric outcome of such digital tests is essential in terms of reliability and validity. Psychometric items include test items such as validity and reliability. Every study and developer concerning psychometric tests is mandated to register their study before enrolment. The participant's characteristics and psychometric properties of the outcome have to be recorded in this platform (Brown & Williams, 2019). In psychological assessment,

computerized assessment has a prospect of enhancing time and accuracy in this field of psychology. These metrics, powered by technology, continue to increase the speed of hiring while providing meaningful information for talent decisions. It is important to ensure these tests are powerful and create a feeling of happiness, as stated by Jones et al. (2018).

5.9   AI-ENHANCED SERVICE DELIVERY AND ACCESSIBILITY

- **Teletherapy: Expanding Access to Mental Health Services**
  AI with real-time feedback can facilitate the quality of teletherapy. During video therapy, AI can identify the emotional state of the patient by analyzing the speech patterns, voice, and facial expressions of the patient. Doctors can utilize information from this analysis and change treatment plans and actions according to the patient's emotional state. This treatment procedure can be enhanced by examining the facial expression and tone of the patient, which will help the doctors comprehend the sentimental state of the patient's mind. Since smart telehealth interventions are problem-based, it has become easier for people living in rural or less developed areas of the world to access mental health services. Customers can be connected to licensed medical professionals via secure, AI-powered videoconferencing to ensure they get all the help they may need wherever they go. It also offers sessions with a view to teletherapy in order that one can obtain psychotherapy within the comfort of their own homes from any geographical point.

- **Digital Platforms: Streamlining Mental Health Services and Appointments**
  Digital platforms have the potential to enhance patient care, including provider continuity of care, and improve results. A few particular uses in mental healthcare are prompts to create a suicide safety plan, general practice referrals for specialist appointments, and standardized risk assessment templates. Electronic health records are widely utilized within clinical services to document clinical treatment. Throughout the course of their treatment, digital platforms can facilitate interaction and communication with service consumers (Larsen et al., 2023). While new platforms like conversational agents have new opportunities, established technologies like text messaging have improved results. Beyond the potential use of these platforms to improve communication, developments in smartphone sensors are creating new opportunities for digital phenotyping, a technique for obtaining objective behavioral measurements. These methods may be used for the measurement of treatment response, the early detection of behavioral changes, and the discovery of new cohorts exhibiting comparable tendencies (Basavarajappa & Chand, 2017). Human aspects and user experience must be taken into account in every digital platform, regardless of its mode or functionality, in order to guarantee user safety and adoption. Applying current quality frameworks and including stakeholders and end users, especially through co-design processes, might help with this. Clinical appointments were scheduled through websites, application-based and automated slot booking were used by the clients moreover clinicians also find this transition for easier way to maintain the client record and follow-ups even more digitalization added advantages are considered in one aspect same way there are certain ethical consequences and issues were arising with professional qualification, experience and license practice or proper educational qualification to take up clients. To avoid certain unethical activities, it should be mapped through regulatory bodies like the American Psychological Association (APA), Rehabilitation Council of India (RCI), or state mental health bodies to monitor the ethical practice to ensure the quality of service and treatment.

5.10   OTHER EFFECTIVE ASSISTIVE CONTRIBUTIONS OF AI

One such very innovative application is in predictive analytics. AI algorithms can analyze large amounts of data that are sourced from several sources, such as electronic health records, social media activity, and wearable devices, to identify the risk of mental health issues quite early. For example, AI systems can pick up on subtle changes in speech patterns, social interactions, and activity levels that may indicate depression or bipolar disorder. The early detection capability brought about by this would enable timely intervention and individualized treatment plans, which would possibly reduce the impact of mental crises even before they have the chance to develop. Another rare but effective role of AI in personalized mental healthcare is basically tied to the points made above.

These therapeutic approaches are then tailored by AI according to the analysis of data from previous interactions, responses to treatment, and personal preferences. For instance, AI systems can recommend special self-help exercises or therapeutic content that would be aligned with a unique mental health profile for a particular individual. Such a level of personalization goes beyond the mere generic treatment plans to a more nuanced and targeted approach, therefore enhancing the effectiveness of mental health interventions. AI also opens up a plethora of opportunities as far as the processing of natural languages is concerned, with its applications in the development of sophisticated tools for mental health.

Advanced models of natural language processing (NLP) can analyze and understand human languages with unbelievable accuracy, creating AI-powered recovery tools that convey meaningful conversations to the end-user. The tools will go on to support CBT by guiding exercises and feedback, and reframing negative thought patterns in the user's mind. Other applications include offering real-time emotional support and coping strategies to make mental healthcare more accessible and interactive. Additionally, its potential can be extended to both augmented reality and virtual reality environments that are in use during exposure therapy.

AI enhances such technologies by creating adaptive and responsive virtual environments, making them more lifelike in simulating scenarios for therapeutic use. For instance, AI-driven VR can immerse individuals in controlled settings, exposing them to fears or anxieties in a very controlled, safe, and manageable way. This enables the tailoring of exposure therapy sessions in real time on an individual user basis, through the manipulation of the level of exposure by the user's responses and progress, for more effectiveness and personality in the treatment of a case.

5.11 ETHICAL AND REGULATORY CONSIDERATIONS

AI in healthcare is advancing quickly, and the topic of controlling this growth is becoming more and more popular. Many AI innovations become the property and domain of private organizations. Due to the way AI is being used, it is possible that governmental agencies, businesses, and clinics will be involved in gathering, using, and safeguarding patient health data more than usual. This brings up privacy concerns about data security and deployment. In light of the reidentification problem, new and enhanced methods of anonymization and data security will be required. In addition to the need for innovation, regulations will be in place to make sure that private data custodians are employing secure and state-of-the-art techniques to safeguard patient privacy. Currently, monitoring and regulation run the risk of lagging behind the technology they are meant to oversee. Since the technology we use today are capable of rapid advancement, we run the risk of falling behind very soon (Murdoch, 2021).

Although there are hazards and difficulties associated with AI assistants, individuals with mental health issues may benefit from them. The substitution of knowledgeable individuals, having a sufficient body of evidence, data usage and security, and the seeming revelation of crimes were the ethical problems we discovered. It is noted that the application of such principles, including where they appear to conflict with one another, requires contextual judgment and provides several ethical recommendations for those who design and deploy AI assistants (Coghlan et al., 2023a). These ethical challenges can be understood and addressed through the five principles of beneficence, non-maleficence, and respect for autonomy, justice, and explicability (transparency and accountability). Although we concentrated on using AI assistants for mental health, the ethical issues apply to AI assistants in a variety of settings and circumstances, particularly those in which the end users are particularly vulnerable.

5.12 DISCUSSION

The findings of this chapter highlight the transformative potential of AI in mental healthcare, particularly in the context of the COVID-19 pandemic. AI technologies have the capacity to revolutionize the way mental health services are delivered, making them more accessible, efficient, and personalized. For example, AI-driven predictive models can help clinicians identify patients at high risk of developing mental health disorders, allowing for early intervention and improved outcomes.

However, the chapter also emphasizes the need for caution in the deployment of AI in mental healthcare. The ethical challenges associated with AI, including the risk of perpetuating biases and the potential for data breaches, must be carefully managed. Furthermore, there is a need for ongoing research to evaluate the long-term impact of AI on mental health outcomes and to develop strategies for mitigating any negative effects.

The findings suggest that while AI has the potential to address some of the challenges posed by the pandemic, it is not a panacea. Human oversight and clinical judgment remain essential components of mental healthcare, and AI should be seen as a tool to augment, rather than replace, these elements.

5.13 CONCLUSION

Overall, there are a variety of possibilities and problems, and AI in mental healthcare after the pandemic showcases the former. It tells of such potential benefits related to AI-driven innovations as better diagnostic accuracy, tailored treatment plans, and greater access to care. However, it also indicates ethical and practical matters that should be developed regarding those technologies in order to provide for an implementation on an equal and efficient basis.

Therefore, in the future, it will require researchers, clinicians, and policymakers to work together on making such guidelines or best practices. We can then effectively utilize the potential of AI for better outcomes in mental health treatment while safeguarding the rights and welfare of the patients.

AI can significantly improve mental healthcare by providing new solutions to persistent problems and raising the general level of care. Early-stage disease detection, personalized treatment, and more precision in diagnostics related to mental health can be provided using all of these through sentiment analysis, predictive modeling, and computerized psychometric tests. Technological advancement drives quality patient care at a lower cost of healthcare resource use. Teletherapy, offered over digital platforms or with the help of AI, may hold the promise of increasing access to mental healthcare by eliminating geographic limits and putting around-the-clock support at the fingertips of patients. High rates of provision for the care of patients and accessibility to interventions, especially in rural areas and others underserved, can be noted in the delivery of treatments for mental health via mHealth technologies (Flynn et al., 2020; Gual-Montolio et al., 2022). However, AI applied in mental healthcare keeps raising important ethical and legal questions. Data privacy, security, openness, and accountability are the bases of enhancing productivity of AI and making the public confidence richer.

Coghlan et al. (2023b) says, "it would be very important that regulatory frameworks evolve in parallel to technological advances, in ensuring safety, efficacy and ethical deployment of AI technologies." We need a middle ground, which shall provide better and more human-centric psychosocial models of care without compromising the precision and power that the data under the AI framework bring about. This would prove helpful in encouraging policymakers to take a more holistic view of social and environmental determinants of mental health and in integrating technological innovation within comprehensive strategies for mental health. AI in mental healthcare will really reshape mental healthcare by enhancing early identification, personalized care, and availability of service.

On that note, AI can help in humanely designing and engineering society in a way that preserves human rights and does not abuse what it means to be human. This can unite the experience of humans with the know-how of AI for equal, open-for-all touch in a new decade of mental health-care. Applying AI in treating mental health is as perilous as it is a revolution in the advancement of the field. It is likely that the grafting together of the human touch and AI will bring into being an all-new era of personalized, on-demand mental healthcare. If such development is to occur through robust ethical norms and well-defined legal frameworks, its benefits will be reaped together with the effective control of potential risks. Individual human rights and well-being must remain in mind during the deluge of considerations that must be taken into account in regard to the unlimited uses and consequences of AI in mental health. Technology should be developed in light of working toward the people whose lives they want to make easier. This should be for the goal of broadening access to mental healthcare and fostering better mental health for all.

REFERENCES

Arias, D., Saxena, S., & Verguet, S. (2022). Quantifying the global burden of mental disorders and their economic value. *E Clinical Medicine*, *54*, 101675. https://doi.org/10.1016/j.eclinm.2022.101675

Bajwa, J., Munir, U., Nori, A., & Williams, V. (2021). Artificial intelligence in healthcare—a bibliometric analysis. *Journal of Hospital Administration*, *10*(2), 1–14.

Basavarajappa, C., & Chand, P. K. (2017). Digital platforms for mental health-care delivery. *Indian Journal of Psychological Medicine*, *39*(5), 703–706. https://doi.org/10.4103/ijpsym.ijpsym_209_17

Berardi, C., Antonini, M., Jordan, Z., Wechtler, H., Paolucci, F., & Hinwood, M. (2024). Barriers and facilitators to the implementation of digital technologies in mental health systems: a qualitative systematic review to inform a policy framework. *BMC Health Services Research*, *24*(1). https://doi.org/10.1186/s12913-023-10536-1

Bouhouita-Guermech, F., Samet, A., Maalel, A., & Bouhlel, S. (2023). Ethics in AI-driven mental health care: a comparative review. *Journal of Ethics and Information Technology*, *25*(1), 89–102.

Brown, A., & Williams, B. (2019). Enhancing recruitment through digitalized psychometric assessments. *Journal of Organizational Psychology*, *45*(2), 123–135.

Chakraborty, A. K., & Das, S. (2023). A comparative study of a novel approach with baseline attributes leading to sentiment analysis of Covid-19 tweets. In *Elsevier eBooks* (pp. 179–208). https://doi.org/10.1016/b978-0-32-390535-0.00013-6

Coghlan, S., Leins, K., Sheldrick, S., Cheong, M., Gooding, P., & D'Alfonso, S. (2023a). To chat or bot to chat: ethical issues with using chatbots in mental health. *Digital Health*, *9*. https://doi.org/10.1177/20552076231183542

Coghlan, S., Miller, T., & Paterson, J. (2023b). Addressing ethical challenges in AI-driven mental health care. *AI & Society*, *38*(2), 311–328.

Flynn, D., Gregory, P., Makki, H., & Gabbay, M. (2020). Expectations and experiences of remote consulting in primary care: a qualitative study. *BJGP Open*, *4*(3), BJGPO.2020.0078. https://doi.org/10.1016/j.ijmedinf.2009.03.008

Galea, S., Merchant, R. M., & Lurie, N. (2020). The mental health consequences of COVID-19 and physical distancing. *JAMA Internal Medicine*, *180*(6), 817. https://doi.org/10.1001/jamainternmed.2020.1562

Gerke, S., Minssen, T., & Cohen, G. (2020). Ethical and legal challenges of artificial intelligence-driven healthcare. In *Elsevier eBooks* (pp. 295–336). https://doi.org/10.1016/b978-0-12-818438-7.00012-5

Gual-Montolio, P., Jaén, I., Martínez-Borba, V., Castilla, D., & Suso-Ribera, C. (2022). Using artificial intelligence to enhance ongoing psychological interventions for emotional problems in Real- or Close to Real-Time: a systematic review. *International Journal of Environmental Research and Public Health/International Journal of Environmental Research and Public Health*, *19*(13), 7737. https://doi.org/10.3390/ijerph19137737

Health, N. L. G. (2020). Mental health matters. *The Lancet Global Health*, *8*(11), e1352. https://doi.org/10.1016/s2214-109x(20)30432–0

Johnson, K. B., Wei, W., Weeraratne, D., Frisse, M. E., Misulis, K., Rhee, K., Zhao, J., & Snowdon, J. L. (2020). Precision medicine, AI, and the future of personalized health care. *Clinical and Translational Science*, *14*(1), 86–93. https://doi.org/10.1111/cts.12884

Johnson, R., et al. (2021). Timeliness and efficiency of digitalized psychometric assessments in high-volume recruitment processes. *Journal of Personnel Selection and Assessment*, *29*(3), 201–215.

Jones, C., et al. (2018). Customization and contextualization of digital psychometric assessments for talent decision-making. *Journal of Applied Psychology*, *103*(4), 567–578.

Langarizadeh, M., Tabatabaei, M., Tavakol, K., Naghipour, M., & Moghbeli, F. (2017). Telemental Health Care, an Effective Alternative to Conventional Mental Care: A Systematic Review. *Acta Informatica Medica*, *25*(4), 240. https://doi.org/10.5455/aim.2017.25.240-246

Larsen, M. E., Vo, L. C., Pratap, A., & Peters, D. (2023). Integrated digital platforms for clinical care. In *Springer eBooks* (pp. 1–19). https://doi.org/10.1007/978-3-030-42825-9_148-1

Lee, P., Abernethy, A., Shaywitz, D., Gundlapalli, A. V., Weinstein, J., Doraiswamy, P. M., Schulman, K., & Madhavan, S. (2022). Digital health COVID-19 impact Assessment: lessons learned and compelling needs. *NAM Perspectives*. https://doi.org/10.31478/202201c

Leka, S., Jain, A., & Centre for Organizational Health & Development, School of Medicine, University of Nottingham. (2014). *Eu Compass for Action on Mental Health and Well-Being: Mental Health in the Workplace in Europe— Consensus Paper*. https://health.ec.europa.eu/system/files/2017–07/compass_2017workplace_en_0.pdf

Marreddy, M., & Mamidi, R. (2023). Learning sentiment analysis with word embeddings. In *Elsevier eBooks* (pp. 141–161). https://doi.org/10.1016/b978-0-32-390535-0.00011-2

MHE. (2024, February 26). *Digitalisation & Mental Health: Navigating the Future*. Mental Health Europe. https://www.mentalhealtheurope.org/what-we-do/digitalisation/

Minerva, F., & Giubilini, A. (2023). Is AI the future of mental healthcare? *Topoi*, *42*(3), 809–817. https://doi.org/10.1007/s11245-023-09932-3

Murdoch, T. B. (2021). Privacy and artificial intelligence: challenges for protecting health information in a new era. *BMC Medical Ethics*, *22*(1). https://doi.org/10.1186/s12910-021-00687-3

Naik, N., Hameed, B. M. Z., Shetty, D. K., Swain, D., Shah, M., Paul, R., Aggarwal, K., Ibrahim, S., Patil, V., Smriti, K., Shetty, S., Rai, B. P., Chlosta, P., & Somani, B. K. (2022). Legal and ethical consideration in artificial intelligence in healthcare: who takes responsibility? *Frontiers in Surgery*, *9*. https://doi.org/10.3389/fsurg.2022.862322

Nilsen, P., Ståhl, C., Roback, K., & Cairney, P. (2022). Never the twain shall meet—a comparison of implementation science and policy implementation research. *Implementation Science*, *17*(1), 1–12.

Stoumpos, A. I., Kitsios, F., & Talias, M. A. (2023a). Digital transformation in healthcare: technology acceptance and its applications. *International Journal of Environmental Research and Public Health/ International Journal of Environmental Research and Public Health*, *20*(4), 3407. https://doi.org/10.3390/ijerph20043407

Tai, M. C. (2020). The impact of artificial intelligence on human society and bioethics. *Tzu-chi Medical Journal/Cí-jì Yīxué*, *32*(4), 339. https://doi.org/10.4103/tcmj.tcmj_71_20

Tam, C. W. C., Pang, E. P. F., Lam, L. C. W., & Chiu, H. F. K. (2004). Severe acute respiratory syndrome (SARS) in Hong Kong in 2003: stress and psychological impact among frontline healthcare workers. *Psychological Medicine*, *34*(7), 1197–1204. https://doi.org/10.1017/s0033291704002247

Teo, A. R., Choi, H., Andrea, S. B., Valenstein, M., Newsom, J. T., Dobscha, S. K., & Zivin, K. (2015). Does mode of contact with different types of social relationships predict depression in older adults? Evidence from a nationally representative survey. *Journal of the American Geriatrics Society*, *63*(10), 2014–2022. https://doi.org/10.1111/jgs.13667

World Health Organization (WHO). (2023, February 6). *Artificial Intelligence in Mental Health Research: New WHO Study on Applications and Challenges*. https://www.who.int/europe/news/item/06-02-2023-artificial-intelligence-in-mental-health-research-new-who-study-on-applications-and-challenges

Yang, C. C. (2022). Explainable artificial intelligence for predictive modeling in healthcare. *Journal of Healthcare Informatics Research*, *6*(2), 228–239. https://doi.org/10.1007/s41666-022-00114-1

6 Leveraging Digital Health Technologies in Health Care Teams

A Discussion of Policy and Practice in Canada

Charlotte Hruczkowski, Ryan Brown, and Tim Konoval

The COVID-19 pandemic fundamentally changed all facets of life. Work, education, and healthcare rapidly shifted to the digital space, which created new challenges and presented new opportunities. Digital health technologies (DHTs) have transformed the way healthcare is delivered, leading to potentially improved patient outcomes and greater access to care. The integration of electronic health records has streamlined the process of storing and accessing patient information, leading to more coordination and efficacy. In addition, telemedicine has made it possible for patients to consult with healthcare providers remotely, which is especially beneficial for those in rural or underserved areas. Wearable devices have also become increasingly popular and, combined with data analytics, have facilitated the monitoring of patient health and the early detection of potential medical issues, ultimately leading to more personalized and proactive care (Butcher & Hussain, 2022; Stoumpos et al., 2023). Furthermore, the adoption of digital technologies is essential for healthcare organizations to stay competitive, providing high-quality, cost-effective care (Haleem et al., 2021). The World Health Organization (WHO) describes this digital transformation of healthcare as disruptive; however, it also notes that technologies can be incorporated to improve health outcomes in a variety of ways:

> Digital transformation of health care can be disruptive; however, technologies such as the virtual care, remote monitoring, artificial intelligence, big data analytics, blockchain, smart wearables, platforms, tools enabling data exchange and storage and tools enabling remote data capture and the exchange of data and sharing of relevant information across the health ecosystem creating a continuum of care have proven potential to enhance health outcomes by improving medical diagnosis, data-based treatment decisions, digital therapeutics, clinical trials, self-management of care and person-centered care as well as creating more evidence-based knowledge, skills and competence for professionals to support health care.
>
> **(WHO, 2021)**

As we have come out of the pandemic and returned to a new state of normal, lessons learned must be embraced, and the use of virtual care in practice settings should be discussed. This chapter will explore the use of DHTs in team-based care, focusing on virtual care and telehealth modalities in the context of interprofessional education and collaborative practice (IPECP) across Canada. Best practices in virtual care, both uniprofessional and interprofessional, prior to the pandemic and steady state post-pandemic will be compared and contrasted, as will differing models of care. Importantly, the underlying framework underpinning this chapter is the National Interprofessional Competency Framework developed by the Canadian Interprofessional Health Collaborative (CIHC) (CIHC, 2024).

DOI: 10.1201/9781003485629-6

This chapter will further explore policy as an enabler and also a barrier to digital health implementation pre- and post-COVID as well as regulatory implications using tangible case studies of implemented digital health initiatives. Each policy and practice recommendation will be reinforced by tangible Canadian case studies focusing on DHTs across teams including primary care and specialist consult service. The path forward is explored using an environmental scan of innovation in Canada, with emerging trends being identified, specifically a patient's role in the healthcare team and patient partner engagement in program design. A summary section includes 3–5 review questions along with a dedicated section for relevant definitions. Resources are provided for the practical application of DHTs in practice settings. A final call to action encourages teams to embrace the use of DHT in the day-to-day processes to enhance the collaboration of healthcare teams and promote the role of the patient on the team.

6.1 SUPPORTING EVIDENCE OF TECHNOLOGY IN HEALTHCARE

Virtual care has become an essential tool in healthcare delivery, especially amid the COVID-19 pandemic (Dave & Patel, 2023). Healthcare centralization in a pandemic is a matter of life and death when dealing with a novel pathogen causing high rates of morbidity and mortality and (early on) limited understanding of its mechanism of action and transmission (Khalili et al., 2023; Zulman & Verghese, 2021). The increased use of virtual care during the pandemic started to support the care of patients diagnosed with COVID-19, including those who were suspected, quarantined, or discharged home (Smith et al., 2020). In this way, care was provided safely to coordinate testing and triage the clinical needs of those infected with the virus, particularly in the outpatient setting (Smith et al., 2020).

In order to ensure the effective implementation of virtual care as a safe proxy to in-person care, healthcare providers must adhere to certain best practices. These best practices involve both the interaction with the patient and the security of patient privacy. While the term "virtual care" encompasses a spectrum ranging from a provider to patient phone, an asynchronous digital exchange or a technologically advanced video appointment, experts agree upon some common tenants for an optimal experience such utilizing secure and reliable technology platforms; ensuring clear communication; adapting workflows and processes; implementing appropriate clinical guidelines; and monitoring and documenting patient data (Segal et al., 2022; Schwamm et al., 2020).

One challenge for the continued adoption of technology into practice is the variability in evidence to support the use of virtual care as a delivery method to monitor and manage other medical issues. This problem derives from several factors: Namely, we have to yet (1) reach a clear understanding of the basic definitions of technology in practice across professions (e.g., difference between telemedicine and telehealth); (2) determine the degree to which success or failure in one application of technology applies to other contexts (e.g., prescription renewals for some but not all conditions, or differences in patients or care settings; von Huben et al., 2022); (3) establish frameworks to ensure reliability when conducting and reporting research on technology use, such as National Institute for Health and Care Excellence (NICE) framework (National Institute for Health and Care Excellence, 2021), MAST (Kidholm et al., 2012), or CONSORT E-HEALTH (Eysenbach & Consort-EHEALTH Group, 2011); and (4) embed implementation strategies that support rapid, on-going changes in technological capabilities.

There is growing literature that supports digital technology use in different ways. This literature ranges from the situations and specific patient conditions that technology is appropriate or not to facilitate care. However, there is variability in the research itself, including describing who the technology is used by and if it is transferable to other members of the care team, as well as what technology was used (such as telephone visits or video-enabled methods) and if the type of visit is appropriate using different types of technology, including whether other asynchronous methods (such as emails or apps) would work in the same way. The literature is also very limited in exploring different types of technology across one setting, such as reviewing telephone, virtual, app-enabled, websites, and social media, and whether this technology could be used the same way across different patient types (e.g., based on age, language, and health concerns).

Literature understanding of how technology can be used to communicate across the team is limited. However, one study reported that technology may result in faster screening and referral to specialist care (and treatment) for certain conditions such as inflammatory arthritis, where a fast diagnosis and treatment is essential for positive patient outcomes (Rogier et al., 2021). Donnelly et al. (2021) also discussed how it could improve team communication across the care continuum, including the ability to consult other providers and those with specialized clinical knowledge. Understanding how technology can be used to improve the efficiencies and communication across the team is limited.

One use of DHT is by providing the patient with more information and facilitating various conversations. Physicians reported that virtual care could be used for advanced directives or health planning, as well as follow-up visits for patients who received regular, on-going care (Gomez et al., 2021; Donaghy et al., 2019), including medication reconciliations (Gomez et al., 2021). There is also support for monitoring chronic diseases (Hasani et al., 2020), including chronic digestive diseases (Cross et al., 2019). Additionally, there is support for patient remote monitoring when patients have the devices to do so (Gomez et al., 2021). There is an opportunity to explore which types of visits (or conversations) can be conducted remotely, including which team members (e.g. physicians, nurses, and pharmacists) can facilitate these conversations to support teamwork and distribute resources.

However, there were mixed feelings about whether virtual care was appropriate to deliver bad news, such as a new cancer diagnosis. Some research supported it (Holstead & Robinson, 2020), and others thought emotional conversations were most appropriate in-person (Donaghy et al., 2019). However, the settings of these practices were different—one being in cancer care and the other general practice, and so understanding the context to which the technology is being used could support certain areas where it is used. For example, delivering bad news may be better suited for acute or outpatient care because important news can be delivered faster. Delivering bad news may be more challenging in general practice because of a different (and often longer-term) relationship providers have with their patients.

A key finding in many articles regarding whether virtual care is appropriate centered around relationship building, including the ability to connect with patient families and provide a more family-centered treatment plan. A key influence of building relationships is nonverbal communication. It was reported that the lack of physical cues and body language, whether to read the patient's reaction, or a response from the provider to show patient support, was considered an important aspect as to whether to use virtual care or not (Gomez et al., 2021; Donaghy et al., 2019; Holstead & Robinson, 2020). And so, if the relationship to the patient is important, then it needs to be considered whether or not relationships can be formed and maintained through technology. This still has yet to be explored.

Due to the evidence of virtual care use being mixed, there is an opportunity to solidify more feedback from providers, technology experts, and patients to support the adoption of technology in practice. Many articles use physician participants (Gomez et al., 2021; Holstead & Robinson, 2020; Hasani et al., 2020) and exclude other team members and patients. This may include a variety of participants in the research that would highlight the dynamics of interprofessional teams and complexity of collaborating across the continuum of care.

6.2 CONSIDERATIONS OF TEAM-BASED CARE USING DIGITAL TECHNOLOGY AND VIRTUAL CARE

DHTs impact the care delivered by healthcare teams more than adjusting the mode of service. The use of technology expands from virtual care to how digital technology is used within and across teams to collaborate and engage patients (Hruczkowski, forthcoming). The transition to use technology in regular practice reflects a societal shift into technology utilization. Prior to the emerging digital health age, there were existing innovations and technologies used in healthcare; however, there has been a change in the mindset of professionals, decision-makers, and patients during the present time that altered the perspectives of using technology as a way to function and coordinate care in a team.

Care across the continuum is delivered by a team of health professionals. The implementation of digital technology into healthcare needs to bridge from policy into practice, which includes educating healthcare teams on how to use it within their team environments. Providers (medicine, nursing, allied health, etc.), adjacent staff (admins, IT, managers, etc.), and patients and support persons should be involved in learning about how and when to use digital technology (Arnaert et al., 2019).

Healthcare teams first learn to work together and then collaborate in practice through a global strategy called Interprofessional Education and Collaborative Practice (IPECP). Interprofessional education (IPE) is a collaborative learning approach where students from different healthcare professions learn together with the goal of optimized patient care (Khalili et al., 2022). IPE is an andragogical strategy that involves learners from two or more professions engaging in interactive learning with the goal of acquiring knowledge and skills to work effectively as a team in collaborative practice (WHO, 2019). Collaborative practice, on the other hand, refers to interprofessional teamwork in which healthcare providers from different professions work together with patients, families, and communities to deliver coordinated and integrated healthcare. Collaborative practice involves the sharing of knowledge, skills, and resources among team members to improve patient outcomes, enhance patient safety, and optimize healthcare delivery (Brewer & Flavell, 2018; MacQuarrie & Brown, 2023). The CIHC has identified six domains that are essential for effective IPECP (CIHC, 2024):

- Team Communication
- Role Clarification and Negotiation
- Relationship-Focused Care/Services
- Collaborative Leadership
- Team Functioning
- Team Differences and Disagreements

These domains of interprofessionalism will be key as we explore the interplay of DHTs and collaborative practice teams at both the policy and practice levels.

6.3   POLICY IMPLICATIONS: DIGITAL CARE IN CANADA

The Canadian healthcare system adjusted care during the pandemic. However, there are ongoing healthcare challenges that began prior to the shift in care delivery. These challenges include inequitable access to care (Digital Health Canada [DHC], 2022), an insatiable demand across the system complemented with continued population growth (Duong & Vogel, 2023), and the ongoing health human workforce crisis with decreased funding (Canadian Academy of Health Sciences, 2023). Although the impact the pandemic had on these issues has not yet been fully discovered, the situation provided new opportunities to problem solve.

Prior to the pandemic, digital health use was limited and not part of common delivery of healthcare. There were many unknowns about how to use it in the safest and most efficient way. The urgency to rapidly implement technology in the pandemic offered the opportunity to challenge our prior beliefs and understanding about using technology. Considering alternatives to care delivery has the possibilities to enhance connections across the continuum, provide improved distribution of services, and ensure the long-term sustainability of care. However, we still need to address funding models, supporting evidence, the ethical and legal implications (including patient data), and navigating the interoperability of technology across teams.

6.4   FUNDING AND PAYMENT MODELS

Canadian healthcare is funded federally and distributed to individual provinces along with a mandate letter to direct how these funds are spent. In 2021, the prime minister of Canada mandated the health minister of Canada to "work in partnership with provinces and territories to [provide] an early increase of investments in primary and virtual care . . ." (Prime Minister of Canada, 2021). It is the responsibility of the province to redistribute the funding to individual care organizations and providers. This means there are overarching directives on how to use the funds; however, individual provinces have their own individual priorities and distribution models, which are outlined by individual provincial premiers and ministers of health in a similar, mandated way. For example, in Alberta, the premier mandated the minister of health to "collaborate with the Minister of Technology and Innovation to perform an independent review of the effectiveness of the information technology systems used throughout Alberta's health system and provide recommendations on how to strengthen Alberta's health-care system through the use of technology and driven by population needs" (Government of Alberta, 2023). The province then works with individual organizations to distribute the funds.

However, the massive pivot to digital health has uncovered interoperability issues between providers in Canada (typically physicians and all others) as physicians are largely independent contractors who bill the public funded system for services rendered. Disparities in the way team members are paid (or not paid) are often a limiting factor in delivering effective care in the digital arena. Nursing and allied health professionals who are salaried employees of health systems can easily pivot based on organizational will, whereas physicians may have no ability to bill these services. The remuneration barrier to using digital modalities in care is not new to the pandemic and was identified as a factor why Canada lagged behind other countries to adopt virtual care in practice (CHI, 2018a, 2018b). From physician perspectives in both primary and specialist areas, having an applicable fee schedule was indicated as a factor (50% and 43%, respectively) that would facilitate the integration of technology into practice (CHI, 2018b). However, this is one of the multiple influencing factors that determine whether or not physicians alter traditional care methods with technology. Others included improved technology (along with an understanding of how best to use the technology), support services (e.g., provided through medical associations and government bodies), and guidelines to ensure privacy and security (CHI, 2018b).

6.5   HEALTH DATA MANAGEMENT: ETHICAL AND LEGAL CONSIDERATIONS

Health data are classified as sensitive personal data and personally identifiable information, which requires a high safety and security standard (WHO, 2021). However, access to health data is an important aspect of involving patients as a member of the team and sharing continual updates with them. This can improve the care of a patient. However, in Canada, patient health information is siloed within care centers and is not readily accessible or exchangeable at the point of care, or to the patients themselves (CHI, 2018a). This inaccessibility not only causes inefficiencies in health resource management and the delivery of care, for example, by creating extra costs (e.g., when tests are duplicated) and uncoordinated and/or delayed treatments. There are also issues with patient data such as ethics and storage capacity.

Some work has been conducted to standardize data, enable greater information exchange, and facilitate seamless access to health information for all Canadians, including working groups at local and provincial levels. Leaders across the healthcare system have advanced digital health transformation across Canada through partnerships, collaboration, and alignment with provinces, territories, pan-Canadian health organizations (e.g., the CIHI [2022], Statistics Canada [StatCan], and Public Health Agency of Canada [PHAC]), Indigenous peoples, the private sector, data and standards experts, and, of course, clinical leaders and patients.

There are ethical and legal considerations of health data management, specifically involving patient privacy. This includes informed consent, data security and confidentiality, data minimization

PATIENT PRIVACY CONSIDERATIONS

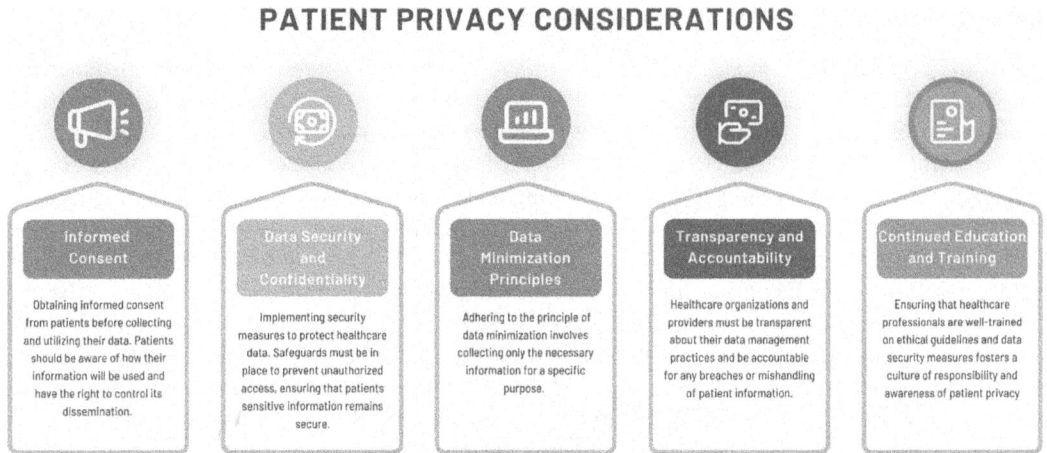

Informed Consent	Data Security and Confidentiality	Data Minimization Principles	Transparency and Accountability	Continued Education and Training
Obtaining informed consent from patients before collecting and utilizing their data. Patients should be aware of how their information will be used and have the right to control its dissemination.	Implementing security measures to protect healthcare data. Safeguards must be in place to prevent unauthorized access, ensuring that patients sensitive information remains secure.	Adhering to the principle of data minimization involves collecting only the necessary information for a specific purpose.	Healthcare organizations and providers must be transparent about their data management practices and be accountable for any breaches or mishandling of patient information.	Ensuring that healthcare professionals are well-trained on ethical guidelines and data security measures fosters a culture of responsibility and awareness of patient privacy

FIGURE 6.1   Privacy Principles regarding Patient Data.

principles, transparency and accountability, and continued education and training (Ozair et al., 2015; Rahman & Jim, 2024; Nittari et al., 2020; see Figure 6.1). As new technology emerges such as the use of artificial intelligence or precision medicine treatments, it is anticipated that there will be more guidelines added to how healthcare providers and stakeholders ethically and legally manage patient data in multiple forms. The move toward commercialization of patient data further complicates these dilemmas and highlights the risks of loss of anonymity, surveillance and marketing, discrimination, and violation of Indigenous data sovereignty (Spithoff et al., 2022). However, in Canada, studies have shown public support for secondary uses of patient data for research, and the outcomes provide clear public benefits, particularly with de-identified data (Spithoff et al., 2022).

6.6   PRACTICE IMPLICATIONS: IMPLEMENTING CHANGE IN CANADA

The majority of Canadians (58%) see at least one other care provider, in addition to a regular doctor (CHI, 2018a). This means there could be conflicts in the care provided across the continuum because provider digital systems do not always communicate with one another (CHI, 2018b). In fact, when reviewing the ability to exchange patient summaries from physicians outside of their clinical location, specialists (19%) and primary care physicians (16%) were able to do so (CHI, 2018b). This creates problems such as the risk for medical error and the ineffective use of healthcare services due to unintended overlap in services. This highlights the need to recognize team communication as a key factor for the implementation of digital technologies in practice.

The integration and implementation of digital technology in care settings require complex thinking and implementation strategies. Healthcare is a complex system and requires change to consider the team across the continuum of care as well as the individual preferences and needs of patients and providers.

6.7   INTEROPERABILITY AND THE CONTINUUM OF CARE

The integration of digital technologies in healthcare has paved the way for the adoption of virtual care, which encompasses a wide range of services delivered remotely, from consultations to monitoring and follow-ups (DHC, 2022). In the context of uniprofessional care, virtual care primarily focuses on enabling a single healthcare provider, such as a physician or a nurse, to deliver care and interact with patients through digital platforms. This approach has proven to be especially beneficial in improving access to care for patients in remote or underserved areas, as well as for individuals

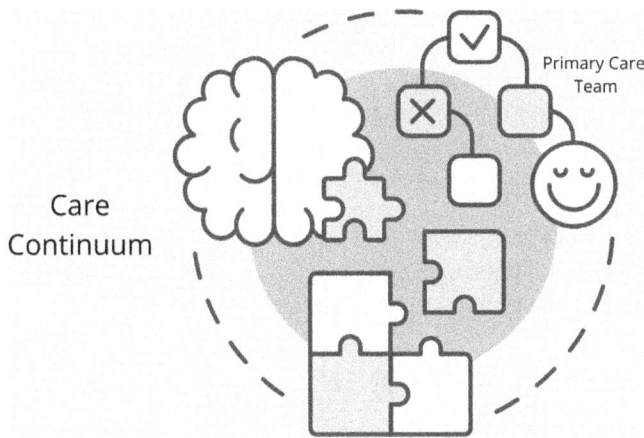

FIGURE 6.2 Care Coordination across a Continuum of Care.

with mobility limitations. On the other hand, interprofessional care in the virtual setting involves a collaborative approach, where multiple healthcare professionals from different disciplines work together to provide comprehensive care to patients. This method allows for a more holistic and multidimensional approach to patient care, leveraging the expertise of various professionals such as physicians, nurses, pharmacists, and allied health professionals (Khalili et al., 2023). The seamless coordination and communication among interprofessional teams through virtual platforms can lead to enhanced care experiences and potentially improved patient outcomes. However, this requires enhancing the coordination of team-based services using digital technologies across the care continuum and within the individual teams (Figure 6.2). Communication in virtual spaces has been noted recently as a central tenet to the success of interprofessional, virtual care teams (Gordon et al., 2020; Gustin et al., 2020).

A consideration of interoperability across teams is the housing, managing, and sharing health data. In Canada, various electronic medical record (EMR) platforms are used for the purposes of storing patient data and conducting administrative procedures such as bookings. The functionality of different platforms includes communicating across the care team—such as between a specialist and a primary care provider. However, there are various limitations to EMRs, specifically that providers report not being able to communicate with one another (CHI, 2018b). There are challenges to streamlining healthcare data across the continuum of care due to the variety of EMR systems used. Many of the different EMR systems are not designed to communicate with one another. There are attempts to standardize systems, but this is a complex issue at both the national and provincial levels.

6.7.1 CASE STUDY: IMPLEMENTING SYSTEMS ACROSS THE CONTINUUM OF CARE

In Alberta, Canada, an initiative to standardize the EMR system began in 2019. The program is called "ConnectCare" and was aimed to reduce the gaps in care across the continuum, including enhancing communication and sharing patient data across teams (Alberta Health Services, 2024). However, the implementation of the system had multiple challenges and unanticipated problems. First, although the program had the capability to store medical records, it was originally created as a scheduling tool. Scheduling systems do not innately store data in a usable form, and so extracting administrative data for research, trending, and projecting opportunities is limited. The second issue was that the program was created outside of Canada, which did not naturally incorporate important contextual practice needs. An example of this is the inability to remove patient allergy "red flag pop-ups." Updated practice guidelines suggest a specific antibiotic can be used with patients who are penicillin allergic; however, there is a warning pop-up if some antibiotics are prescribed. The system developers reported the pop-up is not able to be removed from the system, even if guidelines have been updated. The system is also limited in the way it allows for various health professionals to update patient allergies, and as a result, patients may not necessarily receive the most effective treatment due to being mislabeled (e.g., the difference between a mild, moderate, and severe beta-lactam allergy would change the treatment plan [Center for Disease Control, 2024]). Although it is important to streamline the EMR system used across healthcare systems to facilitate communication across the teams, there are implementation barriers that need to be addressed such as the ability to update guidelines and support practices that are context specific.

6.8   WORKFLOWS CHANGE IN CONTEXT

Implementation strategies are needed for practice changes, particularly when teams are working together to provide care. In a case study observing the adaptations to use DHTs in primary care, teams were observed from different clinic models (medical homes and centralized clinics; Hruczkowski, forthcoming). The case found that the implementation of digital technologies occurred differently between individual providers and that these changes were supported by the availability of system-level resources (Hruczkowski, forthcoming). The findings also highlight how the implementation of DHTs can be used to facilitate team collaboration and patient engagement (Hruczkowski, forthcoming). The outcomes of the work created the basis for a resource to support the development and implementation of practice tools to integrate DHTs into individual teams and practices (MD Connections, n.d.). Drawing on implementation science frameworks (Damschroder et al., 2009; Powell et al., 2015), some of the implementation strategies include the following:

1. **Promote Adaptability:** As the integration of technology is often provider or team specific, create living guidelines that are flexible and transferable to different practice settings.
2. **Develop Educational Materials:** Digital technology continues to evolve, providing simple and on-going educational materials that can support teams to change their delivery methods.
3. **Capture and Share Local Knowledge:** Facilitate ways to share the experience of patients, including their preferences and lived experiences of using digital technology to manage their health at home.
4. **Facilitation:** Promote the use of experts in the field who can consult teams on how to integrate technology to improve practices in specific settings.

6.8.1   Telemedicine Consults: Bridging the Gap to Specialists

In recent years, telehealth has emerged as a promising strategy to address the increasing demand for healthcare services (Cunha et al., 2009). Telemedicine refers to the utilization of tele-communication technology, such as videoconferencing and telephone consultations, to provide virtual remote healthcare services, either synchronously or asynchronously. The COVID-19 pandemic accelerated the adoption and implementation of telemedicine as an essential care delivery modality, ensuring continuity of service in a time of unprecedented uncertainty. Telemedicine has not only enabled access to healthcare services remotely but also provided opportunities for virtual specialist consults from primary care providers (and others), overcoming barriers such as geographical distance and temporal differences.

Virtual telemedicine consults can allow for in-depth discussions between primary care providers and specialists via videoconferencing, telephone, or asynchronous platforms. The most robust services allow specialists to review medical records, conduct thorough assessments, provide personalized treatment recommendations, and even bill the encounter to insurance companies. This level of depth in virtual consultations ensures that patients receive high-quality care, comparable to in-person visits (NQF Projects, 2014; Palen et al., 2012; Pogorzelska & Chlabicz, 2022). The COVID-19 pandemic has acted as a catalyst for the widespread adoption of virtual telemedicine consults in North America, where previously infrastructure, regulatory, and remunerative barriers were present.

Moreover, the collaborative nature of virtual telemedicine consults not only enhances the coordination of care between primary care physicians and specialists but also fosters a multidisciplinary approach to patient management. Through virtual meetings and consultations, specialists from different fields can come together to discuss complex cases, share their expertise, and collectively formulate the most effective treatment plans. This interdisciplinary collaboration often leads to a more holistic and well-rounded approach to patient care, particularly for individuals with multiple comorbid conditions (Cerbo et al., 2015; Green & Johnson, 2015; Kruse et al., 2017).

As telemedicine consults continue to evolve, there is an opportunity to capitalize on the depth of patient education and empowerment. By utilizing interactive platforms and educational resources, specialists can empower patients to become active participants in their own care, fostering a deeper understanding of their health conditions and treatment plans. This depth of patient empowerment contributes to improved adherence to medical recommendations and promotes a proactive approach to health management.

6.8.2   OPERATIONAL AND POLICY-LEVEL BARRIERS

While promising in a number of facets, operational and policy-level barriers to implementing system-level specialist telemedicine consult services available to all do exist. In Canada, physician remuneration poses a number of issues:

1. **Fee-for-Service Model Limitations**: The traditional fee-for-service model, which pays physicians for each patient visit or procedure, may not adequately compensate for the time and effort required for virtual consultations. Virtual care often involves extensive patient record reviews, detailed assessments, and follow-ups, which are not always accounted for in this model.
2. **Inconsistent Billing Codes**: The lack of standardized billing codes for virtual services across different provinces and territories creates confusion and inconsistency. Uncertainty about which services are billable and at what rates leads to reluctance in adopting virtual care practices.
3. **Reimbursement Rates**: Lower reimbursement rates for virtual consultations compared to in-person visits can disincentivize physicians from offering virtual care. This discrepancy fails to recognize the value and potential cost savings of virtual consultations, such as reduced travel time and increased convenience for patients.
4. **Administrative Burden**: Navigating the administrative complexities of billing for virtual care can be cumbersome. Physicians might face additional administrative burden and verification processes, which can be a deterrent, particularly for those already managing heavy workloads.
5. **Lack of Incentives for Collaborative Care**: Virtual care often involves collaboration among multiple healthcare providers. Many current remuneration models typically do not reward this interprofessional approach, which can be essential for comprehensive patient care. Without financial incentives for collaboration, physicians might be less motivated to engage in virtual multidisciplinary consultations.
6. **Investment in Technology**: The initial investment required for setting up and maintaining virtual care infrastructure, such as telemedicine platforms and data analytics tools, can be significant. Current remuneration models do not always cover these costs, leaving physicians to bear the financial burden, which can be a barrier to adopting virtual care.
7. **Variability in Provincial Policies**: Healthcare in Canada is provincially regulated, leading to variability policies and remuneration models. This inconsistency can create disparities

in the availability and quality of virtual care across different regions, affecting both physicians and patients.

8. **Limited Patient Access to Technology**: For virtual care to be effective, patients need access to reliable Internet and appropriate devices. In areas with limited technological infrastructure, this can be a significant barrier, indirectly impacting physicians' ability to offer virtual care and be remunerated for it.

Addressing these barriers requires a comprehensive approach, including updating remuneration models to reflect the true value of virtual care, standardizing billing practices, and providing financial support for technological investments.

6.8.3   LICENSURE CONSIDERATIONS

Addressing the regulatory aspects of physician licensure is also crucial to fully leverage the potential of virtual telemedicine consults. Several key factors need to be considered.

1. **Provincial Licensure Requirements:** Canada's healthcare system is provincially regulated, and each province has its own licensing requirements for physicians. In other words, a physician licensed in one province cannot automatically provide care to patients in another province without obtaining the necessary licensure. This limitation restricts the ability of healthcare providers to offer virtual services across different geographic regions, thereby reducing access to care, especially in underserved areas.

2. **Interprovincial Licensure Compacts:** To address these challenges, Canadian regulators have considered adopting policies similar to interstate licensure compacts seen in other countries. These compacts allow physicians to practice across multiple jurisdictions without obtaining individual licenses for each area. An interprovincial licensure compact would enable Canadian physicians to provide virtual care to patients in any province, thus expanding access to a broader pool of qualified healthcare professionals and enhancing continuity of care. Currently, this type of arrangement only exists in Atlantic Canada (Nova Scotia, Prince Edward Island, and New Brunswick).

3. **Virtual Care Licensure:** Some provinces have started implementing special telemedicine licensure or registration processes to streamline licensing requirements for healthcare providers delivering virtual care, allowing physicians to provide care to patients in multiple provinces without the need for full licensure in each province. This approach helps reduce administrative burdens and promotes the growth of virtual healthcare services.

4. **Standardized Guidelines and Regulations:** The increasing use of telemedicine has highlighted the need for standardized guidelines and regulations to govern virtual care delivery in Canada. These regulations should address licensure requirements, quality assurance, and ethical standards specific to telemedicine practice. Establishing consistent and cohesive regulations across provinces would help ensure patient safety, quality care delivery, and the efficient use of virtual platforms.

5. **National Licensing Framework:** Another potential solution could be the development of a national licensing framework. Such a framework would allow physicians to be licensed to practice across all provinces and territories, simplifying the process and ensuring that regulatory standards are uniformly maintained across the country. This national approach could significantly enhance the accessibility and flexibility of virtual care.

6.8.4   CASE STUDY: VIRTUAL HALLWAY

One such example is the Virtual Hallway platform, a telemedicine specialist consult solution that is redefining how primary care providers (nurse practitioners and physicians) are able to consult specialist and subspecialist services in a region(s) (Nova Scotia, Canada, but available in other Canadian provinces) where there is a critical mass of specialist services in the urban tertiary referral center, but more than half of the population resides in geographically distant rural areas.

The Virtual Hallway platform leverages asynchronous booking of consults to enable primary care providers to seamlessly connect with specialists via a phone call within 24 hours, facilitating expedited and efficient diagnosis and treatment planning for patients without the need for them to travel long distances to access specialized care. Virtual Hallway effectively democratizes access to specialist care on a first-come-first-serve basis, giving community-based providers in remote and rural areas immediate and direct access to specialists who may not be available in their region (Nouveau Health, 2023).

Platforms like Virtual Hallway solve a number of health system problems:

1. As discussed above, increasing the availability of specialist consults bridges the urban and rural divide. In North America, there are significantly fewer specialists per capita in rural areas compared to urban areas (Johnston et al., 2019; Pong et al., 2011). Telemedicine addresses this by decreasing the travel time for patients as 84% of phone consultations mitigate the need for in-person specialist consults (Virtual Hallway, n.d.a).
2. Physician burnout, particularly in primary care, reached record levels during the COVID-19 pandemic (McKay et al., 2023). Interprofessional collaboration and peer support can often bolster resilience in primary care providers who often feel set adrift to deal with multiple complex patient issues. Virtual Hallway allows for increased confidence in care plans and an immediate safety net for primary care, consistently scoring very high in user satisfaction. Furthermore, this type of interaction leads to immediate clinical feedback and learning, which can mitigate the need for consultation in the future on similar presentations (Virtual Hallway, n.d.b).
3. Tied into the point above, resource management in healthcare is always an ongoing concern. Increased confidence of primary care providers leads to a greater proportion of lower acuity patients being managed locally by primary care and leaving specialists and subspecialists with more capacity to manage high acuity cases (Virtual Hallway, n.d.c).
4. Data integration is key for effective continuity of care and is often a pain point for consultation between providers and interprofessional teams. Virtual Hallway securely transfers consult notes back to the referring provider in a format that can seamlessly be imported into most EMR systems. Virtual Hallway can also bill insurance companies directly for the consult on behalf of providers in eligible jurisdictions, reducing administrative burden on physicians.
5. Finally, it is acknowledged that healthcare's carbon footprint is massive, shockingly larger than that of the aviation industry. The shift to forms of predominantly virtual care during the COVID-19 pandemic resulted in significantly reduced greenhouse emissions by health systems broadly as well as due to reduced transportation for consult appointments. This is an unintended, but sustained, benefit of peer-to-peer virtual consult services like Virtual Hallway (Hale et al., 2024; Virtual Hallway, n.d.d).

Platforms such as Virtual Hallway have had transformative effects on the way healthcare is delivered and experienced by both patients and providers alike. While specialist consults are currently only available to family physicians and nurse practitioners, there is a planned expansion to pharmacists, which will further promote care in communities and necessitate further discussions in interprofessional practice.

6.9   PROVIDERS AS KEY STAKEHOLDERS AND THE PATIENT LEADING ROLE

Establishing clear roles and responsibilities is essential for effective digital health implementation. The existing team may have new roles, and the responsibilities that they once had may be evolving with new technologies and ways of doing things being introduced.

The implementation of technology into care has the potential to enhance healthcare practices and improve communication within teams. However, there are gaps in understanding how using virtual care impacts team communication and individual practices. To ensure seamless adoption of new care delivery methods, education and training should be provided to healthcare professionals, clinic staff, and patients. Primary care team members, such as receptionists, administrators, and clinic support staff, require particular attention. A case study conducted in the United Kingdom using mixed methods revealed that receptionists and administrators are pivotal in ensuring patients grasp new virtual consultation methods. Surprisingly, other practice members only sometimes acknowledged or factored in this, and as a result, receptionists are not often given any training. There is a financial investment to train staff members, and often ad hoc or in-house training (or only training physicians) limits how well technology is implemented. Not only is this a significant obstacle to implementation, but it can lead to inconsistency and lack of clarity of virtual care practices, among the care team and between patients and providers.

Patient roles in healthcare are still being understood. However, it is undeniable that one of the major forces to use virtual care involves the patient. The patient perspective is used as part of the decision-making process and often drives the way in which healthcare is delivered (Gilmore et al., 2019). Consistently, their perspectives provide insights into care outcomes and the effectiveness of care (Gilmore et al., 2019), including their involvement in shared decision-making increases compliance with treatment (Deniz et al., 2021).

Patients indicated their perspectives on the availability, use, and interest in technology prior to the pandemic (CHI, 2018a). Surprisingly, some of the interest and desire for technology in care did not focus on virtual care but rather other methods of technology use, such as having asynchronous contact (such as email) with providers and healthcare teams regarding their health issues, the ability to book online, and having access to their health data remotely (CHI, 2018a). Recent research has also highlighted that patients are not feeling part of conversations during virtual visits (Gordon et al., 2020). However, more understanding is needed from the patient perspective. For example, following the pandemic, there was opportunity for practices to go back to the traditional face-to-face methods; however, some patients reported a preference for online visits. Importantly, we must understand that not all patients want or prefer virtual care, but some do, and further, in what situations or conditions this works for them.

We must also know that there are certain visits that are more appropriate for virtual care or telephone visits and that these may be patient or condition specific. Therefore, it is up to the provider delivering care to outline to their patients what works and does not.

Implementing technology in care involves the careful consideration of patients in their context, including population-level statistics or clinic-level demographics. This responsibility of understanding their clientele falls on the providers and healthcare teams that are using technology. Previously to the pandemic, the purpose of virtual care was often to improve access to rural populations. However, our populations are much more complex. Rural patients may live in semi-rural or remote locations. Urban patients could live in the inner city or the suburbs and may not be in close proximity to their care teams. Throughout the nation, we also have populations that are transient that regularly flow in and out of the province for work or leisure. However, there are other demographics and socio-economic factors that may impact the use of technology in either positive or negative ways, including language, culture, technological barriers, or health literacy.

Regarding patients' access to technology, not only does this impact live-virtual visits but also other aspects of digital care. For instance, wearable technologies (e.g., the Apple watch or Fitbit) provide a way for patients to monitor their health independently. However, this technology is expensive and may also require subscription services. A question that is raised is who will pay for these technologies, or will it be left up to the patient.

And then there is linking the remote monitoring with providers. There remains a disconnect between technology and communicating the data to care providers. Although technology has the ability to do so, the seamlessness of it is limited. For example, when Apple launched their watch, they had embedded a function for it to communicate with health providers, but we do not currently see that in many average healthcare clinics in Canada.

6.10   SUMMARY AND CONCLUSION

KEY MESSAGES

- The COVID-19 pandemic accelerated the use of digital technologies across teams and the continuum of care.
- Using technology in healthcare is not limited to virtual visits, but there is opportunity to use various DHTs to facilitate care (e.g., email, apps, and remote monitoring).
- Digital technologies are context-specific, and the implementation of technology in practice needs to happen from the ground up. At the same time, guidelines and financial support need to be provided to support ground-level integration.

6.11   PATH FORWARD AND CALL TO ACTION: IMPLEMENTING DIGITAL HEALTH TOGETHER

The path forward involves establishing research and policy changes that focus on the following:

1. Common targeted initiatives that help advance digital health use that support clinical benefits and achieve better care outcomes.
2. Developing strategies that are contextual and serve both health providers and patients.
3. Standardizing core building blocks to advance the appropriate and best use of digital technologies in care (e.g., reference materials, data standards, standard and recommended frameworks, and patient/provider roles).
4. Establishing joint networks across the health system for an overarching approach.
5. Creating join statements and resources that are applicable to the practice area (for an example consensus statement, see the Canadian Rheumatology Association https://pubmed.ncbi.nlm.nih.gov/35105707/).
6. Updating policies and regulations and matching practice standards to licensing body expectations.
7. Creating federal and provincial plans to help focus and guide the implementation of digital care.
8. Defining the patient's role on the team more clearly, including how to engage with their teams using technology.
9. Providing an interprofessional approach to curriculum integration and alignment across professions.

6.12   CRITICAL THINKING EXERCISES

1. What can the interprofessional team do to enhance communication across the care continuum?
2. What role does the patient play in virtual care?

6.13   RELEVANT DEFINITIONS

- **DHT** is an overarching term that encompasses technology use in health (see Figure 6.3).
- **Virtual Care** is a broad term that includes any interaction between patients and/or members of their circle of care (DHC, 2022). Virtual care encompasses concepts/domains and capabilities to deliver care to patients (see Figure 6.4).

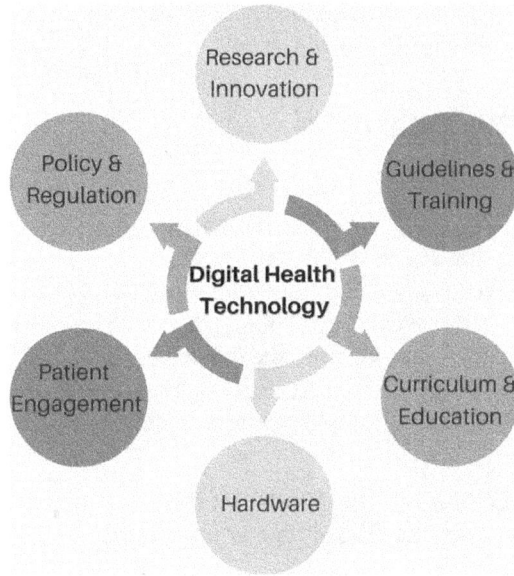

FIGURE 6.3   DHT Umbrella.

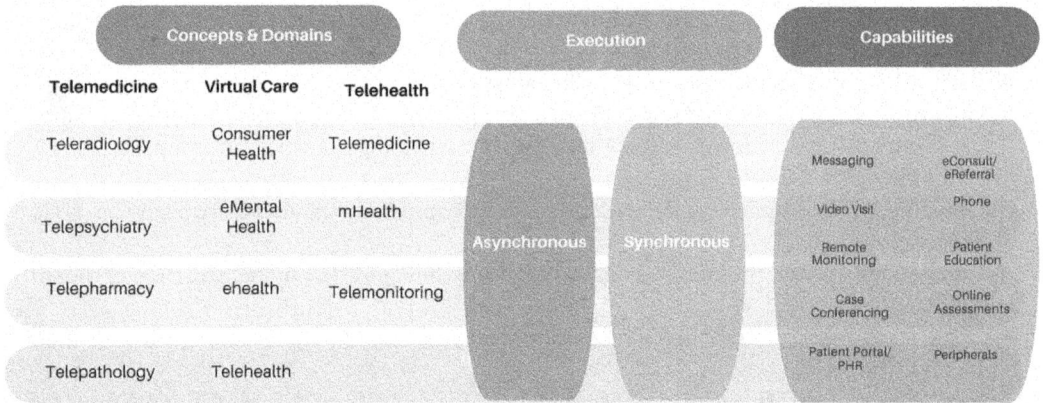

FIGURE 6.4   Canadian Virtual Care Lexicon.

- *Concepts and domains* are types of virtual care.
- *Capabilities* are how virtual care is delivered. This includes remote patient monitoring (RPM) or telehomecare (Canada Health Info way, 2024), which enables healthcare providers to electronically monitor patients outside of conventional clinical settings, such as in the home.

6.14   LEARNING AND PRACTICE RESOURCES

- Accreditation Canada: https://accreditation.ca/assessment-programs/telehealth-rapid-assessment/

- Alberta Health Services: https://krs.libguides.com/timelytopics
- Canadian Agency for Drug and Technologies in Health: https://www.cadth.ca/
- Canada Health Infoway: https://www.infoway-inforoute.ca/en/digital-health-initiatives/virtual-care
- Canadian Institute for Health Information: https://www.cihi.ca/en/virtual-care-in-canada
- Center for Connected Health Policy (USA): https://www.cchpca.org/
- Digital Health Canada (Canada's Health Informatics Association): https://digitalhealth-canada.com/wp-content/uploads/2022/06/Virtual-Care-National-Lexicon-v-JAN2521.pdf
- Health Canada: https://www.canada.ca/en/health-canada/corporate/transparency/health-agreements/bilateral-agreement-pan-canadian-virtual-care-priorities-covid-19/policy-framework.html
- HealthCare Excellence Canada: https://www.healthcareexcellence.ca/
- Health Standards Organization (Global): https://healthstandards.org
- National Institutes of Health Informatics: https://www.nihi.ca/
- Ontario Health: https://www.ontariohealth.ca/providing-health-care/clinical-standards-guidelines/clinically-appropriate-virtual-care-guidance
- Policy Commons (Global): https://policycommons.net
- The Canadian Health Information Management Association: https://www.echima.ca/
- World Health Organization (Global): https://www.who.int/health-topics/digital-health#tab=tab_1

REFERENCES

Alberta Health Services. (2024). *Connect Care: Implementation Timeline*. Retrieved June 6, 2024, from https://www.albertahealthservices.ca/assets/info/cis/if-cis-cc-infographic-site-implementation-timeline.pdf

Arnaert, A., Ponzoni, N., Sanou, H., & Nana, N. G. (2019). Using the BELT framework to implement an mhealth pilot project for preventative screening and monitoring of pregnant women in rural Burkina Faso, Africa. *Telehealth and Medicine Today*. https://doi.org/10.30953/tmt.v4.100

Brewer, M., & Flavell, H. (2018). Facilitating collaborative capabilities for future work: what can be learnt from interprofessional fieldwork in health. *International Journal of Work-Integrated Learning*, *19*(2), 169–180. https://files.eric.ed.gov/fulltext/EJ1182102.pdf

Butcher, C. J., & Hussain, W. (2022). Digital healthcare: the future. *Future Healthcare Journal*, *9*(2), 113–117. https://doi.org/10.7861/fhj.2022–0046

Canada Health Infoway. (2018a). *Connecting Patients for Better Health*. https://www.infoway-inforoute.ca/en/component/edocman/3564-connecting-patients-for-better-health-2018/view-document?Itemid=0

Canada Health Infoway. (2018b). *2018 Canadian Physician Survey*. https://www.infoway-inforoute.ca/en/component/edocman/3643–2018-canadian-physician-survey/view-document?Itemid=103

Canada Health Infoway. (2024). *Digital Health Initiatives*. Retrieved from https://www.infoway-inforoute.ca/en/digital-health-initiatives

Canadian Academy of Health Sciences. (2023). *Canada's Health Workforce: Pathways Forward*. https://cahs-acss.ca/assessment-on-health-human-resources-hhr/

Canadian Institute for Health Information (CIHI). (2022). *Virtual Care in Canada: Strengthening Data and Information*. https://www.cihi.ca/sites/default/files/document/virtual-care-in-canada-strengthening-data-information-report-en.pdf

Canadian Interprofessional Health Collaborative. (2024). *CIHC Competency Framework for Advancing Collaboration 2024*. https://www.cihc.ca

Centers for Disease Control and Prevention. (2024). *Clinical Features of Penicillin Allergy*. Accessed June 6, 2024. https://www.cdc.gov/antibiotic-use/hcp/clinical-signs/index.html#cdc_hcp_clinical_resources-resources

Cerbo, A. D., Morales-Medina, J. C., Palmieri, B., & Iannitti, T. (2015, January 1). Narrative review of tele-medicine consultation in medical practice. *Patient Preference and Adherence*, *9*, 65–75. https://doi.org/10.2147/PPA.S61617

Cross, R. K., Langenberg, P., Regueiro, M., Schwartz, D. A., Tracy, J. K., Collins, J. F., Katz, J., Ghazi, L., Patil, S. A., Quezada, S. M., Beaulieu, D., Horst, S. N., Russman, K., Riaz, M., Jambaulikar, G., Sivasailam, B., & Quinn, C. C. (2019). A randomized controlled trial of TELEmedicine for patients with inflammatory bowel disease (TELE-IBD). *American Journal of Gastroenterology, 114*(3), 472–482. https://doi.org/10.1038/s41395-018-0272-8

Cunha, A. M., Capretz, M. A. M., & Raptopoulos, L. S. C. (2009, September 1). Support systems for telehealth services: critical operational and ICT complementary assets for large-scale provisioning. *Proceedings of the 2009 IEEE Toronto International Conference-Science and Technology for Humanity (TIC-STH)* (pp. 544–550). https://doi.org/10.1109/TIC-STH.2009.5444480

Damschroder, L. J., Aron, D. C., Keith, R. E., Kirsh, S. R., Alexander, J. A., & Lowery, J. C. (2009). Fostering implementation of health services research findings into practice: a consolidated framework for advancing implementation science. *Implementation Science, 4*, 50. https://doi.org/10.1186/1748-5908-4-50

Dave, M., & Patel, N. (2023). Artificial intelligence in healthcare and education. *Springer Nature, 234*(10), 761–764. https://doi.org/10.1038/s41415-023-5845-2

Deniz, S., Akbolat, M., Çimen, M., & Ünal, Ö. (2021). The mediating role of shared decision-making in the effect of the patient–physician relationship on compliance with treatment. *Journal of Patient Experience, 8*, 23743735211018066. https://doi.org/10.1177/23743735211018066

Digital Health Canada. (2022). *Virtual Care in Canada: Lexicon*. Retrieved from https://digitalhealthcanada.com/wp-content/uploads/2022/06/Virtual-Care-National-Lexicon-v-JAN2521.pdf

Donaghy, E., Atherton, H., Hammersley, V., McNeilly, H., Bikker, A., Robbins, L., Campbell, J., & McKinstry, B. (2019). Acceptability, benefits, and challenges of video consulting: a qualitative study in primary care. *British Journal of General Practice, 69*(686), 586–594. https://doi.org/10.3399/bjgp19X704141

Donnelly, C., Ashcroft, R., Bobbette, N., Mills, C., Mofina, A., Tran, T., Vader, K., Williams, A., Gill, S., & Miller, J. (2021). Interprofessional primary care during COVID-19: a survey of the provider perspective. *BMC Primary Care, 22*(1), 1–12. https://doi.org/10.1186/s12875-020-01366-9

Duong, D., & Vogel, L. (2023). Overworked health workers are "past the point of exhaustion". *CMAJ: Canadian Medical Association Journal, 195*(8), E309. https://doi.org/10.46747/cfp.7004224

Eysenbach, G., & Consort-EHEALTH Group. (2011). CONSORT-EHEALTH: improving and standardizing evaluation reports of Web-based and mobile health interventions. *Journal of Medical Internet Research, 13*(4), e1923. https://doi.org/10.2196/jmir.1923

Gilmore, K. J., Pennucci, F., De Rosis, S., & Passino, C. (2019). Value in healthcare and the role of the patient voice. *Healthcare Papers, 18*(4), 28–35. https://doi.org/10.12927/hcpap.2019.26031

Gomez, T., Anaya, Y. B., Shih, K. J., & Tarn, D. M. (2021). A qualitative study of primary care physicians' experiences with telemedicine during COVID–19. *The Journal of the American Board of Family Medicine, 34*, S61–S70. https://doi.org/10.3122/jabfm.2021.S1.200517

Gordon, H. S., et al. (2020). "I'm Not Feeling Like I'm Part of the Conversation" Patients' Perspectives on Communicating in Clinical Video Telehealth Visits. *Journal of General Internal Medicine, 35*, 1751–1758. https://doi.org/10.1007/s11606-020-05673-w

Government of Alberta. (2023). *Minister of Health Mandate Letter*. Retrieved from https://open.alberta.ca/dataset/bf7f9a42-a807-49b3-8ba3-451ae3bc2d2f/resource/6163feb7-8494-4bfe-a1d8-520631d3968b/download/hlth-mandate-letter-health-2023.pdf

Green, B. N., & Johnson, C. D. (2015, March 1). Interprofessional collaboration in research, education, and clinical practice: working together for a better future. *Journal of Chiropractic Education, 29*(1), 1–10. https://meridian.allenpress.com/jce/article/29/1/1/131206/Interprofessional-collaboration-in-research

Gustin, T. S., Kott, K., & Rutledge, C. (2020). Telehealth etiquette training: a guideline for preparing interprofessional teams for successful encounters. *Nurse Educator, 45*(2), 88–92. https://doi.org/10.1097/NNE.0000000000000680

Hale, I., Green, S., Davis, M., & Nowlan, J. (2024). Planetary health lens for primary care: considering environmental sustainability offers benefits to patients and to providers. *Canadian Family Physician, 70*(4), 224–227. https://doi.org/10.46747/cfp.7004224

Haleem, A., Javaid, M., Singh, R. P., & Suman, R. (2021). Telemedicine for healthcare: capabilities, features, barriers, and applications. *Sensors International, 2*(2021). https://doi.org/10.1016/j.sintl.2021.100117

Hasani, S. A., Ghafri, T. A., Al Lawati, H., Mohammed, J., Al Mukhainai, A., Al Ajmi, F., & Anwar, H. (2020). The use of telephone consultation in primary health care during COVID-19 pandemic, Oman: perceptions from physicians. *Journal of Primary Care & Community Health, 11*. https://doi.org/10.2150132720976480

Holstead, R. G., & Robinson, A. G. (2020). Discussing serious news remotely: navigating difficult conversations during a pandemic. *JCO Oncology Practice, 16*(7), 363–368. https://doi.org/10.1200/OP.20.00269

Hruczkowski, C. [forthcoming]. *Impacts of the COVID-19 Pandemic on Primary Care Delivery: A Case Study*. Doctoral Thesis. University of Alberta.

The Impact Artificial Intelligence Has on Telehealth and Medicine. (2021, June 7). Retrieved from https://techsprohub.com/the-impact-artificial-intelligence-has-on-telehealth-and-medicine/

Johnston, K. J., Wen, H., & Joynt Maddox, K. E. (2019). Lack of access to specialist associated with mortality and preventable hospitalizations of rural Medicare beneficiaries. *Health Affairs*, *38*(12), 1993–2002. https://doi.org/10.1377/hlthaff.2019.00838

Khalili, H., Pandey, J., Langlois, S., Park, V., Brown, R., El-Awaisi, A., MacMillan, K., Cohen Konrad, S., Daulton, B., Green, C., Kolcu, G., McCartan, C., Baugh, G., Pfeifle, A., Wetzlmair, L., Kolcu, I., & Breitbach, A. P. (2023). Forward thinking and adaptability to sustain and advance IPECP in healthcare transformation following the COVID-19 pandemic. *The Internet Journal of Allied Health Sciences and Practice*, *22*(1), 18.

Khalili, H., Park, V., Daulton, B., Langlois, S., Wetzlmair, L. C., MacMillan, K. M., El-Awaisi, A., Green, C., Ballard, J., Pandey, J., Konrad, S. C., Frost, J., Başer Kolcu, M. I., Kolcu, G., McCartan, C., Baugh, G., Gaboury, I., Breitbach, A., Brown, R., & Pfeifle, A. (2022). Interprofessional education and collaborative practice (IPECP) in post-COVID healthcare education and practice transformation era—discussion paper. In *Joint Publication by InterprofessionalResearch.Global, American Interprofessional Health Collaborative & Canadian Interprofessional Health Collaborative*. Available at www.interprofessionalresearch.global

Kidholm, K., Ekeland, A. G., Jensen, L. K., Rasmussen, J., Pedersen, C. D., Bowes, A., & Bech, M. (2012). A model for assessment of telemedicine applications: mast. International *Journal of Technology Assessment in Health Care*, *28*(1), 44–51. https://doi.org/10.1017/S0266462311000638

Kruse, C. S., Krowski, N., Rodríguez, B., Tran, L. M., Vela, J., & Brooks, M. (2017, August 1). Telehealth and patient satisfaction: a systematic review and narrative analysis. *BMJ Open*, *7*(8), e016242. https://doi.org/10.1136/bmjopen-2017–016242

MacQuarrie, C., & Brown, R. (2023). Interprofessional simulation in rural healthcare teams: leadership considerations. In *Challenges and Opportunities in Healthcare Leadership: Voices from the Crowd in Today's Complex and Interprofessional Healthcare Environment* (Eds. Angela Lampe, Cindy Constanzo, William Leggio & Timothy Guetterman). Information Age Publishing, Charlotte, NC.

McKay, M., Brown, R., Mallam, K., MacDonald-Green, A., & Bernard, A. (2023). Engaging the collective voice of physicians: optimizing participation in research and policy development in the context of COVID-19 and physician burnout. *Healthcare Management Forum*, *36*(6). https://doi.org/10.1177/08404704231199083

MD Connections. (n.d.). *Tools for Practice*. Retrieved from https://mdconnections.ca/

National Institute for Health and Care Excellence (UK). (2021). *Evidence Standards Framework for Digital Health Technologies*. London, UK: NICE. https://www.nice.org.uk/Media/Default/About/what-we-do/our-programmes/evidence-standards-framework/digital-evidence-standards-framework.pdf

Nittari, G., et al. (2020). Telemedicine practice: review of the current ethical and legal challenges. *Telemedicine and e-Health*, *26*(12), 1427–1437. https://doi.org/10.1089/tmj.2019.0158

Nouveau Health. (2023, January 1). *Telemedicine—Benefits & Definitions*. Retrieved May 20, 2024, from https://nouveauhealth.com/services/telemedicine/telemedicine-benefits-definitions/

NQF Projects. (2014, January 1). Retrieved from https://www.qualityforum.org/ProjectDescription.aspx

Ozair, F. F., Jamshed, N., Sharma, A., & Aggarwal, P. (2015). Ethical issues in electronic health records: a general overview. *Perspectives in Clinical Research*, *6*(2), 73–76. https://doi.org/10.4103/2229–3485.153997

Palen, T. E., Price, D., Shetterly, S., & Wallace, K. (2012, July 8). Comparing virtual consults to traditional consults using an electronic health record: an observational case–control study. *BMC Medical Informatics and Decision Making*, *12*, 65. https://doi.org/10.1186/1472-6947-12-65

Pogorzelska, K., & Chlabicz, S. (2022, May 17). Patient satisfaction with telemedicine during the COVID-19 pandemic—a systematic review. *International Journal of Environmental Research and Public Health*, *19*(10), 6113. https://doi.org/10.3390/ijerph19106113

Pong, R. W., DesMeules, M., Heng, D., Lagace, C., Guernsey, J. R., Kazanjian, A., Manuel, D., Pitblado, J. R., Bollman, R., Koren, I., Dressler, M. P., Wang, F., & Luo, W. (2011). Patterns of health services utilization in rural Canada. *Chronic Disease and Injury in Canada*, *31*(S1), 1–36. https://www.canada.ca/en/public-health/services/reports-publications/health-promotion-chronic-disease-prevention-canada-research-policy-practice/vol-31-no-1–2010/supplement/introduction.html

Powell, B. J., Waltz, T. J., Chinman, M. J., Damschroder, L. J., Smith, J. L., Matthieu, M. M., Proctor, E. K., & Kirchner, J. E. (2015). A refined compilation of implementation strategies: results from the Expert Recommendations for Implementing Change (ERIC) project. *Implementation Science*, *10*(1), 1–14. https://doi.org/10.1186/s13012-015-0209-1

PrimeMinister of Canada. (2021). *Minister of Health Mandate Letter*. Retrieved from https://www.pm.gc.ca/en/mandate-letters/2021/12/16/minister-health-mandate-letter

Rahman, M. A., & Jim, M. M. I. (2024). Addressing Privacy and Ethical Considerations in Health Information Management Systems (IMS). *International Journal of Health and Medical*, *1*(2), 1–13. https://doi.org/10.62304/ijhm.v1i2.127

Rogier, C., Van Dijk, B. T., Brouwer, E., de Jong, P. H., & van der Helm-van, A. H. (2021). Realizing early recognition of arthritis in times of increased telemedicine: the value of patient-reported swollen joints. *Annals of the Rheumatic Diseases*, *80*(5), 668–669. https://doi.org/10.1136/annrheumdis-2020–219513

Schwamm, L. H., Estrada, J., Erskine, A., & Licurse, A. (2020). Virtual care: new models of caring for our patients and workforce. *The Lancet*, *258*, 104–107. https://doi.org/10.1016/S2589–7500(20)30104–7

Segal, J. B., Davis, S., & Dukhanin, V. (2022). Working framework for appropriate use of virtual care in primary care. *Journal of the American Board of Family Medicine*, *35*(3), 629–636. https://www.jabfm.org/content/jabfp/35/3/629.full.pdf

Smith, A. C., Thomas, E., Snoswell, C. L., Haydon, H., Mehrotra, A., Clemensen, J., & Caffery, L. J. (2020). Telehealth for global emergencies: implications for coronavirus disease 2019 (COVID-19). *Journal of Telemedicine and Telecare*, *26*(5), 309–313. https://doi.org/10.1177/1357633X20916567

Spithoff, S., Stockdale, J., Rowe, R., McPhail, B., & Persaud, N. (2022). The commercialization of patient data in Canada: ethics, privacy and policy. *CMAJ*, *194*(3), E95–E97. https://www.cmaj.ca/content/194/3/e95

Stoumpos, A.I., Kitsios, F., & Talias, M.A. (2023). Digital transformation in healthcare: technology acceptance and its applications. *International Journal of Environmental Research and Public Health*, *20*(3407). https://doi.org/10.3390/ijerph20043407

Virtual Hallway. (n.d.a). *Bridging the Rural–Urban Divide: The Role of Virtual Hallway in Improving Equitable Access to Specialist Care*. Retrieved from https://virtualhallway.ca/wp-content/uploads/2023/07/Whitepaper-Bridging-the-Rural-Urban-Divide.pdf

Virtual Hallway. (n.d.b). *Alleviating Primary Care Physician Burnout through Interprofessional Collaboration: A Case for Virtual Hallway*. Retrieved from https://virtualhallway.ca/wp-content/uploads/2023/07/Whitepaper-Alleviating-Primary-Care-Physician-Burnout-Through-Interprofessional-Collaboration-A-Case-for-Virtual-Hallway.pdf

Virtual Hallway. (n.d.c). *Addressing Patient Leakage and Enhancing Retention through Virtual Hallway Phone Consults*. Retrieved from https://virtualhallway.ca/wp-content/uploads/2023/08/Whitepaper-Addressing-Patient-Leakage.pdf

Virtual Hallway. (n.d.d). *Peer Consultation Networks: Bridging Healthcare Efficiency and Carbon Emission Reductions*. Retrieved from https://virtualhallway.ca/wp-content/uploads/2023/10/Whitepaper-Carbon.pdf

von Huben, A., Howell, M., Carrello, J., Norris, S., Wortley, S., Ritchie, A., & Howard, K. (2022). Application of a health technology assessment framework to digital health technologies that manage chronic disease: a systematic review. *International Journal of Technology Assessment in Health Care*, *38*(1), e9. https://doi.org/10.1017/S026646232100063X

World Health Organization. (2010). *Framework for Action on Interprofessional Education & Collaborative Practice*. Retrieved from https://www.who.int/hrh/resources/framework_action/en/

World Health Organization. (2019). *Recommendations on Digital Interventions for Health System Strengthening*. Retrieved from https://apps.who.int/iris/bitstream/handle/10665/311941/9789241550505-eng.pdf?ua=1

World Health Organization. (2021). *Global Strategy on Digital Health 2020–2025*. Retrieved from https://www.who.int/docs/default-source/documents/gs4dhdaa2a9f352b0445bafbc79ca799dce4d.pdf

Zulman, D.M., & Verghese, A. (2021). Virtual care, telemedicine visits, and real connection in the era of COVID-19: Unforeseen opportunity in the face of adversity. *JAMA*, *325*(5), 437–438. https://doi.org/10.1001/jama.2020.21332

7 How Data-Driven Insights Can Improve Patient Outcomes, Public Health Strategies, and Decision-Making

Rafiqul Chowdhury and Sahand Ashtab

7.1 INTRODUCTION

The earlier management information systems and transaction processing systems have evolved to become more sophisticated to help decision-makers configure optimal decisions in a specific context within a specific scope in a timely manner, given the changing nature of the business world. Given the implications of such changes and the need to respond, it is more important than before to utilize a cluster of business intelligence, data visualization, and predictive and prescriptive analytics tools to make effective, efficient, and real-time decisions (Sharda et al., 2018).

The data-driven approach and analytics span various sectors, including manufacturing and healthcare. Predictive analytics tools in the manufacturing sector are effective in estimating the demand or a parameter that can be used as an input for an optimization model to make strategic or tactical decisions (Ashtab &Tosarkani, 2023) or predict a certain outcome such as whether or not a product or service will still be in demand considering different client/customer segmentation (Ashtab & Campbell, 2021). Comparative performance analysis is conducted for different applications in this sector, including applying different algorithms and models to the same dataset to determine the best-performing predicting models (Kharitonov et al., 2022). However, given the difference in goals between manufacturing and healthcare supply chain networks (Toba et al., 2008), predicting outcomes is more crucial in the healthcare sector than it is in the manufacturing sector.

Nowadays, a data-driven approach in the healthcare delivery system contributes to improving patients' experience/outcome, including proactive outreach and wellness follow-ups, as well as enhancing financial management and medical research by utilizing quality data. The data-driven approach uses information gathered from raw data to gain insight and is an effective tool to make informed strategic and tactical decisions in healthcare supply chain networks. In this regard, different machine learning algorithms and models are used to predict a specific patient health outcome (Chaw et al., 2024).

The COVID-19 (SARS-CoV-2) pandemic caused a substantial loss of human life worldwide, requiring an unparalleled challenge to the public health system (Alexander & Grantz, 2021). The economic, psychological, and social disarray generated by the COVID-19 pandemic was devastating (Wang & Mustafa, 2023). This coronavirus pandemic has a global public health and socioeconomic burden, raising unprecedented concern for infectious diseases. The highly infectious COVID-19 transmission process has multiple stages with varying transmission rates (Chen et al., 2020; Wang et al., 2020; Böhmer et al., 2020; Wu et al., 2020). The initial stages of the transmission process showed an exponential increase (Li et al., 2020; Zhao et al., 2020a, 2020b). Thus, describing any infectious disease transmission process to design effective interventions and restrict its spread is a critical scientific issue.

DOI: 10.1201/9781003485629-7

Mathematical models and epidemiological analysis are essential for understanding the dynamics of many chronic diseases, particularly infectious diseases, and designing public health strategies to contain them (Hollingsworth, 2009). The use of mathematical models in studying infectious diseases has been transformed to identify potential public health interventions and assess their impact. Mathematical models proved helpful in advising policy during the severe acute respiratory syndrome (SARS) outbreak in 2003. The trajectory risk prediction of infectious diseases (e.g., COVID-19) based on available covariates will help infectious disease prevention (Chowdhury et al., 2022; Cheung et al., 2024; Chowdhury et al., 2020).

Patient data may be collected on a single occasion or repeatedly from the same patients. For example, patients with a chronic disease may visit primary care providers repeatedly, producing a long sequence of data collected over time. In the Health and Retirement Study (HRS; Islam & Chowdhury, 2017; Sonnega et al., 2014) repeated reporting of functional limitations, mental health, physical condition, health change, healthcare utilization, medical expenditure, income, and wealth among older adults produce a long sequence of longitudinal variables. Another source of extended response and feature sequences is electronic medical records (EMRs) (Pham et al., 2017; Zhao et al., 2019). Health professionals can use EMR data to model health conditions (response) and risk factors (feature variables) to make informed decisions. EMRs are official health documents for individuals, commonly shared across various departments of healthcare facilities and agencies, which enhance patient safety and lessen the administrative burden for healthcare providers (Tripepi et al., 2013). For example, researchers looked at the Electronic Health Records (EHRs) of patients who underwent knee joint replacement to develop a data-driven health management approach using EHRs to identify and visualize overlapping patient groups with similar disease risks (Kriegova et al., 2021). Health analytics can identify treatment patterns, emergency room visits, drug consumption, and hospitalization. This will allow health system administrators to determine emerging healthcare trends and predict system demand. Analyzing patient data in real time can help lower readmission rates, minimize treatment errors, identify at-risk populations, and prevent medical emergencies.

Despite the merits, data-driven healthcare has several challenges, including data security. Cybercriminals constantly target medical records, and these attacks are often successful. Thus, it is crucial to incorporate data protection measures and mechanisms into healthcare systems. In this regard, due to the growing costs of healthcare management, innovative ideas and technologies are critical to maintaining a sustainable healthcare system (Ashtab & Anderson, 2023).

Longitudinally collected disease data may pass through different trajectories (paths; Chowdhury & Islam, 2020). Longitudinal data are useful for analyzing the events of interest in life course research. The most important advantage of using longitudinal data is that it allows for studying individual development over time (Singer & Willett, 2003; Jos & Twisk, 2013). In other words, one can study the individual trajectories (path). Physicians or other primary care providers would be interested in diagnosing the disease progression and regression over time and finding the causes that trigger the disease, leading to a particular trajectory. Healthcare professionals would be interested in seeing the answer to the following questions:

1. What is the risk of a specific condition for a patient at a time point given the risk factors and the history of health conditions?
2. How to estimate the risk of specific conditions over a range of time points given the risk factors and the history of health conditions,
3. How to predict the health condition for the next time point given the risk factors and the history of health conditions (i.e., predicting the future path of the disease),
4. How to measure the main and interaction effects of risk factors (risk factors with historical health conditions), and
5. How to identify historical health conditions between time points.

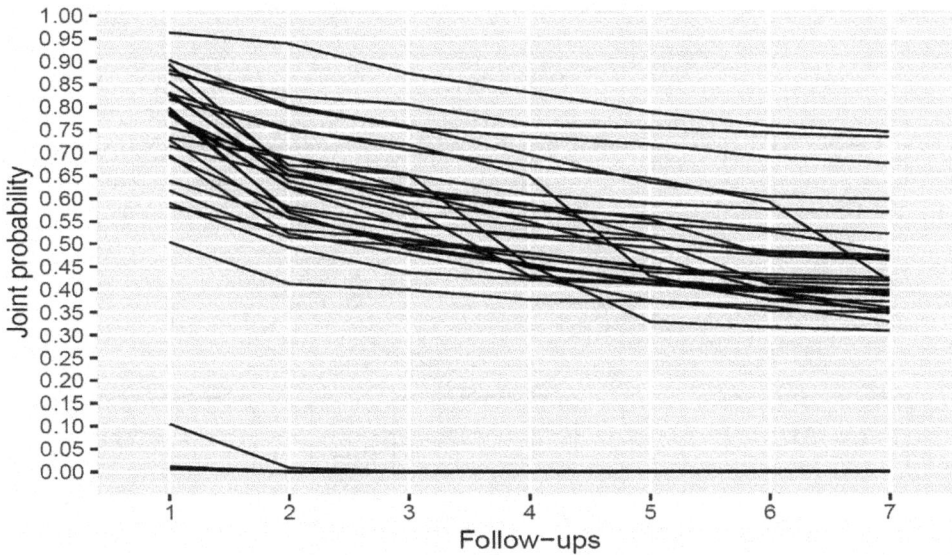

FIGURE 7.1 Activity of daily living (ADL) problem trajectories for selected subjects.

This chapter will develop and adopt a data-driven approach to possibly answer the aforementioned questions predicting the risk at a particular point in time on the trajectories allows healthcare professionals to screen an individual and suggest necessary therapy and preventive measures. This will also help a patient's awareness of the future course of the disease (Tripepi et al., 2013) and compliance with primary care providers' suggestions. For example, Figure 7.1 provides several patients' activity of daily living (ADL) problem trajectories at seven time points. The outcome of interest is the ADL Index among elderly people. The index is categorized as a binary outcome (0 = No ADL problem, 1 = ADL problem). This chapter aims to illustrate a data-driven analytic framework to answer questions 1–5 posed earlier. A literature review is performed to identify recently developed models used as analytic tools for longitudinal data.

The rest of this chapter includes the following sections: **Section 2** expands the problem and develops/extends models to create a data-driven analytical approach. An illustration using HRS data illustrates the developed analytic framework in **Section 3**. Discussions and conclusions are given in **Section 4**. A comprehensive reference list has been added. All the R-codes used for the chapter are provided in an **Appendix**.

7.2 METHODS

For repeated binary outcomes, Islam and Chowdhury (2010) proposed a model for indicating the relationships in unconditional models in terms of underlying conditional models for analyzing longitudinal data. Chowdhury and Islam (2020) demonstrated the trajectory risk prediction for repeated multinomial outcomes, and more recently, they proposed the same for repeated ordinal outcomes (Chowdhury & Islam, 2022). Our illustration will be a special case of Chowdhury and Islam (2020) for repeated binary outcomes.

To illustrate the proposed framework, we use follow-ups of six to eleven data from HRS in the United States. The data are freely available from the HRS website: https://hrs.isr.umich.edu/data-products. The dependent variables considered are the ADL Index, denoted by $y_1, y_2, y_3, y_4, y_5, y_6$, and y_7, where y_1–y_7 are binary outcomes (0 = No ADL problem, 1 = ADL problem) constructed by

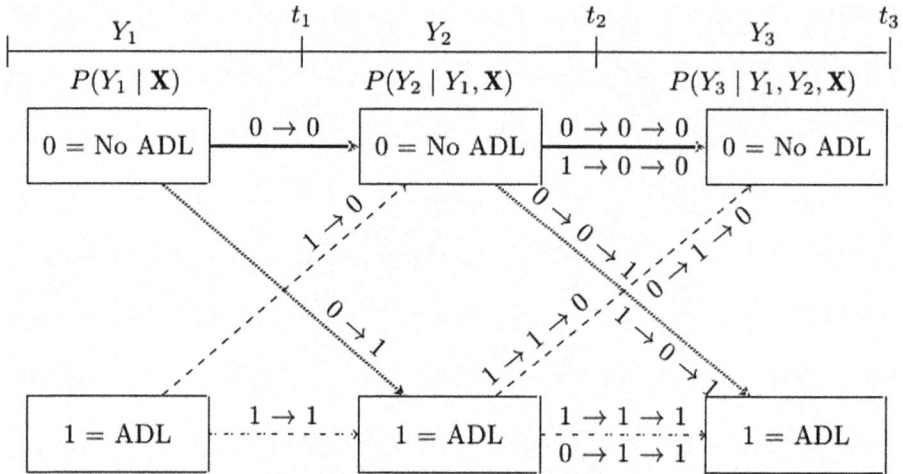

FIGURE 7.2   The possible trajectories of ADL for a subject for three repeated outcomes.

recategorizing the ADL index that scored from 0 to 5. In the original data, the ADL index ranges from 0 to 5, representing the number of tasks a subject has difficulty performing (whether respondents faced difficulties in walking, dressing, bathing, eating, and getting in/out of bed). This dataset contains a large number of variables. We used selected variables for illustration purposes. So far, 20 waves (follow-ups) of data are available. For details, see the HRS codebooks (https://hrs.isr.umich.edu/documentation/codebooks).

Figure 7.2 presents the trajectories from three repeated outcomes (y_1, y_2, and y_3). A total of eight possible trajectories or paths are indicated by the arrows. These trajectories are (1) $0 \rightarrow 0 \rightarrow 0$; (2) $0 \rightarrow 0 \rightarrow 1$; (3) $0 \rightarrow 1 \rightarrow 0$; (4) $0 \rightarrow 1 \rightarrow 1$; (5) $1 \rightarrow 0 \rightarrow 0$; (6) $1 \rightarrow 0 \rightarrow 1$; (7) $1 \rightarrow 1 \rightarrow 0$; and (8) $1 \rightarrow 1 \rightarrow 1$. In the Markov model terminology, these arrows are called transitions, that is, a patient may or may not change the disease status over the follow-ups. If we consider two time points (e.g., $0 \rightarrow 0$ or $0 \rightarrow 1$), then it is the first order; if we consider three follow-ups as in the figure, then it will be the second order; and so on. For trajectory risk prediction, we need to estimate the transition probability by linking the covariate impact on the transition probability.

Here, y, x, and t represent the outcome, vector of frisk factors, and periods, respectively. By modeling these transitions, we can predict likely future trajectories of disease progression and regression to estimate the risk of developing or not developing ADL problems at each time point, given the observed covariates. Then, we can use the Markov chain to link the probabilities of individual transitions from each follow-up to obtain the trajectory probabilities as follows.

$$\hat{P}\left(Y_1 = y_1, Y_2 = y_2, Y_3 = y_3 \mid \mathbf{X} = x\right) = \hat{P}\left(Y_1 = y_1\right) \times \hat{P}\left(Y_2 = y_1 \mid Y_1 = y_1; \mathbf{X} = \mathbf{x}\right)$$
$$\times \hat{P}\left(Y_3 = y_1 \mid Y_1 = y_1; Y_2 = y_2; \mathbf{X} = \mathbf{x}\right) \quad (7.1)$$
$$\text{where } y_1, y_2, y_3 = 0,1 \text{ and } \mathbf{X} = [X_1, X_2, ..., X_p] \text{ is vector of covariates.}$$

The left-hand side of Equation (7.1) is the joint probability (trajectory risk) we are interested in estimating from the data. The joint probability on the left-hand side is estimated for the full sample. The first part of the right-hand side of Equation (7.1) is the marginal probability that needs to be estimated from the first follow-up, and the second and third parts are the conditional probabilities that need to be estimated from the data. These conditional probabilities are estimated by stratifying the sample based on the values of the previous outcomes, that is, from the reduced sample. According to Lindsey and Lamber (1998), repeated measures show how individual responses change over time and are generally conditioned on a subject's previous history (Lindsey & Lamber, 1998). Lee and Nelder (2004) concluded that conditional models are of fundamental interest and that marginal predictions can be made from them (Zhao et al., 2020b). We can use the Markov regression model to estimate these transition probabilities. However, using the Markov models, we cannot assess the impact of the prior outcomes due to the effective stratification of the data in addition to the over-parameterization (Chowdhury & Islam, 2020; Lee & Nelder, 2004). For example, for the three repeated outcomes shown in Figure 7.1, we need to fit a total of seven models: one marginal model, two second-order models, and four second-order models. The total number of models will grow exponentially with increased follow-ups. Also, we cannot include the interaction between previous outcomes and the interaction between previous outcomes and risk factors in the model. Following Chowdhury and Islam (2020), we will use the regressive logistic model to link the risk factors with the transition probabilities and estimate the conditional probabilities shown in Figure 7.1. This approach reduces the over-parameterization by including previous outcomes as covariates. Hence, one needs to fit only one model from each follow-up. The marginal logistic regression model from the first follow-up with the covariate vector can be shown as

$$\hat{P}(Y_1 = y_1 \mid \mathbf{Z}) = \frac{e^{\mathbf{Z}\hat{\beta}}}{1 + e^{\mathbf{Z}\hat{\beta}}}, \text{ where } \mathbf{Z} = \mathbf{X} = [X_1, X_2, ..., X_p], \hat{\boldsymbol{\beta}} = [\hat{\beta}_0, \hat{\beta}_1, ..., \hat{\beta}_p] \text{ is the vector of the} \quad (7.2)$$

regression coefficients.

The first-order regressive logistic regression model with the covariate vector can be shown as

$$\hat{P}(Y_2 = y_2 \mid Y_1 = y_1; \mathbf{X}) = \frac{e^{\mathbf{Z}\hat{\beta}}}{1 + e^{\mathbf{Z}\hat{\beta}}}, \text{ where } \mathbf{Z} = [X_1, X_2, ..., X_p, Y_1], \hat{\boldsymbol{\beta}} = [\hat{\beta}_0, \hat{\beta}_1, ..., \hat{\beta}_p, \hat{\beta}_{p+1}]$$
is the vector of the regression coefficients. $\quad (7.3)$

Similarly, the second-order regressive logistic regression model with the covariate vector is

$$\hat{P}(Y_3 = y_3 \mid Y_1 = y_1; Y_2 = y_2; \mathbf{X}) = \frac{e^{\mathbf{Z}\hat{\beta}}}{1 + e^{\mathbf{Z}\hat{\beta}}}, \text{ where } \mathbf{Z} = [X_1, X_2, ..., X_p, Y_1, Y_2],$$
$$\hat{\boldsymbol{\beta}} = [\hat{\beta}_0, \hat{\beta}_1, ..., \hat{\beta}_p, \hat{\beta}_{p+1}, \hat{\beta}_{p+2}] \text{ is the vector of the regression coefficients.} \quad (7.4)$$

The order of the regressive model is defined as the total number of follow-ups minus one. The models in Equations (7.2) and (7.3) are the first- and second-order regressive models. We need to fit seven models, one marginal model and six conditional models for the data from seven follow-ups. Now, using the fitted models in Equations (7.2) and (7.3), we can predict the necessary marginal and conditional probabilities for Equation (7.1) and estimate the joint probability of trajectory risk, the right-hand side probability of Equation (7.1). For example, to obtain the trajectory risk for a subject with ADL problem for all three follow-ups and specified risk factors, we need to estimate the following probabilities:

$$\hat{P}(Ys_1 = 1, Y_2 = 1, Y_3 = 1 \mid \mathbf{X}^* = x^*) = \hat{P}(Y_1 = 1 \mid \mathbf{X}^* = x^*) \times \hat{P}(Y_2 = 1 \mid Y_1 = 1; \mathbf{X}^* = x^*)$$
$$\times \hat{P}(Y_3 = 1 \mid Y_1 = 1; Y_2 = 1; \mathbf{X}^* = x^*) \quad (7.5)$$

We can obtain the first-order conditional probability by plugging in the value in $\mathbf{Z} = [\mathbf{X}^*, 1]$ in the fitted model in Equation (7.3), the second-order conditional probability by plugging in $\mathbf{Z} = [\mathbf{X}^*, 1, 1]$ in the fitted model in Equation (7.4), and so on. Finally, the marginal probability can be estimated from the marginal model in Equation (7.1) by plugging in the value in $\mathbf{Z} = [\mathbf{X}^*]$. For higher-order conditional probabilities, the general form can be found elsewhere [7].

TABLE 7.1

Distribution of the ADL Index across Follow-ups.

Value	y_1	y_2	y_3	y_4	y_5	y_6	y_7
No ADL (0)	5660	5165	4667	4290	3733	3417	2906
ADL (1)	770	714	740	671	696	640	656
Total	6431	5881	5410	4965	4434	4063	3569

The following list presents the risk factors used for illustration purposes. Table 7.1 presents the frequency distribution of outcomes (ADL) for y_1–y_7. For simplicity, subjects with missing values are removed.

For the illustration, the risk factors considered are

1. Age in years
2. Marital status (Mstat: married/partnered = 1, single/separated = 0)
3. Whether they drink alcohol (yes = 1, no = 0)
4. Gender (male = 1, female = 2)
5. The number of health conditions ever had (Ncond) ranging from 0 to 8
6. Race (White/Caucasian = 1, Black/African American/others = 0)
7. Education in years
8. Veteran status (1 = yes, 0 = no)
9. Body mass index (BMI)
10. Mental health index (CESD) ranging from 0 to 8
11. Large muscle index (Lmuscle) ranging from 0 to 4
12. Total income (Income)
13. Self-rated memory (Memory) ranging from 1 to 5 (1 = excellent, 2 = very good, 3 = good, 4 = fair, 5 = poor)
14. Word recall score (Wrecall) ranging from 0 to 20

The trajectory risk for the seven follow-ups can be estimated using the following equation:

$$\hat{P}\left(Y_1 = y_1, \cdots Y_7 = y_7 \mid \mathbf{Z}^* = \mathbf{z}^*\right) = \hat{P}\left(Y_1 = y_1 \mid \mathbf{X}^* = \mathbf{x}^*\right) \times \hat{P}\left(Y_2 = y_2 \mid Y_1 = y_1; \mathbf{X}^* = \mathbf{x}^*\right)$$
$$\times \cdots \times \hat{P}\left(Y_7 = y_7 \mid Y_1 = y_1, \cdots, Y_6 = y_6; \mathbf{X}^* = \mathbf{x}^*\right) \quad (7.7)$$
$$\text{where } y_1, \cdots y_7 = 0,1.$$

7.3 RESULTS

Table 7.2 shows the estimates of the parameters and their significance levels for the marginal and regressive logistic models, along with the model statistics for all follow-ups. The depression score (CESD) significantly (1% level) increases the risk of ADL problems throughout all the regressive models. The BMI significantly (1% level) increases the risk of ADL problems throughout all the regressive logistic models except for the third- and sixth-order models. The regression coefficients for gender showed a significant inverse relationship with the outcomes for all the models except for fourth- and sixth-order models. This means female subjects have a lower risk than male subjects, as females were coded as 2 compared to males as 1. Other covariates showed associations with outcomes (see Table 7.2.) It is expected and interesting to see that the previous two/three outcomes generally showed significant and positive associations with the current outcome in the regressive logistic models. That means subjects with ADL problems in the past significantly increased the same in current follow-ups.

TABLE 7.2

Estimates of Regressive Logistic Coefficients for Marginal and Six Conditional Models

	Models						
Estimate	Marginal	First order	Second order	Third order	Fourth order	Fifth order	Sixth order
(Intercept)	−5.66	−6.89	−7.00	−7.83	−8.54	−8.06	−10.58
Age	0.02	0.02	0.04a	0.06a	0.07a	0.05a	0.09a
Mstat	−0.11	0.01a	0.15	−0.10	−0.32a	−0.04	−0.04
Ncond	0.18a	0.19	0.15a	0.15a	0.08	0.07	0.11b
Drink	−0.37a	−0.08	−0.01	0.03	0.06	−0.06	0.05
Gender	−0.26b	−0.51a	−0.32b	−0.21	−0.50a	−0.27	−0.38b
Race	−0.14	−0.14	−0.23	0.22	−0.24	−0.19	0.04
Educ	0.00	0.05a	0.03	0.01	−0.01	0.03	−0.02
Veteran	−0.12	−0.46a	−0.10	−0.09	0.10	0.06	−0.14
BMI	0.04a	0.05a	0.03a	0.01	0.03a	0.02a	0.01
CESD	0.18a	0.15a	0.15a	0.12a	0.14a	0.14a	0.18a
Lmuscle	1.01a	0.80a	0.72a	0.71a	0.84a	0.75a	0.75a
Income	0.00	0.00a	0.00	0.00	0.00	0.00	0.00
Memory	0.16	0.20	0.16	0.01	−0.03	−0.08	0.08
Wrecall	−0.07a	−0.01	−0.09a	−0.08a	−0.08a	−0.07a	0.01
Y_1		1.77a	1.04a	0.81a	0.17	0.33	0.10
Y_2			1.72a	0.77a	0.69a	0.36b	0.13
Y_3				1.56a	0.93a	0.43a	0.49a
Y_4					1.44a	1.01a	0.29
Y_5						1.47a	1.13a
Y_6							1.78a
	a Significant at 1% level; b Significant at 5% level						
Akaike information criterion	2987.1	2634.9	2549.1	2343.5	2262.8	2120.5	1956.0
Bayesian information criterion	3088.6	2741.7	2661.2	2460.7	2384.3	2246.7	2085.7
Log-likelihood	−1478.5	−1301.4	−1257.5	−1153.7	−1112.4	−1040.3	−957.0

As a case study, let's compare two subjects with some variations in the risk factors to understand how a data-driven approach can help various health professionals educate patients and convince them to adhere to treatment plans. Consider an elderly subject 1 who has problems with the ADL at all seven time points (first to seventh follow-ups). For this subject, all time-invariant risk factors (Mstat, Ncond, Drink, Gender, Race, Education, and Veteran) remain unchanged for all seven follow-ups. Meanwhile, seven time-variant risk factors change (Table 7.4). The risk (joint probabilities) for all seven follow-ups for this subject are 0.96, 0.94, 0.87, 0.83, 0.79, 0.76, and 0.74, respectively (Table 7.5, second part, first row). These joint probabilities are the risks for all elderly, with the same value of all fourteen risk factors in the sample. This means subjects like this will face ADL problems through the seven follow-ups. Notably, conditional probabilities (in Table 7.5) are for the reduced sample.

Now consider another elderly subject 2, whose Wrecall scores for all follow-ups are 20, compared to subject 1, whose Wrecall scores differ (8, 7, 6, 5, 7, 8, and 6). The high Wrecall score of 20

TABLE 7.3

Estimated Marginal, Conditional, and Joint Probabilities for Selected Elderly

			Conditional Probabilities					
ID	Y1–Y7	P(Y1)	PY2| Y1	Y3|Y1 ...Y2	Y3|Y1 ...Y3	$Y3\|Y1$ ...$Y4$	$Y3\|Y1$ ...$Y5$	$Y3\|Y1$ ...$Y6$
1	0...0	0.01	0.01	0.01	0.01	0.01	0.01	0.01
2	0...0	0.10	0.08	0.04	0.00	0.03	0.02	0.04
3	0...0	0.01	0.00	0.01	0.01	0.01	0.02	0.02
4	0...0	0.01	0.01	0.01	0.01	0.01	0.02	0.01
5	0...0	0.01	0.00	0.02	0.00	0.04	0.02	0.01
6	0...0	0.01	0.01	0.04	0.02	0.03	0.01	0.03
7	1...1	0.76	0.91	0.90	0.93	0.98	0.95	0.98
8	1...1	0.96	0.97	0.93	0.95	0.95	0.96	0.98
9	1...1	0.86	0.79	0.97	0.93	0.97	0.98	0.99
10	1...1	0.88	0.90	0.95	0.97	0.98	0.96	0.98
11	1...1	0.90	0.89	0.94	0.92	0.91	0.95	0.99
12	1...1	0.87	0.94	0.98	0.94	0.99	0.98	0.99
			Joint probabilities					
ID	Y1 to Y7	P(Y1)	Y1, Y2	Y1...Y3	Y1...Y4	Y1...Y5	Y1...Y6	Y1...Y7
1	0...0	0.01	0.00	0.00	0.00	0.00	0.00	0.00
2	0...0	0.10	0.01	0.00	0.00	0.00	0.00	0.00
3	0...0	0.01	0.00	0.00	0.00	0.00	0.00	0.00
4	0...0	0.01	0.00	0.00	0.00	0.00	0.00	0.00
5	0...0	0.01	0.00	0.00	0.00	0.00	0.00	0.00
6	0...0	0.01	0.00	0.00	0.00	0.00	0.00	0.00
7	1...1	0.76	0.69	0.62	0.57	0.56	0.53	0.52
8	1...1	0.96	0.94	0.87	0.83	0.79	0.76	0.74
9	1...1	0.86	0.67	0.65	0.61	0.59	0.58	0.57
10	1...1	0.88	0.80	0.75	0.73	0.72	0.69	0.68
11	1...1	0.90	0.80	0.76	0.70	0.63	0.60	0.60
12	1...1	0.87	0.82	0.81	0.76	0.75	0.74	0.73

means for each task, the number of correctly recalled words is scored, with higher scores indicating better performance. All other risk factors for this subject are the same as those of subject 1. Now, the risk (joint probabilities) for all seven follow-ups for this subject are 0.92, 0.89, 0.70, 0.59, 0.52, 0.47, and 0.46, respectively (Table 7.5, second part, fourth row). This indicates that this subject will gradually be free from the ADL problem as the risk for sixth and seventh follow-ups is reduced to 0.47 and 0.46, respectively, below the cut-off value of 0.50 to have an ADL problem. These reductions are expected, as we can see from the fact that most of the estimated coefficients for Wrecall are significant and inversely associated (Table 7.2) with the dependent variable (ADL). We can compare the predicted risks between different subjects with different values of risk factors. The modeling framework shown here can be used to develop more comprehensive and fully parameterized models as long as data permit.

Next, we estimated the conditional and joint probabilities for all the samples using the fitted models in Table 7.2. The estimated conditional and joint probabilities for 12 subjects for all the follow-ups using the fitted marginal and regressive logistic model are shown in Table 7.3. It is worth

TABLE 7.4

Outcomes and Covariate of a Selected Subject for All Seven Follow-Ups

ID	Follow-up	Adla	Age	Mstat	Ncond	Drink	Gender	Race
1	1	1	64	0	7	0	2	0
1	2	1	66	0	7	0	2	0
1	3	1	67	0	7	0	2	0
1	4	1	69	0	7	0	2	0
1	5	1	72	0	7	0	2	0
1	6	1	73	0	7	0	2	0
1	7	1	75	0	7	0	2	0
Educ	**Veteran**	**BMI**	**CESD**	**Lmuscle**	**Income**	**Memory**	**Wrecall**	
10	0	58.4	6	4	8484	1	8	
10	0	58.4	5	4	7536	0	7	
10	0	55.6	1	3	10812	1	6	
10	0	53.9	1	4	11976	1	5	
10	0	47.6	2	3	18948	1	7	
10	0	47.6	1	4	18266.83	1	8	
10	0	47.8	4	4	5844	1	6	

mentioning that the marginal and conditional probabilities are estimated based on the observed independent variables and the responses at the previous time points for these 12 subjects. These probabilities are different because their covariate patterns are different. The first six subjects (1–6) have no ADL problems for all seven follow-ups, while the second six subjects (7–12) have ADL problems for all seven follow-ups. We can see that for first six subjects, the conditional probabilities are very small, as their outcomes for all seven follow-ups are zero. For subjects 7–12, the conditional probabilities of having ADL positive consistently remain over 0.80 for all of the seven follow-ups. So previous ADL episodes significantly increased the current episodes as their coefficients were found to be statistically significant (Table 7.2). The corresponding joint risks of developing ADL problems across the seven time points are also very high (above 0.50).

Table 7.4 presents the covariate values and outcomes for a particular subject for all seven follow-ups. Table 7.2 shows that BMI, CESD, and Wrecall (word recall) variables showed significant associations with all the outcomes. We want to compare the trajectory risk of five new patients with different values of these three independent variables with that of the patients from Table 7.4. To do this, we used five new patients not in the sample and compared their trajectories with the subjects shown in Table 7.4. Among the new subjects, in the first sample with ID 2, only the CESD scores for all follow-ups are set to zero compared to those covariates in Table 7.4. Similarly, in the second sample with ID 3, only the Wrecall scores for all follow-ups are set to zero compared to those covariates in Table 7.4. In the third sample with ID 4, only the Wrecall scores for all follow-ups are set to 20 compared to those covariates in Table 7.4. Again, in the fourth sample with ID 7, only the CESD scores for all follow-ups are set to eight compared to those covariates in Table 7.4. Finally, in the fifth sample with ID 8, only the CESD scores for all follow-ups are set to eight compared to those covariates in Table 7.4.

Table 7.5 presents the predicted marginal conditional and joint probabilities for all five new subjects and the subject with ID 1 shown in Table 7.4. The trajectories of all six subjects are shown in Figure 7.2. The trajectory for the subject with ID 1 shown in Table 7.4 is the third line from the top of the figure. The trajectory for the new subject with ID 2 is the fourth line from the top of the figure. This subject's CESD scores are zero for all follow-ups compared to higher values of CESD (1–6) for the subject with ID 1. Due to the CESD score of zero, the trajectory showed much lower risks for

TABLE 7.5

Marginal, Conditional, and Joint Probabilities for New Subjects

Subject	Marginal Probability 1	Conditional Probabilities at Different Follow-Ups					
		2	3	4	5	6	7
1	0.96	0.97	0.93	0.95	0.95	0.96	0.98
2	0.90	0.95	0.92	0.95	0.93	0.96	0.97
3	0.98	0.98	0.96	0.97	0.97	0.98	0.98
4	0.92	0.97	0.78	0.85	0.87	0.91	0.98
7	0.97	0.98	0.97	0.98	0.98	0.98	0.99
8	0.85	0.87	0.83	0.93	0.88	0.93	0.97
	Marginal Probability 1	Joint Probabilities at Different Follow-Ups					
		2	3	4	5	6	7
1	0.96	0.94	0.87	0.83	0.79	0.76	0.74
2	0.90	0.85	0.78	0.74	0.69	0.66	0.64
3	0.98	0.96	0.92	0.89	0.86	0.84	0.83
4	0.92	0.89	0.70	0.59	0.52	0.47	0.46
7	0.97	0.96	0.93	0.91	0.89	0.88	0.87
8	0.85	0.74	0.61	0.57	0.50	0.46	0.45

the trajectory. For the trajectory of the new subject with ID 3, Wrecall values for all follow-up are set to zero; those are the lowest compared to the values for the subject with ID 1. Hence, trajectory risks in the second line from the top of the graph are higher compared to the subject with ID 1 for all follow-ups. On the other hand, a higher Wrecall score shall decrease the trajectory risk, as shown by the second line from the bottom of the graph with subject ID 4. The Wrecall value for this subject is 20 for all the follow-ups. Over the follow-ups, the probabilities went below 0.50. This means this subject is going to be free from ADL problems. The top line of the graph for the subject with ID 7 with a CESD score of 8 for all the follow-ups increased the trajectory risk close to 1. Finally, the first trajectory from the bottom of the graph is for subject ID 8, where BMI values are set to 20 for all the follow-ups. While for the subject with ID 1, in Table 7.4 BMI values are much higher, which is in the obese category. Hence, the subject with ID 8 showed a sharp decrease in the trajectory risk. This subject is quickly going toward ADL problem-free states.

Trajectories for many other subjects with various covariate values can be compared and shown graphically (Figure 7.2). Next, we compared the trajectory of the subject with ID 1 (Table 7.4) with a new subject with ID 9, whose outcomes and covariate vector are the same as those of the subject in Table 7.4, except the CESD was set to zero, Wrecall was set to 20, and BMI was set to 20 for all follow-ups. These two trajectories are shown in Figure 7.3. We can see that there is a very sharp decline in the trajectory of the new patient starting from the second follow-up and going to be free from ADL problems from the third follow-up onward because the probabilities from the third follow-up onward were reduced by 0.50, which is below the threshold level of the ADL problem cut-off. Appendix Figure A4 displays the graph for the conditional probabilities for those six subjects, as shown in Figure 7.2.

In Table 7.2, we present the fitted regressive logistic model with the main effects only. Fitting the regressive logistic model with the main effects and their pairwise interaction terms is possible. We can fit the fully parameterized regressive logistic model if the data permit. We can include

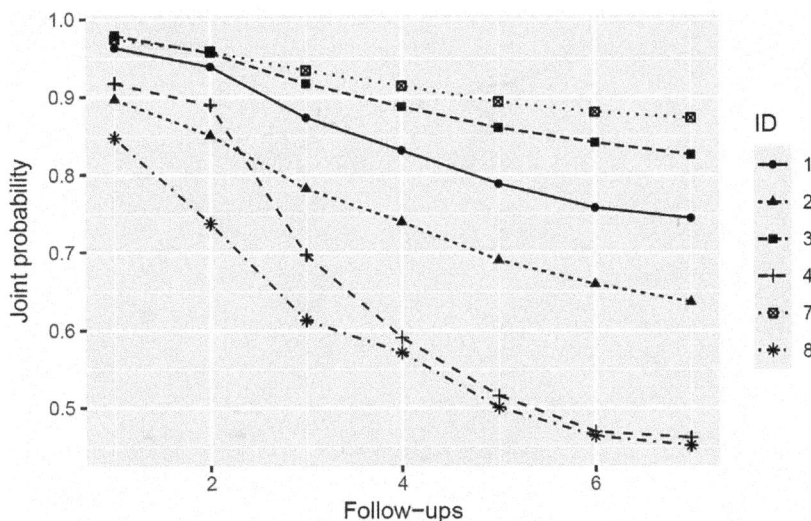

FIGURE 7.3 ADL trajectories of seven subjects with varying covariate values.

the interaction between feature variables within a regressive model between feature variables and responses from previous follow-ups and between responses from prior follow-ups. This may provide better predictive models.

7.4 DISCUSSION AND CONCLUSIONS

We proposed an analytical framework using a series of regressive logistic regression models to predict conditional and joint probabilities for trajectories given a sequence of binary responses (ADL conditions) that pass through different phases over time. The framework is applied to longitudinal data from the US HRS. This approach significantly reduces the over-parameterization compared to the Markov models. A series of conditional models are linked using the Markov chain to estimate trajectory risks. This framework allows us to answer various questions we raised in the introduction. The first follow-up data are used to fit the marginal model, while the subsequent follow-ups provide data to fit the conditional models. Using the Markov models, we cannot assess the impact of the prior outcomes due to the effective stratification of the data.

Disease trajectory risk prediction for a patient using the given risk factors is very useful for healthcare professionals. The risk of 0.90 for developing a condition compared to the risk of 0.51 has a deep implication. Both will classify the disease condition as positive using 0.50 as the probability threshold. Our interest is to find models that better predict the probability of risk of developing the disease. Healthcare professionals may screen individuals to suggest necessary therapy and preventive measures using the predicted risk at a particular follow-up and the trajectories. Risk prediction may also make a patient aware of the future course of the disease (Islam & Chowdhury, 2017). In various areas, categorical dependent and independent variables are observed at different time points over time. For example, longitudinal studies often collect a long sequence of responses and independent variables that are measured repeatedly over time (Islam et al., 2013). Patients with a chronic disease may visit physicians repeatedly, producing a long sequence of data collected over time. EMRs (Tripepi et al., 2013; Zhao et al., 2019) are another source of repeated measures allowing health professionals to model health conditions (response) and risk factors. Clinicians might be interested in understanding the disease progression and regression over follow-ups and finding the causes of the disease to be directed to a particular trajectory. Disease trajectories can be very useful in convincing patients to adhere to treatment plans and primary care providers' suggestions.

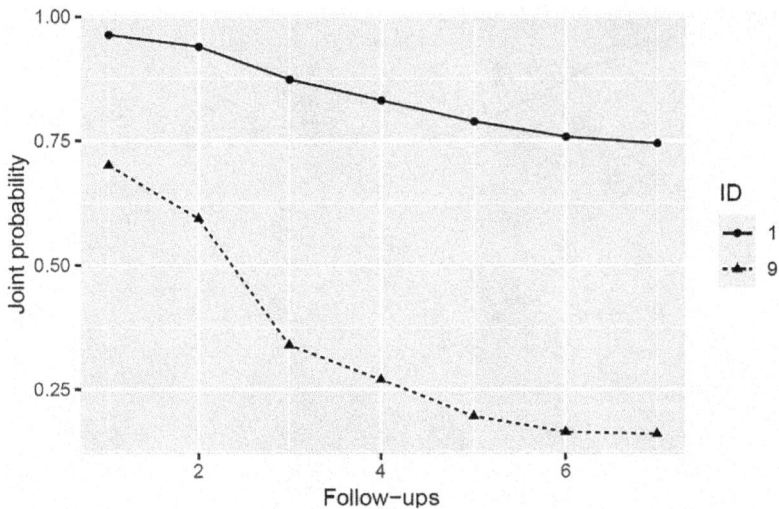

FIGURE 7.4 ADL trajectories of two subjects with different CESD scores.

A computerized system that can produce patient trajectories with various scenarios would be very convincing for a patient and useful for healthcare professionals.

7.5 ACKNOWLEDGMENTS

The authors acknowledge the National Institute on Aging of the University of Michigan for sharing the US HRS data.

REFERENCES

Alexander, D. B., & Grantz, K. H. (2021). Development and dissemination of infectious disease dynamic transmission models during the COVID-19 pandemic: what can we learn from other pathogens and how can we move forward. *Lancet Digit Health*, 3, e41–50 Published Online 2020 December 7, https://doi.org/10.1016/S2589–7500(20)30268–5

Ashtab, S., & Anderson, W. (2023). Differences in manufacturing and healthcare supply chain management: an overview. *International Journal of Health Technology and Management*, 20(3), 232–248.

Ashtab, S., & Campbell, R. (2021). Explanatory analysis of factors influencing the support for sustainable food production and distribution systems: results from a rural Canadian community. *Sustainability*, 13(9), 5324.

Ashtab, S., & Tosarkani, B. M. (2023). Scenario-based multi-objective optimisation model based on supervised machine learning to configure a plastic closed-loop supply chain network. *International Journal of Business Performance and Supply Chain Modelling*, 14, 106–128.

Böhmer, M. M., et al. (2020). Investigation of a COVID-19 outbreak in Germany resulting from a single travel-associated primary case: a case series. *The Lancet Infectious Diseases*, 20(8), 920–928. https://doi.org/10.1016/S1473-3099(20)30314-5

Chaw, J. K., Chaw, S. H., Quah, C. H., Sahrani, S., Ang, M. C., Zhao, Y., & Ting, T. T. (2024). A predictive analytics model using machine learning algorithms to estimate the risk of shock development among dengue patients. *Healthcare Analytics*, 5, 100290.

Chen, T.-M., Rui, J., Wang, Q.-P., Zhao, Z.-Y., Cui, J.-A., & Yin, L. (2020). A mathematical model for simulating the phase-based transmissibility of a novel coronavirus. *Infectious Diseases of Poverty*, 9(1), 1–8. https://doi.org/10.1186/s40249-020-00640-3

Cheung, Y. B., Ma, X., Lam, K. F., Yung, C. F., & Milligan, P. (2024). Estimation of trajectory of protective efficacy in infectious disease prevention trials using recurrent event times. *Statistics in Medicine*, 43(9), 1759–1773. https://doi.org/10.1002/sim.10049

Chowdhury, R. I., Hasan, M. T., & Sneddon, G. (2022). Regressive class modelling for predicting trajectories of COVID-19 fatalities using statistical and machine learning models. *Bulletin of the Malaysian Mathematical Sciences Society*, 45(Suppl 1), 235–250. https://doi.org/10.1007/s40840-022-01287-z

Chowdhury, R. I., & Islam, M. A. (2020). Regressive models for risk prediction for repeated multinomial outcomes: an illustration using health and retirement study (HRS) data. *Biometrical Journal*, 1–18. http://dx.doi.org/10.1002/bimj.201800101

Chowdhury, R. I., & Islam, M. A. (2022). Predictive models for trajectory risks prediction from repeated ordinal outcomes. *Bulletin of the Malaysian Mathematical Sciences Society*, *45*(Suppl 1), 161–209. https://doi.org/10.1007/s40840-022-01277-1

Chowdhury, R. I., Sneddon, G., & Hasan, M. T. (2020, September 14). Analyzing the effect of duration on the daily new cases of COVID-19 infections and deaths using bivariate Poisson regression: a marginal conditional approach. *Mathematical Biosciences and Engineering*, *17*(5), 6085–6097. https://doi.org/10.3934/mbe.2020323

Hollingsworth, T. D. (2009). Controlling infectious disease outbreaks: lessons from mathematical modelling. *Journal of Public Health Policy*, *30*(3), 328–341. http://dx.doi.org/10.1057/jphp.2009.13

Islam, M. A., & Chowdhury, R. I. (2010). Prediction of disease status: a regressive model approach for repeated measures. *Statistical Methodology*, *7*, 520–540.

Islam, M. A., & Chowdhury, R. I. (2017). *Analysis of Repeated Measures Data*. Singapore 189721, Singapore: Springer Nature. http://dx.doi.org/10.1007/978-981-10-3794-8

Islam, M. A., Chowdhury, R. I., & Huda, S. (2013). A multistate transition model for analyzing longitudinal depression data. *The Bulletin of the Malaysian Mathematical Sciences Society Series 2*, *36*, 637–655.

Jos, W. R., & Twisk. (2013). *Applied Longitudinal Data Analysis for Epidemiology*. Cambridge University Press.

Kharitonov, A., Nahhas, A., Pohl, M., & Turowski, K. (2022). Comparative analysis of machine learning models for anomaly detection in manufacturing. *Procedia Computer Science*, *200*, 1288–1297.

Kriegova, E., et al. (2021). A theoretical model of health management using data-driven decision-making: the future of precision medicine and health. *Journal of Translational Medicine*, *19*, 68. https://doi.org/10.1186/s12967-021-02714-8

Lee, Y., & Nelder, J. A. (2004). Conditional and marginal models: another view. *Statistical Science*, *19*, 219–238.

Li, Q., et al. (2020). Early transmission dynamics in Wuhan, China, of novel coronavirus–infected pneumonia. *New England Journal of Medicine*, *382*, 1199–1207.

Lindsey, J. K., & Lamber, P. (1998). On the appropriateness of marginal models for repeated measurements in clinical trials. *Statistics in Medicine*, *17*, 447–469.

Pham, T., Tran, T., Phung, D., & Venkatesh, S. (2017). Predicting healthcare trajectories from medical records: a deep learning approach. *Journal of Biomedical Informatics*, *69*. http://dx.doi.org/10.1016/j.jbi.2017.04.001

Sharda, R., Denle, D., & Turban, E. (2018). *Business Intelligence, Analytics, and Data Science: A Managerial Perspective*. Pearson.

Singer, J. D., & Willett, J. B. (2003). *Applied Longitudinal Data Analysis: Modeling Change and Event Occurrence*. Oxford University Press. https://doi.org/10.1093/acprof:oso/9780195152968.001.0001

Sonnega, A., Faul, J. D., Ofstedal, M. B., Langa, K. M., Phillips, J. W., & Weir, D. R. (2014). Cohort profile: the health and retirement study (HRS). *International Journal Epidemiology*, *43*(2), 576–585. http://dx.doi.org/10.1093/ije/dyu067

Toba, S., Tomasine, M., & Yang, Y. H. (2008). Supply chain management in hospital: a case study. *California Journal of Operations Management*, *6*, 49–55.

Tripepi, G., Heinze, G., Jager, K. J., Stel, V. S., Dekker, F. W., & Zoccali, C. (2013). Risk prediction models. *Nephrology Dialysis Transplantation*, *28*(8), 1975–1980.

Wang, C., & Mustafa, S. A. (2023). Data-driven Markov process for infectious disease transmission. *PLoS One*, *18*(8), e0289897. https://doi.org/10.1371/journal.pone.0289897

Wang, H., et al. (2020) Phase-adjusted estimation of the number of coronavirus disease 2019 cases in Wuhan, China. *Cell Discovery*, *6*(1), 1–8. https://doi.org/10.1038/s41421-020-0148-0

Wu, J. T., et al. (2020). Estimating clinical severity of COVID-19 from the transmission dynamics in Wuhan, China. *Nature Medicine*, *26*(4), 506–510. https://doi.org/10.1038/s41591-020-0822-7

Zhao, J., et al. (2019). Learning from longitudinal data in electronic health records and genetic data to improve cardiovascular event prediction. *Scientific Reports*, *9*. http://dx.doi.org/10.1038/s41598-018-36745-x

Zhao, S., et al. (2020a). Estimating the unreported number of novel coronavirus (2019-nCoV) cases in China in the first half of January 2020: a data-driven modelling analysis of the early outbreak. *Journal of Clinical Medicine*, *9*(2), 388.

Zhao, S., et al. (2020b). Preliminary estimation of the basic reproduction number of novel coronavirus (2019-nCoV) in China, from 2019 to 2020: a data-driven analysis in the early phase of the outbreak. *International Journal of Infectious Diseases*, *92*, 214–217.

Appendix

R-PROGRAMS FOR TRAJECTORY ANALYSIS

The dataset used in this chapter is a subset of the HRS data. For efficient analysis, we used a long-file data format structure to rearrange previous outcomes as covariates, and we exploited multiple cores (CPU) to perform parallel computing. Because of the lengthiness of the steps and programs, we could provide them with this chapter. The models are fitted using R software, for which the programs are available from the authors upon request. Additionally, they will be available from the Research Gate (https://www.researchgate.net/profile/Rafiqul-Chowdhury-2/research).

Appendix Table A1 presents a long-format data file for some subjects. The columns Y_1 to Y_6 are added to use the previous outcomes as covariates. Out of the seven follow-ups, the last model is the sixth-order regressive logistic model, where the outcome from the seventh follow-up is the dependent variable. So, for this last model, we can use only the previous six outcomes as covariates along with other independent variables.

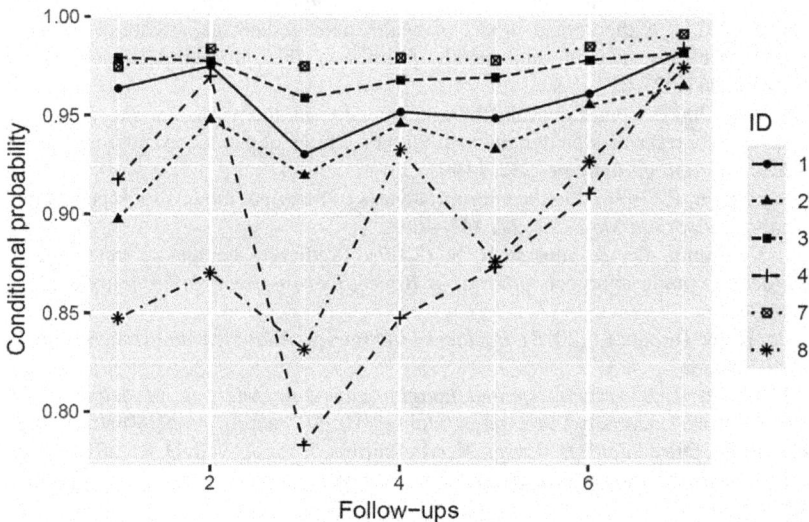

Appendix Figure 1   Comparison of ADL trajectories of conditional probabilities for several subjects.

TABLE A1
Data Structure to Fit Models

hhidpn	Adla	Age	Mstat	Ncond	Drink	Gender	Race
10001010	0	62	0	0	0	1	1
10001010	0	64	0	0	0	1	1
10001010	0	66	0	0	0	1	1
10001010	0	69	0	0	1	1	1
10001010	0	71	0	0	0	1	1
10001010	0	72	0	0	0	1	1
10001010	0	74	0	0	0	1	1

hhidpn	Adla	Age	Mstat	Ncond	Drink	Gender	Race
Educ	Veteran	BMI	CESD	Lmuscle	Income	Memory	Wrecall
12	0	24.4	1	0	6276	0	10
12	0	22.4	1	0	9588	0	12
12	0	21.7	1	0	10188	1	13
12	0	22.3	1	0	10260	1	12
12	0	21.3	1	0	14400	0	11
12	0	20.2	1	0	12000	1	11
12	0	20.9	0	0	12000	0	12

Y1	Y2	Y3	Y4	Y5	Y6	Wave
NA	NA	NA	NA	NA	NA	1
0	NA	NA	NA	NA	NA	2
0	0	NA	NA	NA	NA	3
0	0	0	NA	NA	NA	4
0	0	0	0	NA	NA	5
0	0	0	0	0	NA	6
0	0	0	0	0	0	7

Following is the R program used to fit all the models:

```
indvars <- c("Age", "Mstat", "Ncond", "Drink", "Gender", "Race", "Educ",
        "Veteran", "BMI", "CESD", "Lmuscle", "Income", "Memory", "Wrecall")

## indvars <- c("Age", "Mstat", "Ncond", "Drink", "Gender", "Race", "Educ",
##      "Veteran", "Mobility", "BMI", "CESD", "Lmuscle", "Income", "Memory",
##      "Gindex", "Wrecall")

idvar <- "hhidpn"
depvar <- "Adla"
b        <- 15  ## total number of covariates and previous outcomes
totfol <- 7   ## total number of follow-ups
system.time(
Lo1 <- foreach(i = 1:totfol, .packages=c('MASS','data.table')) %dopar% {
        mdlongN <- allDataBook[allDataBook$Wave==i,][,1:(i+b)]

            fitmod <- glm(Adla~., data = mdlongN[,2:dim(mdlongN)[[2]]],
            family = binomial("logit"))
            prob <- predict(fitmod, newdata = mdlongN, type="response")
            Yh <- ifelse(prob > 0.50, 1, 0)
            prob <- as.data.frame(cbind(hhidpn=mdlongN$hhidpn,
                Y=mdlongN$Adla,Yh,prob,Type=mdlongN$Type))
            mls <- list(fitmod,prob)
            })
stopImplicitCluster()
```

8 Genomics and Personalized Medicine
An Insight from the Healthcare Perspective

Tabsum Chhetri, Saurav Kumar Mishra, Anagha Balakrishnan, Sneha Roy, Kusum Gurung, and John J. Georrge

8.1 INTRODUCTION

The healthcare sector has experienced tremendous growth in the last few years, driven by increased patients, research, and the development of novel drugs. This is because new tools and techniques have been introduced (Chejara et al., 2018). Not only have these methods and tools made it easier to study human illness, but they have also simplified operations in the healthcare sector. Integrating genomics into the healthcare system is one of these significant developments. Traditional, "one-size-fits-all" medicine is replaced by a more patient-centered strategy that tailors interventions to each individual's needs (Lal et al., 2013). Human genomics is transitioning from a research-driven activity to one driven and funded by healthcare (Birney et al., 2017). Genomics, the branch of molecular biology that deals with the study of the complete set of DNA of organisms, including all of its genes, has transformed our understanding of health and disease (https://www.genome.gov/genetics-glossary/genomics). Technological advancements like next-generation sequencing (NGS) and genome-wide association studies (GWAS) have allowed investigators to recognize genetic variants related with various illnesses, drug targets, and patient responses to medications. This newfound knowledge is paving the way for developing personalized therapies with improved efficacy and reduced side effects (Satam et al., 2023; Uffelmann et al., 2021). Personalized medicine offers a multitude of advantages. By analyzing an individual's genetic profile, healthcare professionals can design targeted treatment plans that maximize therapeutic benefit while minimizing the risk of adverse reactions. This patient-centric approach eliminates the need for trial-and-error medication prescribing, streamlining treatment and reducing unnecessary costs associated with diagnostics and ineffective therapies (Cruz-Correia et al., 2018). Furthermore, personalized medicine allows for early disease identification and intervention. Healthcare professionals can implement targeted screening strategies and preventive measures by identifying genetic markers associated with specific diseases. For instance, individuals with a genetic predisposition for conditions like cancer or inherited disorders can undergo testing to assess their risk and take proactive steps to manage the disease progression (Harvey et al., 2012). Pharmacogenomics, a field in modern medicine that helps investigate an individual genetic makeup and the response to certain types of drugs, also paves the way for more individualized treatments catered to each patient's unique genetic profile by identifying the genetic variables affecting medication response, safety, and effectiveness. This results in clinical trials that are more likely to be successful but are also smaller, more effective, and more economical (Nebert et al., 2008; Sadee & Dai, 2005). The economic benefits of genomic medicine are significant, as it enhances genetic diagnosis, making it more efficient and cost-effective (Figure 8.1) by reducing genetic testing to a single analysis. This streamlined approach notifies persons during their lives, enabling more operative intensive care and personalized treatments (Frank et al., 2013).

DOI: 10.1201/9781003485629-8

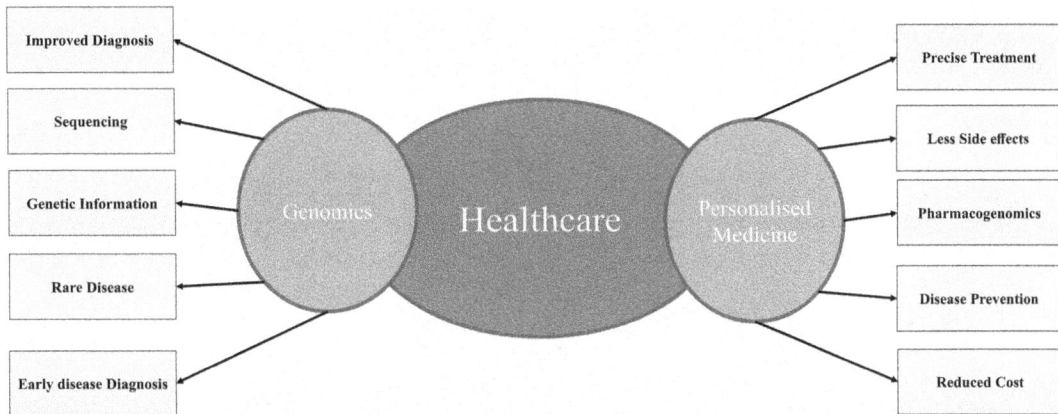

FIGURE 8.1 Basic Overview of Genomics and Personalized Medicine Involvement in Healthcare.

The broader economic impact of genomic medicine includes reducing healthcare costs, increasing productivity, and creating new medical information industries (Payne et al., 2018). However, integrating genomics into clinical practice presents several challenges. The successful implementation of personalized medicine requires healthcare professionals to possess the expertise to interpret and utilize complex genomic data. Additionally, ethical considerations regarding confidentiality, data safety, and possible judgment based on genetic evidence need to be wisely addressed (Rose, 2013).

Despite these hurdles, the convergence of genomics and personalized medicine holds immense promise for the future of healthcare. This dynamic field offers the potential for tailored solutions, improved healthcare delivery efficiency, and reduced healthcare disparities. As research and technology continue to advance, personalized medicine is poised to become the cornerstone of a more effective and patient-centered healthcare system. This study delves deeper into the evolving landscape of genomics and personalized medicine. It explores the development of this field, analyzes the latest advancements in personalized medicine and genomic technologies, and evaluates the impact these advancements have on healthcare delivery.

8.2 GENOMICS IN HEALTHCARE

Genomics studies a genome's structure, function, and its characteristics. It is an interdisciplinary field that emphasizes the molecular characterization and quantification of all the genes in an organism, their interactions, and their impact on the organism. The genome makes up the entire collection of DNA, including all of its genes and its three-dimensional, hierarchical structural arrangement (Stark et al., 2019). Applying genomics to healthcare has transformed the industry by adding new insights into human health and illness. Its significance comes from its capacity to customize care to each patient's unique genetic profile, making therapies more focused and efficient. Genomic screening, which involves population-level screening for early discovery of genetic predispositions, is a component of disease prevention and risk assessment (McCarthy et al., 2013; Pattan et al., 2021). Based on statistical analysis of big datasets, risk prediction models employ genetic data to forecast an individual's likelihood of contracting an illness. Clustered Regularly Interspaced Short Palindromic Repeats (CRISPR) and gene editing technologies promise to treat genetic diseases by manipulating an individual's DNA sequence. Initially, it was challenging to integrate genomics into healthcare as most of the data related to humans was yet to be explored (Li et al., 2020; McCarthy et al., 2013). The Human Genome Project (HGP), launched in 1990, was groundbreaking research that paved the way for genomics in the medical industry. It was completed in 2003, and the HGP laid the foundation for personalized medicine by providing a comprehensive understanding of the

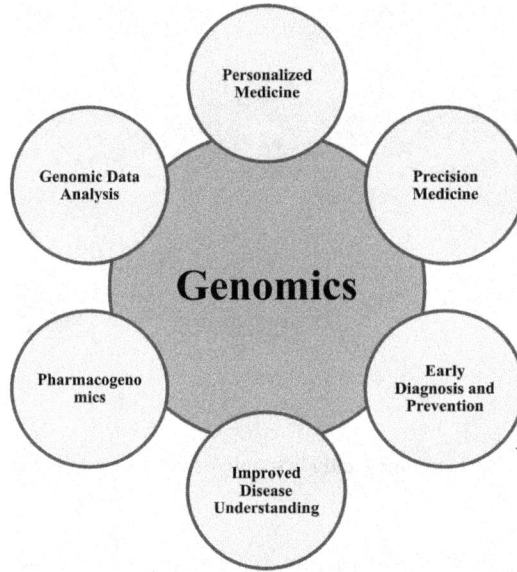

FIGURE 8.2   Basic Overview of Genomics Involvement in Healthcare.

human genome, enabling the development of targeted treatments tailored to an individual's unique genetic profile (Green et al., 2020). Genomic data from the HGP has improved disease diagnosis by identifying genetic markers associated with specific diseases. Integrating genomic data with healthcare services has allowed the growth of targeted treatments and preventive measures, allowing for early intervention and prevention (Carrasco-Ramiro et al., 2017; Stark et al., 2019). After the HGP, NGS was introduced, further aiding genomics' contribution to healthcare. By enabling high-throughput sequencing of entire genomes, NGS technologies have transformed the ground of genomics and improved the speed, accuracy, and affordability of genomic analysis (Weymann et al., 2022). A thorough study of genetic data can be performed with several NGS technologies, which can help with illness diagnosis, treatment, and prevention. With the ability to sequence several genes simultaneously, NGS offers a comprehensive insight into a person's genetic composition. The discovery of variations linked to disease is made possible by this thorough genomic profile, which supports targeted medicines and personalized medicine (Zhang et al., 2011). Clinical oncology is a prevalent field that uses NGS to sequence tumors and match patients to targeted medicines that address genetic changes driving tumor growth (Stadler et al., 2014; Werner, 2010).

Since every person reacts differently to medications, NGS (Figure 8.2) focuses on how genetic variants affect a person's drug reaction, which helps improve medicine safety and efficacy and reduce medical costs. Moreover, early disease detection made possible by genetic profiling can lead to more effective patient outcomes through prompt interventions and individualized treatments (Horner et al., 2010; Kumar & Khurana, 2014).

By examining the complete genome in a single test, NGS provides the best chance of identifying uncommon illnesses. With focused treatments, this method can help find the source of undiagnosed rare diseases, cutting down on pointless testing and hospital stays for patients and their families. Ultimately, this will improve patient outcomes and transform the medical industry. A single test that analyses the complete genome can also diagnose rare diseases (Casolino et al., 2024; Vinksel et al., 2021). Various kinds of NGS technologies are currently being utilized in healthcare. One of the most common is whole-genome sequencing (WGS), wherein all the DNA is sequenced, including its mitochondrial and chromosomal material. It is used in diagnosing cancer. Another type of NGS used is whole exome sequencing (WES), used to find the genetic variation associated with the disease. This focuses mainly on an organism's encoding areas, which comprise approximately 1% of the human genome (Foo et al., 2012; Grody et al., 2013). Transcriptome sequencing is another type of sequencing that can be utilized in healthcare as it sequences a cell's whole RNA transcript assembly. This can be used to understand gene expression in diseased and normal individuals and find the genes that are expressed more, which can be used in identifying diseases before the onset. Single gene testing, which finds mutations or variants linked to a specific ailment, and gene panel testing, which finds mutations associated with various disorders, are two further applications of NGS technologies (Hong et al., 2020; Supplitt et al., 2021). Similarly, genetic variations that are associated with specific diseases can be extracted using a technique called GWAS. The tool searches for single-nucleotide polymorphisms (SNPs) associated with specific diseases, leading to enhanced disease prediction, genetic risk factors, and drug development (Uffelmann et al., 2021).

Through WGS, the integration of multi-omics data, and the development of new technologies like long-read genome sequencing and optical genome mapping, genomics has dramatically enhanced the detection of rare disorders (Turro et al., 2020). Extensive genomic research initiatives such as the 100,000 Genomes Project have exhibited the efficacy of WGS in diagnosing uncommon illnesses within standard healthcare environments. International data sharing and collaboration are essential for improved variant interpretation, particularly for ultra-rare illnesses. Numerous novel molecular diagnostics have been discovered, thanks to bioinformatic techniques honed by extensive genomic research (Kernohan & Boycott, 2024; Wright et al., 2023).

The advancement in genomics has facilitated NGS and gene editing (Figure 8.2) technologies such as CRISPR-Cas9, which has tremendously aided in healthcare. CRISPR is a technology that enables precise gene editing in living organisms (Subica, 2023). Through gene editing, this may help treat human disease. It is based on a naturally occurring defense mechanism in bacteria called CRISPR, which allows the organism to snip off viral DNA to shield itself against viral infections. With the aid of an enzyme known as Cas (CRISPR-associated protein), CRISPR technology cuts DNA at a precise spot to enable the insertion or deletion of genes. The Cas enzyme and guide RNA (gRNA) are the two primary parts of the CRISPR system. The gRNA binds a particular DNA sequence, and the Cas enzyme then slices the DNA at that exact spot (Kaboli & Babazada, 2018). Gene editing, gene therapy, biotechnology, and fundamental research are just a few of the many uses of CRISPR. It can transform several fields because it makes precise and effective gene editing possible (Grissa et al., 2009). This technology has made it possible to research and address various genetic disorders like sickle cell anemia and hemophilia. It has also been used to create models for diseases such as Alzheimer's and leukemia. This has further helped healthcare professionals understand and navigate the treatment of the diseases (Liu et al., 2021; Subica, 2023).

Thus, it can be said that the advancement of precision and personalization, target discovery and validation, clinical trial design, and patient selection resulting from genomic medicine substantially impacted drug development (Ward, 2001). Promising therapeutic targets can be identified by accurately identifying genetic variations and biological pathways linked to diseases through genomic methods. Another application of genomics in medicine is the validation of pharmacological targets and the prediction of therapeutic effects on biomarkers and clinical outcomes through the use of genomic data (Emilien et al., 2000).

Additionally, it has been seen that certain patients may respond well to medications that have previously failed; for this reason, genomic analysis can be performed to repurpose pharmaceuticals. Furthermore, genetic medicine may save healthcare expenses, lessen productivity losses, and promote industry innovation (Li & He, 2023; Bisson, 2012).

Integrating genomics in healthcare, despite having such advantages, has some disadvantages. First, genomics face numerous difficulties and ethical challenges, including data security and privacy, informed consent, genetic prejudice, the implications of genetic information, and equitable access. Prioritizing genetic data within the electronic health records (EHR) system is crucial for seamless integration into clinical workflows. The magnitude and complexity of gene test findings make integrating genomic data into EHRs difficult and call for data warehousing solutions (Sperber et al., 2017). Second, physicians might require further instruction and training to properly comprehend and embrace genomic medicine. Healthcare professionals must ensure that everyone has an equal chance to benefit from these advances by addressing gaps in access to genomics. A multistep process is needed to integrate genomics into clinical practice (Kho et al., 2013). Third, implementing patient participation measures such as patient advisory boards and education is crucial for the success of genomic efforts. This includes teaching patients the fundamentals of genomics, creating plans for integrating genomic data into patient care, and offering instruction and training on interpreting and using genomic data. Fourth, few policy frameworks and clinical standards integrate digital health tools with genomics (Howard et al., 2013). It is necessary to establish strong evidence to show the value and influence of genomic medicine on patient outcomes and healthcare efficiencies because there are evidentiary gaps in clinical effectiveness and cost-effectiveness. These obstacles must be overcome to successfully integrate genomics into healthcare organizations and revolutionize the provision of healthcare (Brlek et al., 2024; Marzban et al., 2022). Thus, genetic medicine has the potential to transform healthcare by tackling these issues and guaranteeing that all individuals have equitable access to genetic services. Apart from that, the utilization of the genomics concept along with bioinformatics and advanced computational biology was also increasing for the accurate therapeutic design that can also contribute to the improvement of the healthcare system (Mishra & Georrge, 2024; Mishra et al., 2024a; Mishra et al., 2023; Vakhariya et al., 2023a, 2023b; Vinjoda et al., 2024).

8.3 PERSONALIZED MEDICINE IN HEALTHCARE

Personalized medicine (PM) customizes medical action to an individual patient's exceptional character. The plan is founded on systematic advancement, namely, knowing each person's unique molecular and genetic profile, which makes them prone to particular diseases. It not only increases the ability to treat and diagnose the condition, but it also has the potential to detect the disease earlier in its progression. PM is driven by advancements in technology, such as DNA sequencing, proteomics, and wireless monitoring devices, which enable the detection of interindividual variations in disease processes (Dey et al., 2023; Illert et al., 2023). However, precision medicine allows for a more in-depth study of individuals' genetic variants, which can lead to the development and selection of medications and care pathways that reduce side effects and result in better outcomes. Treating individual patients based on their unique features stretches back around 2,400 years, but recent technological breakthroughs in the 21st century boosted its dominant position (Delpierre & Lefèvre, 2023).

Furthermore, high-throughput technologies have accelerated its evolution in biology and medicine. From 2003 to 2008, the term predictive, preventive, and personalized medicine (3P medicine) was used in the scientific area in conjunction with genomics, system biology, and pharmacology, with PM projects demonstrating their benefit to the healthcare system. The notion of 3P medicine evolved as a vision for constructing an innovative, complex, and linked approach to healthcare, which is crucial for evidence-based therapy and health risk prediction (Bajinka et al., 2024; Zhang et al., 2023). The evolution of 3P medicine into P4 medicine incorporates the term "participatory" in the framework, emphasizing patients' active involvement in their healthcare. This P4 medicine presents a step toward recognizing the significance of the physical environment, empowering patient–provider communication, creating a collaborative approach to healthcare, and leading to greater treatment adherence, improved outcomes, and increased patient satisfaction (Brehio, 2024; Delpierre & Lefèvre, 2023). This highlights the greater necessity for the concept of 5P medicine, which represents population-based components. This addition may provide crucial information on pharmacological therapies' therapeutic usefulness and long-term efficacy in real-world settings. In recent times, PM has had a more progressive approach to personalized healthcare, which increased a variety of individual traits, including lifestyle, environment, and personal preferences (Blobel et al., 2024). Personalized healthcare emphasizes preventative efforts to maintain health and reduce

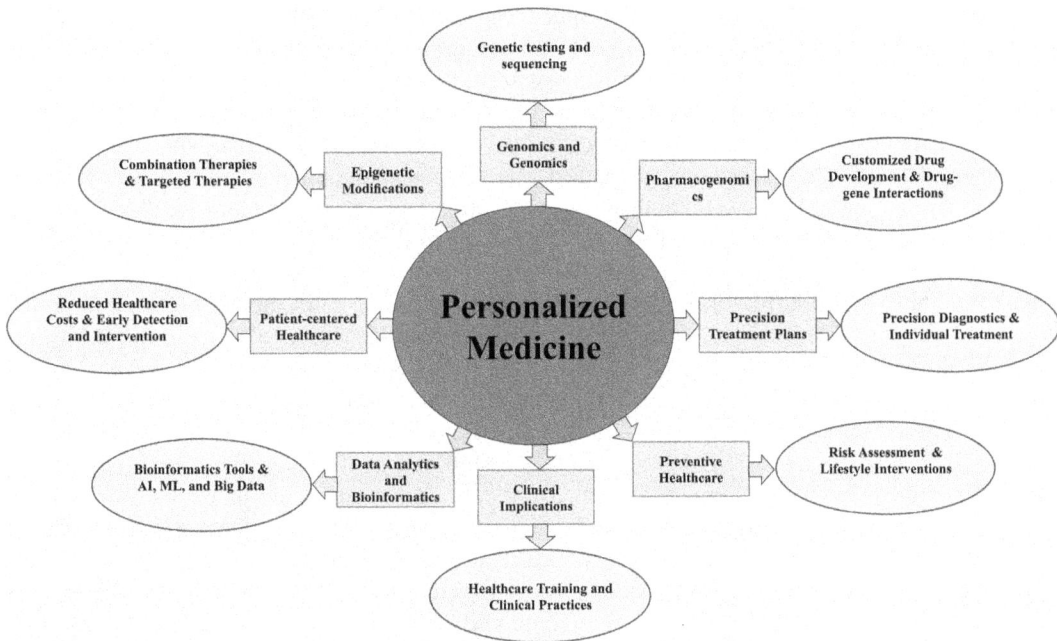

FIGURE 8.3 Involvement in PM Aspects in Healthcare.

illness risk and population-level elements that enable fair access to high-quality care. The emphasis on personalized healthcare shifts from care to prevention and health-enabling progress, including increasing life expectancy, reducing health disparities, and investing in novel treatments. PM and personalized healthcare are two closely connected concepts that reflect transformational approaches to healthcare and go beyond medical treatment to include preventive interventions and lifestyle suggestions. However, using new technologies such as genomics, big data, artificial intelligence (AI), PM, and healthcare can forecast health risks, assist in early diagnosis, and optimize treatment approaches, resulting in more effective and efficient healthcare delivery (Stefanicka-Wojtas & Kurpas, 2023; Sugandh et al., 2023).

Along with health and disease, various factors influence personalized healthcare (Figure 8.3), including genomics, which allows for healthcare customization based on an individual's genetic profile. Recent studies combine genetic linkage, genome-wide association, and whole genome expression data to uncover new insights and propose novel therapeutic solutions for illness mitigation and prevention. Genomics' most significant contributions to PM are in illness prediction and prevention, where genome scanning can identify people at high risk for specific genetic disorders and chronic diseases (Delpierre & Lefèvre, 2023; Tawfik et al., 2023).

The research and use of targeted medicines through genetics is the most popular in PM. However, the impact of the genome on predicting medicine response is one of the most promising topics in PM, known as pharmacogenomics, which employs genomics technology to investigate the impacts of genes on drug behavior through gene expression. Pharmacogenomics has quickly adopted genomic knowledge to detect molecular activity, drug character, and pharmacological targets and generate biomarkers of medication response with potential medical applications. Pharmacogenomics aids in determining the best medicine and dose for individuals while reducing adverse drug reactions and enhancing therapeutic outcomes. It also highlights the risks of severe side effects, allowing the avoidance of dangerous drugs and the selection of safer alternatives (Abad-Santos et al., 2024; Stratton & Olson, 2023). Pharmacogenomics has a significant impact on the healthcare system. It has led to the creation of personalized therapies based on biomarkers, which are rapidly gaining food and drug agency (FDA) clearance. Pharmacogenomics has also influenced clinical trial design and execution, focusing on identifying predictive biomarkers for specific patient groups.

Cancer treatment has advanced significantly with the emergence of pharmacogenomics, which plays a vital role in finding genetic alterations in tumors that certain medications can target. However, pharmacogenomics can alter healthcare by enabling extra personalized, actual, and safe therapies (Kabbani et al., 2023). Furthermore, genomics- and pharmacogenomics-based personalized drug development has hastened the creation of more effective and safer medicines in PM. The most frequent tools employed in this procedure are genomic profiling and biomarker discovery, which detect genetic mutations and changes associated with diseases. Focusing on these precise alterations makes designing and optimizing lead compounds possible using high-throughput screening and structure-based drug design. Furthermore, personalized drug development aims to avoid adverse drug interactions, optimize drug dosing, and allow for the creation of customized medical goods based on individual needs. Not only does PM accelerate clinical trials, improve success rates, enable focused medicines, and raise development costs (Detroja et al., 2024; Jogani et al., 2024; Johny & Mishra, 2023; Maru et al., 2023; Mehta et al., 2023; Sunildutt et al., 2023; Tosca et al., 2023), But personalized medication development is changing healthcare by tailoring therapies to individual patients based on genetic, molecular, and clinical characteristics. One of the most serious characteristics of personalized treatment advances is the realization that people can react significantly differently to the same treatment. Genetic variants can influence how the body metabolizes, transports, and interacts with medicine, resulting in significant variances in efficacy and safety. The potential benefits include enhancing clinical outcomes, lowering the likelihood of adverse drug responses, and making better use of scarce healthcare resources. However, in recent years, the introduction of personalized diagnostics in PM to drug development has sparked a movement to develop new drugs and diagnostic tests in healthcare, where big data and AI play a critical role through data integration analysis, predictive modeling, patient monitoring support, and many other applications. However, various tools and technologies are used to analyze specific patient features and personalize treatment, such as genetic testing, NGS, and molecular imaging (Chintala, 2023). The application of AI and data analytics in healthcare not only enhances patient outcomes by enabling personalized treatment but also contributes to making healthcare more affordable, efficient, and compliant with regulatory needs and ensures data confidentiality and privacy, which are critical for winning patient trust. However, PM is a transformative approach in healthcare that leverages genomic information, advanced data analytics, and tailored therapies to deliver more precise, effective, and AI-driven analytics and big data; healthcare providers can develop personalized treatment strategies that optimize therapeutic outcomes while minimizing the negative effects (Gupta & Kumar, 2023). However, PM enables customized approaches in healthcare and has demonstrated significant benefits in addressing a variety of illnesses such as cancer, cardiovascular diseases, neurological disorders, and age-related diseases. This approach allows healthcare providers to develop targeted therapies, optimize medication, and implement preventive strategies tailored to each patient's needs.

8.4 ADVANCEMENT AND CHALLENGES

All patients diagnosed with the same medical condition will not have the same reaction to the treatments due to the different genetic makeup of every individual. Therefore, with PM, one can find treatments based on their requirement. Genomics studies an organism's whole gene pool or genome and how those genes function and interact with one another and the environment. It includes aspects of genetics and mainly focuses on characterizing every gene in an organism. Today, genomics is a critical field of medical science; genomics, along with bioinformatics tools, can sequence the entire genome or exome, WES to target protein-coding genes, providing a balance between cost and benefit compared to WGS. WES generates big data that require new computational approaches and AI for analysis. Genomics studies the entire individual genome, making it possible to diagnose rare diseases and tumors quickly and accurately, allowing for PM approaches. With wider biotechnological applications, genomics facilitates the creation of synthetic bacterial genomes and oral plant vaccines. Also, genomic analysis is used in conservation biology to assess genetic diversity, find evolutionary trends, and create plans for the conservation of particular species, and also biomarkers related to certain diseases can be identified (McCarthy et al., 2013; Pattan et al., 2021; Sperber et al., 2017). In order to better comprehend genetic and genomic information, the evolutionary aspects of molecular biology, and the structure of biological pathways and networks, genomics and bioinformatics collaborate to analyze and interpret biological data. One of the most important advantages of genomic studies today is the introduction of PM: it is a growing area, also called precision medicine, which makes judgments about illness prevention, diagnosis, and therapy based on a patient's genetic profile, as genomics plays a very central role in the advancement of PM (Stark et al., 2019; Stefanicka-Wojtas & Kurpas, 2023; Stratton & Olson, 2023).

Furthermore, early disease detection and prevention is one of the critical functions of PM. Every person has a different genetic profile and set of molecular traits that affect how quickly a disease develops, how well it responds to treatment, and how susceptible they are to disease. Because of these individual variances, a one-size-fits-all treatment method frequently falls short of expectations. With the help of genomics, a person's genetic profile can be ascertained, making illness prevention, diagnosis, and treatment more accurate. Finding genetic variants that affect drug response, treatment efficacy, and illness susceptibility is part of this, enabling pharmacogenomics (i.e., studying how an individual's genomic makeup impacts their reaction to medications. It integrates the science of pharmacology with genomics to generate more efficient and safer drugs matched to an individual genetic profile.) to determine the suitable drug and quantity for a patient based on their genetic profile, enhancing the effectiveness of therapy and minimizing side effects. When aware of their genetic and environmental factors, patients can make more informed decisions regarding lifestyle choices, treatment alternatives, and disease management techniques. This promotes improved adherence and overall well-being. More than 25% of newly approved pharmaceuticals are personalized, targeted therapies created based on a patient's molecular profile, particularly in oncology; especially in children who are suffering from very rare genetic diseases, rapid genome sequencing can be used to identify the condition and give the correct personalized treatment with minimum side effects (Mishra et al., 2019; Pattan et al., 2021; Sperber et al., 2017). One of the most important advantages of PM and treatments is they can lower long-term healthcare expenditures by preventing advanced and chronic illnesses through early identification, avoiding unneeded therapies, and identifying the most effective treatments, all while requiring an upfront investment. With all the advancements and developments in PM, researchers in this field are encouraged to create or develop new technologies, such as targeted therapies and enhanced analytics. These technologies can enhance early detection and the development of more effective treatments for the future.

With all the great achievements in the field, numerous risks and challenges are associated with relying on PM. One of the most challenging tasks is data management, where AI and bioinformatics tools are used. Still, it is difficult to convert the rapidly expanding amount of data in the healthcare industry into clinically useful information for patients. Using the increased amount of medical data that have been gathered to provide tailored care, therapies, and prognostic diagnoses is the difficult part; ensuring accuracy and reliability is another task. Also, because of the intricacy of genetic connections and the requirement for sophisticated bioinformatics techniques, interpreting the functional impact of genomic variants is a substantial challenge. It is crucial but difficult to guard patient data concealment and the privacy of genetic evidence, particularly when more and more data are gathered, saved, and shared. Although the long-term cost savings from tailored treatment may be substantial, the initial expenses may be substantial. Certain individuals may find obtaining genetic testing and other customized treatments challenging due to their high cost. Precision medicine and physicians' training to deliver individualized care are still relatively new. This may prevent certain patients from receiving precision medicine, especially those who live in remote places or have low incomes (Mishra et al., 2024a, 2024b; Rose, 2013; Uffelmann et al., 2021; Weymann et al., 2022; Wright et al., 2023). PM suggests that cancer therapy targeting dysregulated pathways can be transformational. However, the efficacy of these medications on overall cancer survival has been limited, possibly due to the adaptive nature of cancer. One risk factor is that the application of precision medicine raises ethical questions. Genetic testing can provide private health information that can be used against a patient in discriminatory ways, such as when applying for jobs or getting insurance. Most importantly, there are worries that genetic information could be exploited, leading to insurance firms refusing to cover individuals with specific genetic predispositions. Although PM can potentially improve the understanding of rare diseases and uncover new therapeutic targets, it is unlikely to improve risk estimate, dynamic behavior, cost-effectiveness, and public well-being outcomes for common illnesses.

8.5 CONCLUSION

Overall, genetic techniques in healthcare have hugely favored PM as they give us tailored diagnoses, treatments, and prevention grounded on an entity's genomic makeup, environmental factors, and routine. Targeted screening and preventive actions can be conducted by identifying genetic markers linked to the disease. For example, an individual susceptible to certain diseases, such as cancer or inherited disorders, can be tested, their risks can be evaluated, and action can be taken early in the illness's progression. By identifying the most effective course of action, including the right drugs, doses, and treatment plans, the personalized approach helps maximize therapeutic efficacy and minimize side effects. Beyond the clinical context, PM can revolutionize healthcare by promoting holistic approaches, considering the social and biological factors determining disease. Despite the challenges, combining genetics and PM will be extremely important to healthcare delivery in the future because it provides solutions tailored to each patient's specific needs, improves healthcare delivery efficiency, and reduces healthcare disparities.

REFERENCES

Abad-Santos, F., Aliño, S. F., Borobia, A. M., García-Martín, E., Gassó, P., Maroñas, O., & Agúndez, J. A. (2024). Developments in pharmacogenetics, pharmacogenomics, and personalized medicine. *Pharmacological Research*, 200, 107061.

Bajinka, O., Ouedraogo, S. Y., Golubnitschaja, O., Li, N., & Zhan, X. (2024). Energy metabolism as the hub of advanced non-small cell lung cancer management: a comprehensive view in the framework of predictive, preventive, and personalized medicine. *EPMA Journal*, 1–31.

Birney, E., Vamathevan, J., & Goodhand, P. (2017). Genomics in healthcare: GA4GH looks to 2022. *BioRxiv*, 203554.

Bisson, W. (2012). Drug repurposing in chemical genomics: can we learn from the past to improve the future? *Current Topics in Medicinal Chemistry*, 12(17), 1883–1888.

Blobel, B., Oemig, F., Ruotsalainen, P., Brochhausen, M., & Giacomini, M. (2024). The representational challenge for designing and managing 5P medicine ecosystems. In *pHealth 2024* (pp. 3–13). IOS Press.

Brehio, T. L. (2024). The age of scientific wellness: why the future of medicine is personalized, predictive, data-rich, and in your hands. *Family Medicine*, 56(1), 60.

Brlek, P., Bulić, L., Bračić, M., Projić, P., Škaro, V., Shah, N., Shah, P., & Primorac, D. (2024). Implementing whole genome sequencing (WGS) in clinical practice: advantages, challenges, and future perspectives. *Cells*, 13(6), 504.

Carrasco-Ramiro, F., Peiró-Pastor, R., & Aguado, B. (2017). Human genomics projects and precision medicine. *Gene Therapy*, 24(9), 551–561.

Casolino, R., Beer, P. A., Chakravarty, D., Davis, M. B., Malapelle, U., Mazzarella, L., Normanno, N., Pauli, C., Subbiah, V., & Turnbull, C. (2024). Interpreting and integrating genomic tests results in clinical cancer care: Overview and practical guidance. *CA: A Cancer Journal for Clinicians*, 74(3), 264–285.

Chejara, D. R., Badhe, R. V., Kumar, P., Choonara, Y. E., Tomar, L. K., Tyagi, C., & Pillay, V. (2018). Rethinking drug discovery and targeting after the genomic revolution. *Genomics-Driven Healthcare: Trends in Disease Prevention and Treatment*, 1–17.

Chintala, S. (2023). AI-driven personalised treatment plans: the future of precision medicine. *Machine Intelligence Research*, 17(02), 9718–9728.

Cruz-Correia, R., Ferreira, D., Bacelar, G., Marques, P., & Maranhão, P. (2018). Personalised medicine challenges: quality of data. *International Journal of Data Science and Analytics*, 6(3), 251–259.

Delpierre, C., & Lefèvre, T. (2023). Precision and personalized medicine: what their current definition says and silences about the model of health they promote. Implication for the development of personalized health. *Frontiers in Sociology*, 8, 1112159.

Detroja, K., Sharma, K., Mishra, S. K., & Georrge, J. J. (2024). Phytochemical profiling of Tamarindus indica: a medicinal plant for snakebite. In *Herbal Formulations, Phytochemistry and Pharmacognosy* (pp. 413–421). Elsevier.

Dey, A., Mitra, A., Pathak, S., Prasad, S., Zhang, A. S., Zhang, H., Sun, X.-F., & Banerjee, A. (2023). Recent advancements, limitations, and future perspectives of the use of personalized medicine in treatment of colon cancer. *Technology in Cancer Research & Treatment*, 22, 15330338231178403.

Emilien, G., Ponchon, M., Caldas, C., Isacson, O., & Maloteaux, J. M. (2000). Impact of genomics on drug discovery and clinical medicine. *Qjm*, 93(7), 391–423.

Foo, J.-N., Liu, J.-J., & Tan, E.-K. (2012). Whole-genome and whole-exome sequencing in neurological diseases. *Nature Reviews Neurology*, 8(9), 508–517.

Frank, M., Prenzler, A., Eils, R., & Graf von der Schulenburg, J.-M. (2013). Genome sequencing: a systematic review of health economic evidence. *Health Economics Review*, 3, 1–8.

Green, E. D., Gunter, C., Biesecker, L. G., Di Francesco, V., Easter, C. L., Feingold, E. A., Felsenfeld, A. L., Kaufman, D. J., Ostrander, E. A., & Pavan, W. J. (2020). Strategic vision for improving human health at The Forefront of Genomics. *Nature*, 586(7831), 683–692.

Grissa, I., Vergnaud, G., & Pourcel, C. (2009). Clustered regularly interspaced short palindromic repeats (CRISPRs) for the genotyping of bacterial pathogens. *Molecular Epidemiology of Microorganisms: Methods and Protocols*, 105–116.

Grody, W. W., Thompson, B. H., & Hudgins, L. (2013). Whole-exome/genome sequencing and genomics. *Pediatrics*, 132(Supplement_3), S211–S215.

Gupta, N. S., & Kumar, P. (2023). Perspective of artificial intelligence in healthcare data management: a journey towards precision medicine. *Computers in Biology and Medicine*, 107051.

Harvey, A., Brand, A., Holgate, S. T., Kristiansen, L. V., Lehrach, H., Palotie, A., & Prainsack, B. (2012). The future of technologies for personalized medicine. *New Biotechnology*, 29(6), 625–633.

Hong, M., Tao, S., Zhang, L., Diao, L.-T., Huang, X., Huang, S., Xie, S.-J., Xiao, Z.-D., & Zhang, H. (2020). RNA sequencing: new technologies and applications in cancer research. *Journal of Hematology & Oncology*, 13, 1–16.

Horner, D. S., Pavesi, G., Castrignano, T., De Meo, P. D. O., Liuni, S., Sammeth, M., Picardi, E., & Pesole, G. (2010). Bioinformatics approaches for genomics and post genomics applications of next-generation sequencing. *Briefings in Bioinformatics*, 11(2), 181–197.

Howard, H. C., Swinnen, E., Douw, K., Vondeling, H., Cassiman, J.-J., Cambon-Thomsen, A., & Borry, P. (2013). The ethical introduction of genome-based information and technologies into public health. *Public Health Genomics*, 16(3), 100–109.

Illert, A. L., Stenzinger, A., Bitzer, M., Horak, P., Gaidzik, V. I., Möller, Y., Beha, J., Öner, Ö., Schmitt, F., & Lassmann, S. (2023). The German Network for personalized medicine to enhance patient care and translational research. *Nature Medicine*, 29(6), 1298–1301.

Jogani, R., Mishra, S. K., Sharma, K., & Georrge, J. J. (2024). Metabolite profiling of Rauvolfia serpentina: an antivenom plant. In *Herbal Formulations, Phytochemistry and Pharmacognosy* (pp. 255–260). Elsevier.

Johny, A., & Mishra, S. K. (2023). Pharmacological effects of bioactive compounds from allium sativum. In *Pharmacological Benefits of Natural Agents* (pp. 13–30). IGI Global.

Kabbani, D., Akika, R., Wahid, A., Daly, A. K., Cascorbi, I., & Zgheib, N. K. (2023). Pharmacogenomics in practice: a review and implementation guide. *Frontiers in Pharmacology*, 14, 1189976.

Kaboli, S., & Babazada, H. (2018). CRISPR mediated genome engineering and its application in industry. *Current Issues in Molecular Biology*, 26(1), 81–92.

Kernohan, K. D., & Boycott, K. M. (2024). The expanding diagnostic toolbox for rare genetic diseases. *Nature Reviews Genetics*, 1–15.

Kho, A. N., Rasmussen, L. V., Connolly, J. J., Peissig, P. L., Starren, J., Hakonarson, H., & Hayes, M. G. (2013). Practical challenges in integrating genomic data into the electronic health record. *Genetics in Medicine*, 15(10), 772–778.

Kumar, R., & Khurana, A. (2014). Functional genomics of tomato: opportunities and challenges in post-genome NGS era. *Journal of Biosciences*, 39, 917–929.

Lal, J., Sudbrak, R., Lehrach, H., & Brand, A. (2013). Functional dynamics: from biological complexity to translation and impact in healthcare systems. *Journal of Computer Science and Systems Biology*, 6(2), 88–92.

Li, C., & He, W.-Q. (2023). Global prediction of primary liver cancer incidences and mortality in 2040. *Journal of Hepatology*, *78*(4), e144–e146.

Li, H., Yang, Y., Hong, W., Huang, M., Wu, M., & Zhao, X. (2020). Applications of genome editing technology in the targeted therapy of human diseases: mechanisms, advances and prospects. *Signal Transduction and Targeted Therapy*, *5*(1), 1.

Liu, W., Li, L., Jiang, J., Wu, M., & Lin, P. (2021). Applications and challenges of CRISPR-Cas gene-editing to disease treatment in clinics. *Precision Clinical Medicine*, *4*(3), 179–191. https://doi.org/10.1093/pcmedi/pbab014

Maru, H., Sharma, K., & Mishra, S. K. (2023). A comprehensive review of ethnomedical uses, phytochemical studies, and properties of Holy Basil (*Ocimum sanctum* Linn.). *Pharmacological Benefits of Natural Agents*, 49–68.

Marzban, S., Najafi, M., Agolli, A., & Ashrafi, E. (2022). Impact of patient engagement on healthcare quality: a scoping review. *Journal of Patient Experience*, *9*, 23743735221125439. https://doi.org/10.1177/23743735221125439

McCarthy, J. J., McLeod, H. L., & Ginsburg, G. S. (2013). Genomic medicine: a decade of successes, challenges, and opportunities. *Science Translational Medicine*, *5*(189), 189sr184–189sr184.

Mehta, H. J., Mishra, S. K., & Sharma, K. (2023). Phytochemical studies of *Piper nigrum* L: a comprehensive review. *Pharmacological Benefits of Natural Agents*, 31–48.

Mishra, S. K., & Georrge, J. J. (2024). Tools and platform for allergenicity prediction. In *Reverse Vaccinology* (pp. 165–178). Elsevier.

Mishra, S. K., Jeba Praba, J., & Georrge, J. J. (2024a). An emerging trends of bioinformatics and big data analytics in healthcare. *Digital Transformation in Healthcare 5.0: Volume 2: Metaverse, Nanorobots and Machine Learning*, 159.

Mishra, S. K., Pandya, M., Bhatt, T., & Georrge, J. J. (2024b). Reverse vaccinology 2.0: computational resources for B-cell epitope prediction. In *Reverse Vaccinology* (pp. 203–216). Elsevier.

Mishra, S. K., Priya, P., Rai, G. P., Haque, R., & Shanker, A. (2023). Coevolution based immunoinformatics approach considering variability of epitopes to combat different strains: a case study using spike protein of SARS-CoV−2. *Computers in Biology and Medicine*, *163*, 107233.

Mishra, V., Chanda, P., Tambuwala, M. M., & Suttee, A. (2019). Personalized medicine: an overview. *International Journal of Pharmaceutical Quality Assurance*, *10*(2), 290–294.

Nebert, D. W., Zhang, G., & Vesell, E. S. (2008). From human genetics and genomics to pharmacogenetics and pharmacogenomics: past lessons, future directions. *Drug Metabolism Reviews*, *40*(2), 187–224.

Pattan, V., Kashyap, R., Bansal, V., Candula, N., Koritala, T., & Surani, S. (2021). Genomics in medicine: a new era in medicine. *World Journal of Methodology*, *11*(5), 231–242. https://doi.org/10.5662/wjm.v11.i5.231

Payne, K., Gavan, S. P., Wright, S. J., & Thompson, A. J. (2018). Cost-effectiveness analyses of genetic and genomic diagnostic tests. *Nature Reviews Genetics*, *19*(4), 235–246.

Rose, N. (2013). Personalized medicine: promises, problems and perils of a new paradigm for healthcare. *Procedia-Social and Behavioral Sciences*, *77*, 341–352.

Sadee, W., & Dai, Z. (2005). Pharmacogenetics/genomics and personalized medicine. *Human Molecular Genetics*, *14*(suppl_2), R207–R214.

Satam, H., Joshi, K., Mangrolia, U., Waghoo, S., Zaidi, G., Rawool, S., Thakare, R. P., Banday, S., Mishra, A. K., Das, G., & Malonia, S. K. (2023). Next-generation sequencing technology: current trends and advancements. *Biology (Basel)*, *12*(7). https://doi.org/10.3390/biology12070997

Sperber, N. R., Carpenter, J. S., Cavallari, L. H., L, J. D., Cooper-DeHoff, R. M., Denny, J. C., Ginsburg, G. S., Guan, Y., Horowitz, C. R., Levy, K. D., Levy, M. A., Madden, E. B., Matheny, M. E., Pollin, T. I., Pratt, V. M., Rosenman, M., Voils, C. I., K, W. W., Wilke, R. A., Ryanne Wu, R., & Orlando, L. A. (2017). Challenges and strategies for implementing genomic services in diverse settings: experiences from the Implementing GeNomics In pracTicE (IGNITE) network. *BMC Med Genomics*, *10*(1), 35. https://doi.org/10.1186/s12920-017-0273-2

Stadler, Z. K., Schrader, K. A., Vijai, J., Robson, M. E., & Offit, K. (2014). Cancer genomics and inherited risk. *Journal of Clinical Oncology*, *32*(7), 687–698. https://doi.org/10.1200/JCO.2013.49.72710

Stark, Z., Dolman, L., Manolio, T. A., Ozenberger, B., Hill, S. L., Caulfied, M. J., Levy, Y., Glazer, D., Wilson, J., & Lawler, M. (2019). Integrating genomics into healthcare: a global responsibility. *The American Journal of Human Genetics*, *104*(1), 13–20.

Stefanicka-Wojtas, D., & Kurpas, D. (2023). Personalised medicine—implementation to the healthcare system in Europe (Focus Group Discussions). *Journal of Personalized Medicine*, *13*(3), 380.

Stratton, T. P., & Olson, A. W. (2023). Personalizing personalized medicine: the confluence of pharmacogenomics, a person's medication experience and ethics. *Pharmacy*, *11*(3), 101.

Subica, A. M. (2023). CRISPR in public health: the health equity implications and role of community in gene-editing research and applications. *American Journal of Public Health*, *113*(8), 874–882. https://doi.org/10.2105/AJPH.2023.307315

Sugandh, F., Chandio, M., Raveena, F., Kumar, L., Karishma, F., Khuwaja, S., Memon, U. A., Bai, K., Kashif, M., & Varrassi, G. (2023). Advances in the management of diabetes mellitus: a focus on personalized medicine. *Cureus*, *15*(8).

Sunildutt, N., Parihar, P., Chethikkattuveli Salih, A. R., Lee, S. H., & Choi, K. H. (2023). Revolutionizing drug development: harnessing the potential of organ-on-chip technology for disease modeling and drug discovery. *Frontiers in Pharmacology*, *14*, 1139229.

Supplitt, S., Karpinski, P., Sasiadek, M., & Laczmanska, I. (2021). Current achievements and applications of transcriptomics in personalized cancer medicine. *International Journal of Molecular Sciences*, *22*(3). https://doi.org/10.3390/ijms22031422

Tawfik, S. M., Elhosseiny, A. A., Galal, A. A., William, M. B., Qansuwa, E., Elbaz, R. M., & Salama, M. (2023). Health inequity in genomic personalized medicine in underrepresented populations: a look at the current evidence. *Functional & Integrative Genomics*, *23*(1), 54.

Tosca, E. M., Ronchi, D., Facciolo, D., & Magni, P. (2023). Replacement, reduction, and refinement of animal experiments in anticancer drug development: the contribution of 3D in vitro cancer models in the drug efficacy assessment. *Biomedicines*, *11*(4), 1058.

Turro, E., Astle, W. J., Megy, K., Gräf, S., Greene, D., Shamardina, O., Allen, H. L., Sanchis-Juan, A., Frontini, M., & Thys, C. (2020). Whole-genome sequencing of patients with rare diseases in a national health system. *Nature*, *583*(7814), 96–102.

Uffelmann, E., Huang, Q. Q., Munung, N. S., De Vries, J., Okada, Y., Martin, A. R., Martin, H. C., Lappalainen, T., & Posthuma, D. (2021). Genome-wide association studies. *Nature Reviews Methods Primers*, *1*(1), 59.

Vakhariya, S., Mishra, S. K., & Georrge, J. J. (2023a). Identification of Novel Curcumin Analogues to Inhibit Mitogen-Activated Protein Kinase 1 Using In Silico Combinatorial Library Design and Molecular Docking Approach. *Available at SSRN 4649193*.

Vakhariya, S., Mishra, S. K., Sharma, K., & Georrge, J. J. (2023b). Designing of a novel curcumin analogue to inhibit mitogen-activated protein kinase: a cheminformatics approach. *Journal of Phytonanotechnology and Pharmaceutical Sciences*, *3*(1), 37–47.

Vinjoda, P., Mishra, S. K., Sharma, K., & Georrge, J. J. (2024). In silico identification of novel drug target and its natural product inhibitors for herpes simplex virus. In *Nanotechnology and In Silico Tools* (pp. 377–383). Elsevier.

Vinksel, M., Writzl, K., Maver, A., & Peterlin, B. (2021). Improving diagnostics of rare genetic diseases with NGS approaches. *Journal of Community Genetics*, *12*(2), 247–256. https://doi.org/10.1007/s12687-020-00500-5

Ward, S. J. (2001). Impact of genomics in drug discovery. *Biotechniques*, *31*(3), 626–634.

Werner, T. (2010). Next generation sequencing in functional genomics. *Briefings in Bioinformatics*, *11*(5), 499–511.

Weymann, D., Dragojlovic, N., Pollard, S., & Regier, D. A. (2022). Allocating healthcare resources to genomic testing in Canada: latest evidence and current challenges. *Journal of Community Genetics*, *13*(5), 467–476.

Wright, C. F., Campbell, P., Eberhardt, R. Y., Aitken, S., Perrett, D., Brent, S., Danecek, P., Gardner, E. J., Chundru, V. K., & Lindsay, S. J. (2023). Genomic diagnosis of rare pediatric disease in the United Kingdom and Ireland. *New England Journal of Medicine*, *388*(17), 1559–1571.

Zhang, J., Chiodini, R., Badr, A., & Zhang, G. (2011). The impact of next-generation sequencing on genomics. *Journal of Genetics and Genomics*, *38*(3), 95–109.

Zhang, Y., Li, N., Yang, L., Jia, W., Li, Z., Shao, Q., & Zhan, X. (2023). Quantitative phosphoproteomics reveals molecular pathway network alterations in human early-stage primary hepatic carcinomas: potential for 3P medical approach. *EPMA Journal*, *14*(3), 477–502.

9 Preferences and Selection of Vaccines by Healthcare Consumers

Antonio Pesqueira, Andréia de Bem Machado, and Maria José Sousa

9.1 INTRODUCTION

The ongoing global pandemic has highlighted the critical importance of vaccines and the necessity for efficacious vaccination campaigns in our increasingly interconnected world (Bouguerra et al., 2022).

Global pandemic crisis has highlighted the necessity for international collaboration in order to rapidly identify, prevent, and control the dissemination of infectious diseases. Vaccines represent a vital instrument in the fight against infectious diseases, and the success of vaccination campaigns hinges on individuals receiving the necessary vaccinations (Prasert et al., 2022).

In light of the increasing demand for accessible and affordable healthcare products, it is imperative to gain insight into HC behavior in order to guarantee the sustainability and equitable distribution of pharmaceutical products, including vaccines. This understanding is pivotal to addressing the intricate challenges confronting the healthcare industry (Schoch-Spana et al., 2021).

Notwithstanding recent advances in the utilization of predictive technologies and managerial dynamic capabilities (MDC) in intricate healthcare domains such as HC vaccine preferences and selection, there is a paucity of studies that focus on the prediction of customer purchase behavior and the impact of predictive technology on HC preferences and vaccine selection in healthcare (Thompson et al., 2021).

MDC, such as the capacity to sense, capture, and reconfigure resources in response to HC needs, have emerged as pivotal factors in shaping behaviors and driving the adoption of new technologies within the healthcare sector (Eisenhardt & Martin, 2000).

Other factors, such as sustainability, mass media, efficacy determinants, and product knowledge, also contribute to HC preferences and behavioral choices. However, there is a growing number of research investigating the connections between predictive technology, MDC, and HC preferences in healthcare (Teece, 2010; Teece, 2014).

This chapter aims to identify and examine the principal relationships between predictive technology, MDC, and HC preferences through a literature review based on the TCCM framework. This study evaluates the opportunities and challenges that arise from these interconnections and investigates the role of MDC in shaping HC behaviors and technology adoption in healthcare.

The findings of this study may inform future research and the implementation of MDC and technology in complex areas such as HC preferences and vaccine selection. This research explores the interconnections between micro-MDC, particularly in the domains of sensing and seizing market opportunities, and the preferences and behavioral patterns of HC when selecting and choosing vaccines.

By examining the existing literature on predictive technology and MDC, this study provides valuable insights for policymakers and healthcare providers.

The objective of this preliminary literature review is to examine and integrate existing research on the factors influencing vaccine distribution and HC behavior during the ongoing pandemic. Other secondary objectives aim to examine the impact of trust on vaccine uptake and assess the

DOI: 10.1201/9781003485629-9

potential of predictive technologies to enhance vaccine distribution strategies. By examining these key areas, the chapter seeks to provide a foundation for understanding the challenges and opportunities in optimizing vaccine distribution and improving public health outcomes. Furthermore, it assesses operational efficiency, sustainability, and the relationship between predictive technology and managerial dynamic capabilities. Conducted from an academic standpoint that is independent of any commercial or industrial interests related to the pharmaceutical or healthcare industries, the objective of this research is to provide unbiased, evidence-based insights that can inform healthcare policymakers and providers in their decision-making processes.

9.2 PRELIMINARY LITERATURE REVIEW

9.2.1 VACCINE DISTRIBUTION AND HC BEHAVIOR

In the context of the global pandemic caused by severe acute respiratory syndrome coronavirus 2 (SARS-CoV-2), it was vital for industries and governments to work together to address supply chain disruptions and optimize the distribution of vaccines (Baumgaertner et al., 2018).

The accelerated development, production, and distribution of vaccines during the pandemic were made possible through unprecedented cross-sector and cross-border collaboration. However, this process was beset with challenges, including maintaining the integrity of supply chains and ensuring the timely delivery of vaccines and related supplies (Betsch et al., 2018).

The surge in demand resulting from the pandemic not only disrupted retail markets but also had broader economic repercussions. This phenomenon, in conjunction with the documented psychological responses of fear and uncertainty among HCs, illustrates the intricate relationship between HC behaviors and the occurrence of public health crises (Bouguerra et al., 2022).

The global health crisis precipitated by SARS-CoV-2 has had a profound impact on healthcare systems around the world, underscoring the vital importance of effective vaccine distribution strategies. One notable consequence of the pandemic was the phenomenon of panic purchasing, which not only disrupted retail markets but also had broader negative effects on economies. These behaviors were driven by psychological reactions to the uncertainty and fear associated with infectious disease outbreaks, as extensively documented by scholars (Jiang et al., 2021).

In the context of the ongoing crisis, vaccines have emerged as a crucial instrument in the fight against the spread of the virus, offering substantial financial and health benefits. However, they also introduced challenges, such as the need to manage the risks of drug interactions and to ensure correct dosing (Cifuentes-Faura, 2022).

The pandemic has highlighted the intricate interrelationship between HC behavior, trust in healthcare systems, and the technological innovations that can facilitate vaccine distribution. By focusing on these interconnected elements, healthcare systems can better prepare for future public health challenges, ensuring the equitable and efficient distribution of vaccines across populations (Zhong et al., 2020).

9.2.2 THE ROLE OF TRUST AND POLITICAL INFLUENCE ON VACCINE ACCEPTANCE

A number of factors, including trust, the perceived altruism of pharmacists, knowledge, and the quality of customer service, have been identified as having a significant influence on the behavior of HCs. It is of the utmost importance that these elements be given careful consideration when developing strategies for the selection and distribution of vaccines (Shepherd et al., 2020).

This was due to the central role played by trust in healthcare professionals (HCPs), past experiences, and perceived efficacy and safety of vaccines. The level of trust in vaccines, particularly during the ongoing pandemic, has been significantly shaped by political forces and public policies, notably in the United States. As Dubé et al. (2013) observe, vaccine hesitancy frequently arises from a multifaceted interaction of factors, including political, cultural, and social contexts. This was evident during the COVID-19 pandemic, where public confidence in vaccines fluctuated based on the perceived transparency and integrity of the vaccine development process (Funk & Tyson, 2020). Furthermore, Jaiswal and Halkitis (2020) discuss how medical mistrust, which has its roots in historical injustices and is intensified by contemporary political discourse, has resulted in an increase in vaccine hesitancy among marginalized communities. Furthermore, Latkin et al. (2021) highlight that trust in vaccines is shaped by a social-ecological framework, whereby political narratives, social influences, and individual beliefs converge, often resulting in varied acceptance levels across different demographic groups (Tran et al., 2019).

The role of misinformation, as discussed by Salali and Uysal (2020), must also be considered, as it has been a significant factor in undermining trust in vaccines, particularly when coupled with politicized narratives about the pandemic.

The level of trust placed in healthcare professionals and the perceived safety and efficacy of vaccines had a significant impact on HC decisions regarding treatment options. The establishment and preservation of trust constituted a pivotal element in the success of vaccination campaigns. The implementation of targeted strategies to mitigate vaccine hesitancy and foster acceptance has been identified as a critical priority in public health efforts, as highlighted by the World Health Organization (2018).

It is of the utmost importance that public health campaigns educate the public about the significance of vaccination. In order to improve vaccine uptake, it is essential that these campaigns proactively address the pervasive misconceptions that exist. By focusing on the benefits of herd immunity and the role that individuals play in disease control, tailored communication strategies can effectively overcome vaccine hesitancy and encourage acceptance (Pesqueira et al., 2020).

9.2.3   PREDICTIVE TECHNOLOGIES AND MDC IN VACCINE DISTRIBUTION

The application of predictive technology in the field of vaccine preferences and selection has the potential to contribute to more effective distribution management (Cifuentes-Faura, 2022). The advancement of predictive technologies has the potential for HC preferences, vaccine selection, and cognitive attitudes (Sousa & Costa, 2022).

The effective alignment of vaccine selection with HC preferences and behavioral patterns requires the deployment of dynamic capabilities, particularly in the sensing and capitalization of emerging market opportunities (Smith et al., 2020).

The development of vaccines tailored to meet market demands could be enhanced by adapting to these changes. The utilization of individual dynamic capabilities has the potential to enhance the efficacy of vaccine campaigns. This may be achieved by predicting and analyzing HC behavior data, and subsequently adapting campaigns to align with evolving preferences. The fostering of trust and collaboration between healthcare providers and HCs, with an emphasis on individual choices in achieving herd immunity and controlling disease spread, has the potential to result in more effective public health interventions (Gebhardt et al., 2022).

The implementation of efficient distribution strategies, digital technology utilization, and personalized marketing campaigns serves to enhance awareness and facilitate access to vaccines. The alignment of vaccine offerings with HC preferences has been demonstrated to enhance uptake rates. It is incumbent upon HCPs to prioritize the establishment of trust and the delivery of patient-centered care in order to foster positive relationships with HCs (Sasaki et al., 2022).

The pandemic highlighted the significance of individual dynamic capabilities in influencing healthcare preferences and behavioral patterns (Dash et al., 2019). By leveraging these capabilities, stakeholders are able to design bespoke vaccine campaigns that address the specific HC needs and preferences. This will result in an improvement in vaccine uptake rates and public health outcomes (Salali & Uysal, 2020).

Although the extant literature has examined a range of dimensions pertaining to MDC and predictive technologies, notable deficiencies persist in our comprehension of the long-term influence of these variables on vaccine distribution strategies. Moreover, the majority of existing research has concentrated on Western healthcare systems, with little attention paid to the distinctive challenges encountered by emerging markets. Furthermore, there is a paucity of studies examining the intersection of cultural and socioeconomic factors with HC vaccine preferences, particularly in diverse populations. It is imperative that these gaps be addressed if more inclusive and effective vaccine distribution strategies are to be developed that are sensitive to the nuances of different demographic groups (Rubin & Wessely, 2020).

The ongoing research and development of predictive technologies has the potential to further refine HC preferences, enhance vaccine selection, and improve cognitive attitudes toward vaccination. The combination of these technologies with strategic investments in community pharmacies and healthcare providers has the potential to optimize vaccine distribution and administration. Such investments guarantee that HCs receive not only the most appropriate vaccines but also the most effective ones currently available (Shujahat et al., 2019).

Predictive technologies encompass a range of tools and methods designed to analyze vast datasets and generate forecasts about future trends and behaviors. In the context of vaccine distribution, these technologies can predict demand, optimize supply chains, and tailor communication strategies to different HC segments. The most commonly used predictive technologies include machine learning (ML) algorithms, artificial intelligence (AI), big data analytics (BDA), and geospatial analysis. A variety of predictive technologies have been utilized in the healthcare sector, particularly during the pandemic, with the objective of optimizing the distribution of vaccines and enhancing HC engagement. Each technology possesses distinctive strengths and is best suited to particular contexts (Ratzan & Moritsugu, 2020).

The application of ML algorithms has been instrumental in the development of predictive technologies in healthcare. ML models are capable of analyzing large datasets in order to identify patterns and make predictions regarding future vaccine demand. To illustrate, during the rollout of the vaccine against the novel coronavirus, ML algorithms were employed to forecast the uptake of the vaccine in different regions, thereby enabling the proactive allocation of doses to areas with anticipated high demand. This technology is particularly effective in scenarios where a substantial corpus of historical data is available, as it can continuously refine its predictions based on new data. Furthermore, AI has played a pivotal role in the personalization of vaccine outreach efforts. AI-driven chatbots and virtual assistants have been implemented to provide HC with tailored information about vaccines, address concerns, and schedule appointments. These tools are capable of analyzing HC behavior and preferences in order to tailor messaging, thereby increasing vaccine acceptance and reducing hesitancy. Furthermore, BDA encompasses the processing and analysis of extensive and intricate datasets to derive actionable insights. In the context of vaccine distribution, BDA platforms have been employed to monitor vaccine storage conditions, track distribution progress, and identify logistical constraints (Jiang et al., 2021).

These analytics are vital for guaranteeing the punctual and efficient delivery of vaccines, particularly in extensive immunization campaigns (Prasert et al., 2022).

9.3 METHODOLOGY

9.3.1 METHODOLOGICAL APPROACH

In this literature review, an exploratory search was conducted across a range of academic databases with the aim of identifying relevant studies. Although the intention was to be comprehensive, the review did not adhere to a systematic approach with regard to the specific inclusion and exclusion criteria or the detailed screening processes. Accordingly, the findings presented should be interpreted as a broad overview of the existing literature, rather than as a systematic synthesis. In order to gain a deeper insight into HC buying behavior, cognitive attitudes and purchasing habits, a comprehensive review of the existing literature was conducted, as illustrated in the figure below (Figure 9.1).

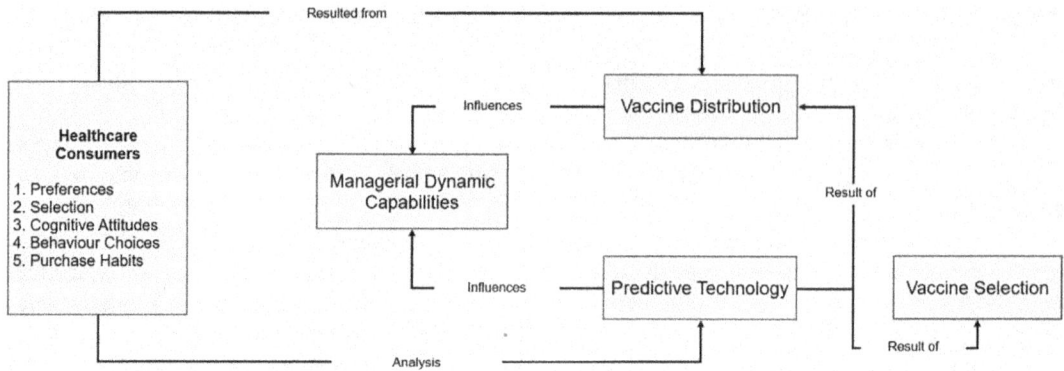

FIGURE 9.1   Conceptual Mapping.

In accordance with established theoretical frameworks, constructs, contexts, and methods, the Theory, Context, Characteristics, and Methods (TCCM) methodology was selected for a systematic and comprehensive review. The analysis of the data collected from the literature review was enabled by the use of R Studio 4.2.0 software and VosViewer. To this end, techniques were employed, including co-occurrence analysis, association strength analysis, network graphs, author analysis, citation network analysis, and co-link matrix analysis (Paul et al., 2021).

The utilization of bibliometric techniques was pivotal to the data analysis process, as it facilitated the identification of pertinent keywords and data points. Furthermore, these techniques enabled the mapping and reorganization of the interconnections between academic articles (Sousa & Costa, 2022; Pesqueira et al., 2020).

The review included publications from PubMed, Scopus, and Web of Science, with 119 publications initially selected for data extraction and analysis. Following rigorous validation and quality control procedures, 58 publications were deemed to meet the requisite standards and were retained for further examination. The study's methodological design was based on scientific network analysis and co-occurrence mapping, which were constructed using the frequency of terms and citation patterns in the relevant literature. The maps were constructed using bibliographic indicators derived from the selected articles (Nguyen & Vuong, 2021).

The review process was conducted in accordance with the following steps: A comprehensive search was conducted across a range of databases, including PubMed, Scopus, and Web of Science. The search terms included a combination of keywords, including "vaccine distribution," "predictive technology," "consumer preferences," "vaccine hesitancy," and "Covid–19."

In regard to the criteria for inclusion and exclusion, studies were included if they met the following criteria: The search yielded peer-reviewed articles published between 2000 and March 2023, studies conducted in healthcare settings, and research focusing on vaccine distribution, predictive technologies, and HC behavior. The exclusion criteria included the following: (1) non-peer-reviewed sources, (2) articles not available in English, and (3) studies focusing on non-healthcare-related topics.

Furthermore, a standardized form was used to extract data from the included studies for the purposes of data synthesis. This form captured details on study design, population, interventions, outcomes, and key findings. The results were synthesized thematically in order to identify patterns and gaps in the existing literature.

The study's comprehensive search was structured around four primary themes: healthcare HC preferences, vaccine selection, technology, and MDC. However, due to the paucity of resources that included all search terms, the selection criteria were broadened by omitting the combination of managerial and dynamic capabilities. The implementation of the TCCM methodology yielded effective results, leading to the generation of robust and consistent findings. By means of

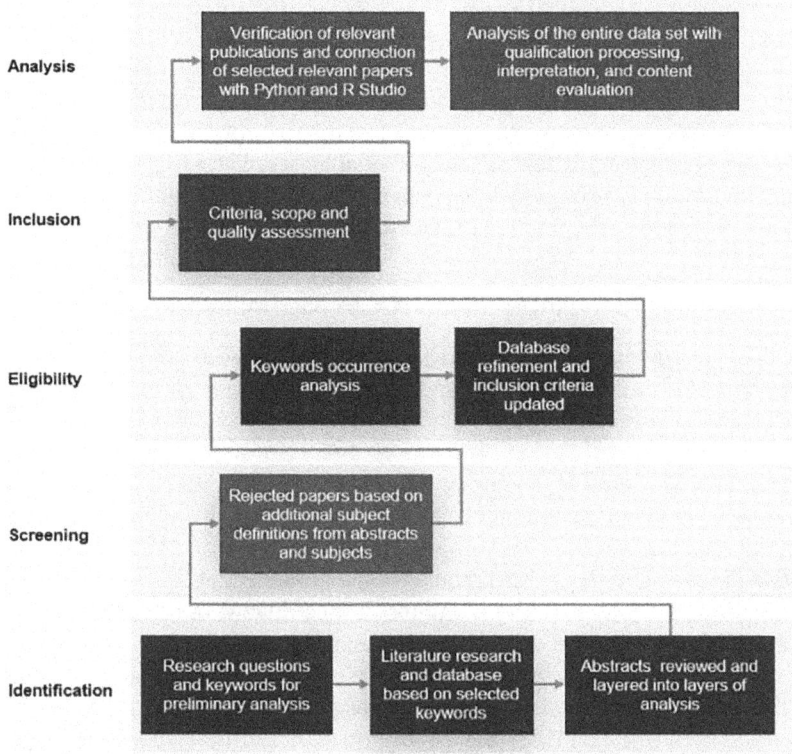

FIGURE 9.2   Applied Methodology.

bibliometric networks, the connections between the most pertinent papers, articles, and publications were elucidated. The networks provided insights into the growth of our research field, enabling the identification of significant trends and patterns. This information proved instrumental in informing our research decisions. The construction of these bibliometric networks facilitated a more nuanced comprehension of the relationships between various publications. Furthermore, it offered insight into the sustained evolution of the research domain (Olivera Mesa et al., 2021).

The visualization revealed the existence of multiple clusters of research, with a particular focus on domains such as predictive algorithms, behavior analysis, and MDC. The analysis encompassed a number of different techniques, including co-occurrence analysis, association strength analysis, network graphs, citation network analysis, and co-authorship relationships. The findings were mapped using bibliographic indicators and binary counting in order to determine the presence or absence of relevant terms (Prahalad & Hamel, 2009).

The study offers valuable insights into significant studies and collaboration patterns. The research process is illustrated in Figure 9.2, which depicts the application of search terms and exclusion criteria in the selected databases.

The data obtained through this clearly defined methodology can inform future research directions and the strategic allocation of resources. Furthermore, the analysis highlights the intrinsic interdisciplinary character of research on predictive technology and vaccine preferences. Acknowledging the links between different fields empowers researchers to design more specific research plans that take into account potential synergies among a range of disciplines.

This strategy allows researchers to focus their efforts on the most promising sectors, thereby increasing the probability of success in their research. The selection criteria for the literature included in this review were designed to ensure the inclusion of high-quality, peer-reviewed studies that are directly relevant to the research questions. The publications were evaluated based on three criteria: methodological rigor, relevance of findings to the study's aims, and contribution to the broader field of healthcare management and vaccine distribution. Studies that did not meet the requisite quality benchmarks or were published in non-peer-reviewed sources were excluded from further consideration. Furthermore, to mitigate potential biases, a cross-validation process was conducted. This entailed multiple reviewers independently assessing the quality and relevance of each study before it was included in the final analysis (Lindholt et al., 2021).

9.3.2 EXPLANATION AND APPLICATION OF THE TCCM METHODOLOGY

In conducting this literature review, the TCCM methodology was employed, which provides a comprehensive framework for synthesizing and analyzing research across various domains. The TCCM framework, originally developed, is designed to guide researchers in conducting a systematic review of the literature by focusing on four key dimensions: The four key dimensions of the TCCM framework are theory, context, characteristics, and methods. Each of these dimensions is of significant importance in comprehending the extant body of research and in identifying avenues for future investigation.

The "Theory" dimension of the TCCM framework entails the identification and synthesis of the theoretical foundations that underpin the literature. In this review, our focus was on theories pertaining to HC behavior, the adoption of predictive technology, and MDC. By analyzing the theoretical foundations of the studies, we were able to map the evolution of key concepts and identify gaps in the current theoretical landscape that require further exploration (Gebhardt et al., 2022).

The "Context" dimension examines the environmental, cultural, and situational factors that influence the phenomena under study. In our review, we examined the influence of diverse contexts, including the global impact of the SARS-CoV-2 pandemic and the variability of healthcare systems, on research pertaining to vaccine distribution and HC preferences. This analysis enabled to comprehend the manner in which contextual factors contribute to the variability in findings and to emphasize the significance of situational specificity in the application of predictive technologies. The "Characteristics" dimension entails an examination of the attributes of the studies included in the review, including the study design, population, and research focus. The characteristics of the studies were analyzed in order to identify both commonalities and differences in the manner in which research on vaccine distribution and HC behavior has been conducted. This dimension facilitated the categorization of the literature into meaningful clusters, thereby providing insights into the methodological strengths and weaknesses of the existing research (Greene et al., 2014).

The "Methods" dimension of the TCCM framework is concerned with the research methodologies deployed in the literature. A review of the methodological approaches employed in the studies was conducted, encompassing quantitative, qualitative, and mixed-methods research. An evaluation of the methods employed enabled us to assess the robustness of the findings and identify methodological trends and gaps in the literature. This dimension also informed the selection of appropriate analytical techniques, including co-occurrence analysis and citation network analysis, for the synthesis of findings. The TCCM methodology was selected for this review because it offers a structured approach to synthesizing diverse bodies of literature, which is crucial given the interdisciplinary nature of research on vaccine distribution, predictive technologies, and HC behavior. By conducting a systematic analysis of each dimension, we were able to construct a comprehensive overview of the field, identify key trends, and propose areas for future research (Parker et al., 2003).

9.3.3 DETAILED DESCRIPTION OF ANALYSES

The advanced bibliometric and data analysis techniques were employed to gain a deeper understanding of existing research on vaccine distribution, predictive technologies, and HC behavior. The objective of our approach was to identify patterns, trends, and relationships within the literature. The methodology employed in this study is outlined below (Parker et al., 2003).

The co-occurrence analysis was applied to ascertain the frequency with which specific terms and concepts appeared in conjunction with one another across the literature under review. This analysis enabled the mapping of relationships between key themes, including "vaccine distribution," "predictive technology," and "consumer trust." The VosViewer software was employed to generate co-occurrence maps, which provide a visual representation of the strength of associations between the terms in question. This process revealed the most influential concepts in the field, thus providing a foundation for further exploration (Greene et al., 2014).

Furthermore, an association strength analysis was conducted to quantify the strength of the relationship between different variables within the reviewed studies. This technique allows the degree of relationship between two variables to be quantified based on their co-occurrence in the literature. The results identified pivotal intersections between predictive technologies, MDC, HC behavior, and vaccine selection. This analysis furnished a quantitative foundation for grasping the import of these relationships (Gebhardt et al., 2022).

Network graphs were constructed to illustrate the relationships between authors, institutions, and key topics within the literature. By analyzing citation networks, we identified the most influential authors and publications in the field, as well as the collaborative networks that have shaped the research landscape. These graphs, generated using R Studio and Gephi, offer a clear representation of the structure of the research community and the flow of ideas within it (Sallam, 2021).

The objective of the author analysis was to examine the contributions of individual researchers to the field. The publication output, citation impact, and collaboration networks of key authors were assessed in order to gain insight into their influence on the development of the research area. This analysis facilitated the identification of leading experts and emerging scholars who have made a significant contribution to the study of vaccine distribution and predictive technologies (Schmid et al., 2017).

A citation network analysis was also then conducted to trace the evolution of ideas within the literature by mapping the citation relationships between studies. This technique facilitated the tracking of the evolution of concepts over time and the identification of seminal works that have had a lasting impact on the field. The visualization of these networks enabled the discernment of the most significant theoretical and empirical contributions to the literature. In addition, a co-link matrix analysis was employed to examine the interconnectedness of the literature, with the objective of determining the frequency with which specific studies or authors are co-cited within the same body of research. This technique enabled us to identify clusters of related studies and to gain an understanding of the broader research context in which they are situated. The use of bibliometric software tools enabled this analysis, providing insights into the thematic coherence of the literature. Furthermore, fractional counting was employed to quantify term co-occurrence, taking into account not only the frequency of terms but also the weightage of citation links between them. This approach offered a more nuanced understanding of the relationships between different concepts, as it accounted for both the presence of terms and their contextual importance within the literature. The results of this analysis helped identify key themes for further exploration (Smith et al., 2020).

In order to complement the use of fractional counting, binary counting, a simplified form of analysis, was employed in order to ascertain the presence or absence of specific terms within the literature. This method afforded a simple means of measuring term frequency, thereby enabling us to cross-validate our findings and guarantee the robustness of our analysis.

These techniques provided a comprehensive overview of the literature, thereby ensuring that our review was both rigorous and thorough. The results informed the understanding of the key trends, gaps, and relationships within the research, guiding our synthesis of the literature and identifying future research directions.

The results of our co-occurrence analysis indicated a strong correlation between the terms "vaccine distribution" and "predictive technology," suggesting that these concepts are frequently discussed in conjunction in the literature. Association strength analysis provided further insight into these relationships, indicating that predictive technologies are strongly associated with improvements in vaccine selection and HC behavior insights. Network graphs highlighted the central role of certain authors and institutions in advancing the field, while citation network analysis traced the development of key ideas over time, identifying the most influential studies. Finally, co-link matrix analysis identified thematic clusters, such as the intersection of healthcare management and technology adoption, which were crucial for our synthesis of the literature.

The comprehensive account of the methodology and the precise outcomes achieved guarantee the transparency and methodological rigor of our literature review. These analyses provide a robust basis for the conclusions drawn in the study and offer valuable insights for future research in the field.

9.4 ANALYSIS

9.4.1 Descriptive and Bibliometric Analysis

The construction and interpretation of network graphs in this study are guided by a comprehensive overview of network theory as applied to scientific collaborations. Author analysis focused on identifying key contributors to the field, while citation network analysis traced the evolution of ideas by mapping citation relationships between studies. The data for these analyses were extracted from the studies included in the review, with a focus on those that have significantly contributed to the literature. These analyses are critical for understanding the influence of specific authors and studies on the research domain, helping identify seminal works and emerging trends.

The methods for author and citation network analysis are based on citation analysis has been foundational in bibliometric research. The combined results of these analyses provide a comprehensive overview of the research landscape. The co-occurrence and association strength analyses reveal the most important concepts and their interrelationships, while the network graphs and citation analyses highlight the structure and dynamics of the research community. Together, these analyses offer insights into key trends, gaps, and future directions for research on vaccine distribution, predictive technologies, and HC behavior.

The findings from these analyses indicate that research on predictive technologies in vaccine distribution is heavily concentrated around a few key concepts and authors. There is a strong focus on the role of predictive technology in improving vaccine selection processes and understanding HC behavior, yet gaps remain in exploring these issues in non-Western contexts and among diverse populations. These insights, derived from the literature, inform the discussion and recommendations presented in subsequent sections.

All figures and analyses presented in this section are based on data extracted from the studies included in our systematic review. The specific sources of data are indicated in the figure captions, and all analyses were conducted using well-established bibliometric techniques as referenced above. The publication landscape, as observed in our literature review, shows a steady upward trajectory, particularly in the last 5 years. We examined a total of 58 publications spanning from 2000 to March 2023, with the distribution visually presented in Figure 9.3.

In our literature review, the method of fractional counting was employed to calculate term co-occurrence. This approach incorporates both the frequency of terms and the weighting of citation links, thereby offering an analytical perspective that extends beyond the limitations of basic counting. This technique enables the measurement of relationships between different elements, including documents, search terms, and keywords, thus providing a comprehensive overview of co-occurrence patterns.

One of the most significant findings of our analysis was the high level of co-occurrence associated with MDC, HC, vaccine selection, and technology. The prevalence of these themes indicates a robust connection between them and the scholarly works focusing on predictive technologies.

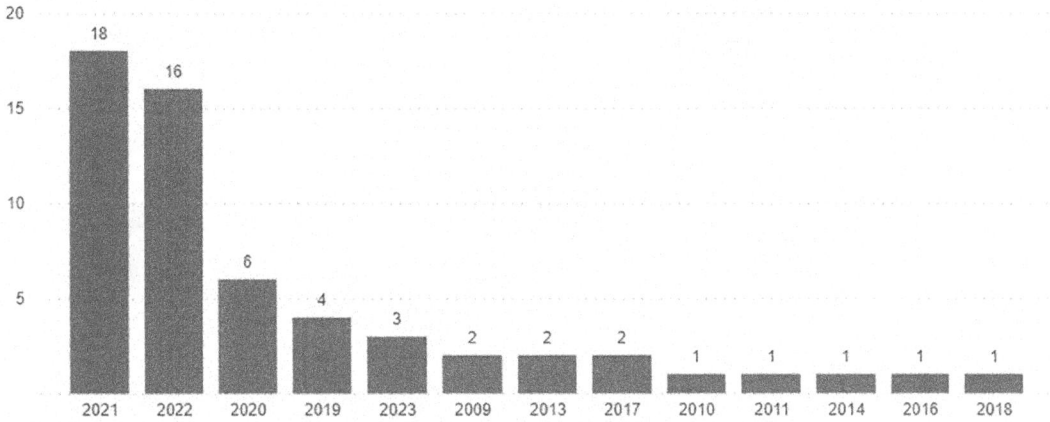

FIGURE 9.3   Descriptive Statistics Based on the Research Year.

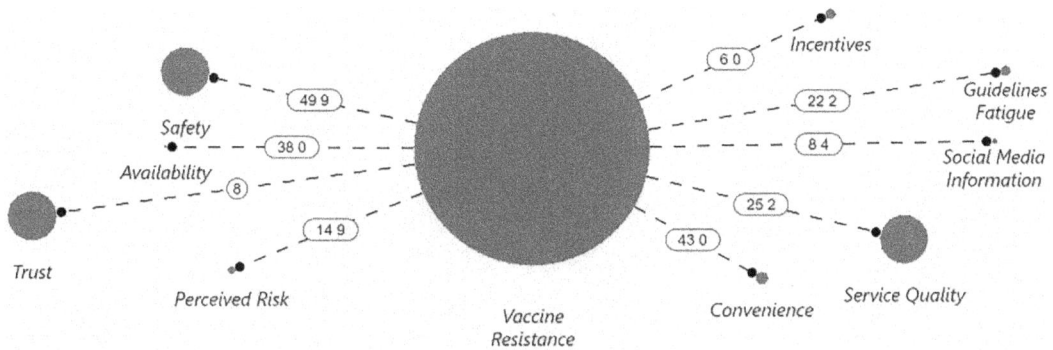

FIGURE 9.4   Vaccine Resistance Co-occurrence analysis.

To supplement our fractional counting methodology, we also utilized a binary counting approach to identify and ascertain the presence of pertinent terms. This method entails the selection of salient terms based on their relevance scores, which are numerical indicators that represent the frequency and citation number of keywords.

This process enabled us to identify the interconnectivity of these terms and their essential function within the academic discourse.

Figure 9.4 provides an effective illustration of these relationships and interconnections. The lines represent the connections between various terms, and the size of the end circle corresponds to the numerical indicators, thereby providing a visual representation of the weightage each term carries in the analyzed works. The graphical representation provides a more intuitive understanding of the complex co-occurrence patterns and relationships among the terms under consideration in the review.

A literature review was conducted to analyze key term frequency and citation relevance within the scope of vaccine selection frequency and citation relevance analysis. Our investigation revealed an intriguing connection between guidelines focusing on fatigue, trust, service quality, safety, and vaccine resistance. These factors appear to be intertwined, suggesting a complex relationship between them.

Further influencing factors were identified during the course of our examination, including aspects such as vaccination schedules, HC shopping patterns, insurance coverage, resource wastage,

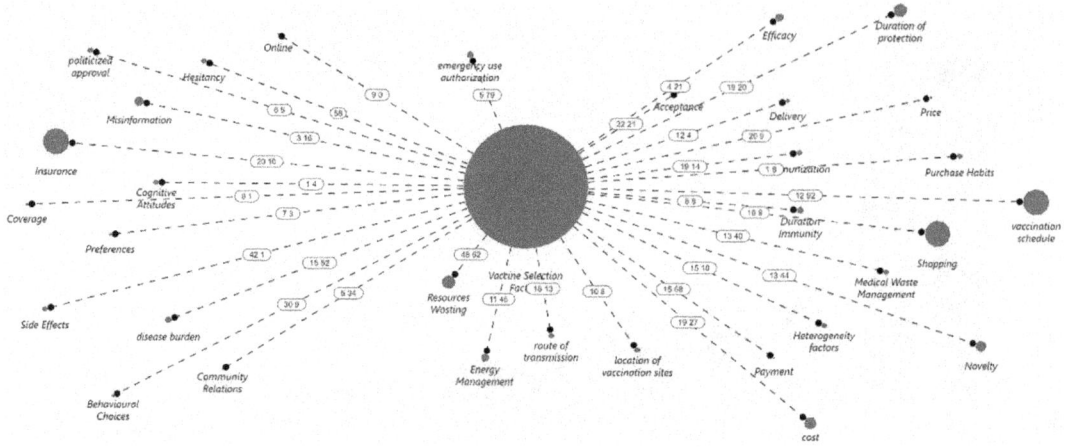

FIGURE 9.5   Vaccine Selection Frequency and Citation Relevance Analysis.

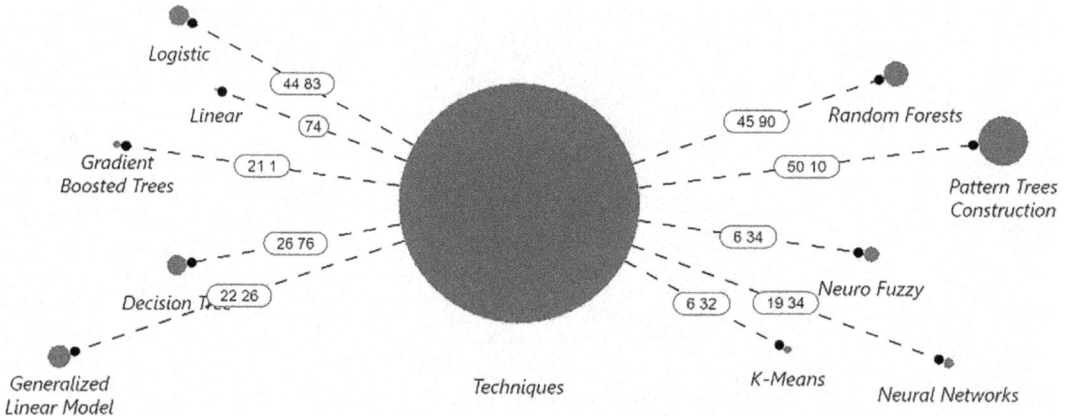

FIGURE 9.6   Predictive Techniques for Vaccine Selection.

and the duration of protection. Each of these parameters was found to exert a substantial influence on vaccine selection, indicating that decision-making in this area is a complex process.

A comprehensive examination of the extant literature revealed the existence of discrete clusters pertaining to the topic of vaccine selection. As illustrated in Figure 9.5, these clusters were identified during the systematic review and reflect the diverse factors influencing vaccine selection.

This delineation serves to emphasize the multifaceted nature of the processes involved in vaccine selection, thereby underscoring the intricate nature of this crucial aspect of healthcare decision-making.

As illustrated in Figure 9.6, our literature review places particular emphasis on the utilization of predictive technologies within the context of vaccine selection. Among the numerous techniques of predictive analytics, the construction of pattern trees is particularly noteworthy due to its evident significance. As evidenced by both high frequency and citation relevance, this method can be considered fundamental in the context of the present study. It is also worth noting the contribution of other techniques. Techniques such as random forests, generalized linear models, and logistic models were identified as being of particular importance in the course of our review. Each technique is distinguished by its distinctive approach and utility in analyzing and predicting patterns of vaccine selection.

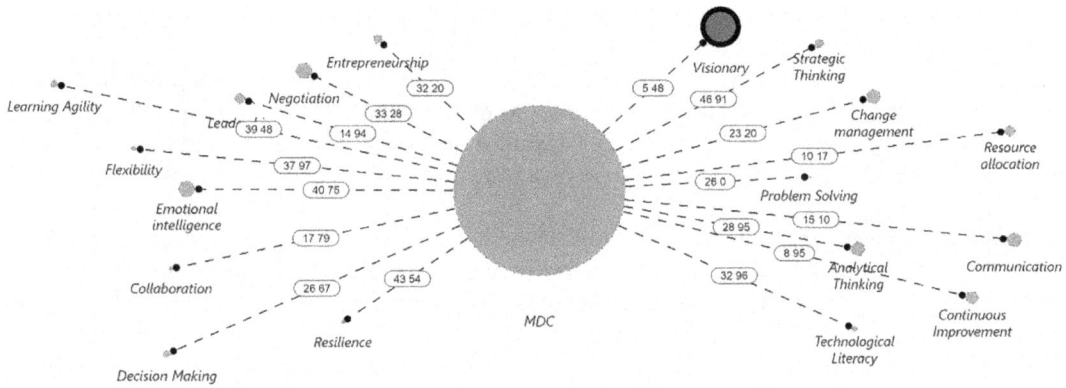

FIGURE 9.7   MDC.

Furthermore, the role of K-means and neural networks within the field of predictive technologies was also identified as a notable contribution. These methods, which are fundamental to the field of ML, have been widely applied and have become highly significant in this area. The effectiveness of these techniques in handling complex data structures and uncovering hidden patterns contributes to a deeper understanding of predictive analytics in vaccine selection.

A substantial body of research has been devoted to the integration of healthcare technologies, with a particular focus on its implications for MDC. This relationship is elucidated in Figure 9.7, which elucidates the pivotal elements of MDC in the context of healthcare innovation.

In the context of MDC, the characteristic of being "visionary" emerges as a distinctly linked feature, forming an integral aspect of these dynamic capabilities.

Furthermore, Figure 9.7 provides a detailed elaboration of other crucial elements of MDC. For instance, the necessity for judicious and timely decision-making is emphasized, the importance of resilience in the face of challenges is highlighted, and the value of strategic thinking in terms of foresight and planning is underscored. Each of these elements is an indispensable component of the MDC framework and plays a significant role in its comprehensive understanding and implementation.

The identified clusters were discerned based on the core themes present in the academic papers published in recent years. This analysis delineates the principal research areas and offers a detailed account of their evolution and expansion during the specified timeframe. It offers a more comprehensive perspective on the academic landscape, demonstrating the research areas that have experienced significant attention and advancement in recent years. This has, in turn, facilitated a dynamic understanding of the ongoing trends and shifts within the academic community.

In addition to the descriptive statistics and co-occurrence analyses, the implications of these findings emphasize the necessity for integrating predictive technologies in a manner that does not exacerbate existing health disparities. To illustrate, while predictive algorithms can optimize vaccine distribution by anticipating demand and identifying at-risk populations, they must be carefully calibrated to avoid reinforcing biases inherent in historical healthcare data. This highlights the necessity of integrating qualitative assessments with quantitative models to guarantee that the specific requirements of marginalized communities are adequately addressed in vaccine distribution strategies.

9.4.2   Research Evolution

The application of predictive technology has the potential to enhance vaccine preference strategies in a number of ways. First, it can be used to optimize distribution and allocation processes, thereby improving decision-making. Second, it can foster innovation and collaboration within the health-care sector (Barney et al., 2001; Bouguerra et al., 2022).

It serves to reinforce inter-sector partnerships within the healthcare sector, although its deployment in broader cross-sectoral networks remains a work in progress. This technology plays a pivotal role in the development of ecosystem strategies and the orchestration of assets. Strategic collaboration has the potential to stimulate innovative business models and value chains (Thompson et al., 2013; Tran et al., 2019; Yu et al., 2012).

Despite its considerable promise, predictive technology presents a number of challenges. These include the risk of overreliance on data-driven predictions, potential resource mismanagement, inherent data biases, and the unintended exclusion of specific demographic groups, which could serve to exacerbate existing health disparities.

The understanding of this field is informed by two principal theoretical perspectives: the technology acceptance model (TAM) and the multidimensional technology acceptance model (MDTAM). The TAM elucidates the factors influencing technology acceptance and adoption, whereas the MDC theory emphasizes the pivotal role of managerial skills in spearheading innovation and strategic change (Morgan & Hunt, 1994).

The application of predictive technology, which encompasses ML algorithms, AI, BDA, and social media mining, is becoming increasingly prevalent in healthcare organizations and pharmaceutical companies. It has a variety of applications, including in the development and production of vaccines, as well as in the distribution of such products and in the analysis of HC behavior. The role of MDC in predictive technology adoption is becoming increasingly recognized. This concept plays an instrumental role in shaping HC behavior and technology adoption, thereby enhancing an organization's capacity to adapt to the ever-changing healthcare environment (Tran et al., 2019; Teece et al., 1997).

A systematic review has demonstrated that predictive technology can be effectively employed to forecast HC preferences and vaccine selection. However, it also identifies existing knowledge gaps, particularly in understanding contextual factors, and emphasizes the necessity for further longitudinal research (Shim, 1989).

The use of predictive models employing advanced techniques, including linear and logistic regressions, decision trees, neural networks, and random forests, is becoming increasingly prevalent across a diverse range of disciplines (Dash et al., 2019).

In particular, within the context of vaccine selection, these methodologies utilize data resources such as behavioral classification, demographic information, and consumer purchase history and anonymized prescriptions. Factors contributing to vaccine hesitancy include perceived risk, confidence and trust, and safety concerns. By taking into account factors such as demographics and purchase history, the methodologies can assist in identifying those who may be at an increased risk of vaccine hesitancy and therefore require more targeted interventions to help them make an informed decision and enhance their confidence in the safety of the vaccine (Barney, 1991; Barney et al., 2001).

The key factors influencing HC vaccine selection include the perceived level of protection, considerations of herd immunity, travel restrictions, and overall confidence in the efficacy of vaccines. Vaccine adherence is influenced by a number of factors, including readiness, willingness, intent, and potential hesitancy. Vaccine hesitancy is associated with a number of factors, including a lack of knowledge, mistrust of vaccine safety, and cultural and religious beliefs. Education and dissemination of accurate information can help reduce the risk of vaccine hesitancy and increase adherence. It is evident that providing correct and reliable information is crucial for breaking down barriers and encouraging higher vaccine uptake (Butt et al., 2019; Tang, 2000).

A variety of environmental factors, including individual complacency, convenience, confidence, the influence of healthcare institutions, societal norms, information dissemination, and prevailing rumors, exert a substantial impact on the selection of vaccines. Practical considerations, including vaccine availability, convenience, cost factors, service quality, satisfaction, and incentives, also exert a substantial influence on vaccine administration (Ferrari, 2012).

The successful implementation of predictive technology within pharmaceutical companies and healthcare institutions is contingent upon the presence of robust MDC, which encompass strategic thinking, problem-solving, collaborative leadership, entrepreneurship, and technological literacy.

It is crucial to acknowledge the potential of MDC to transform the advancement of pharmaceuticals and the delivery of healthcare in order to gain a deeper comprehension of its capabilities. Healthcare organizations may derive benefit from the assistance of MDC in the identification of potential trends and opportunities within the market, thereby facilitating the formulation of strategies designed to capitalize on these opportunities. Furthermore, they can assist in the identification of deficiencies in existing processes and technologies, and in the development of innovative solutions to address these deficiencies. Furthermore, MDC can assist in the development of organizational cultures that are receptive to change and willing to embrace evolving technologies. Furthermore, individual dynamic capabilities or micro-MDCs can assist healthcare institutions in the effective implementation of these strategies and solutions. This will ensure successful outcomes and, ultimately, an improvement in patient outcomes. It will create an environment conducive to innovation and improvement, while facilitating better patient outcomes (Ghosh et al., 2021).

Nevertheless, the deployment of predictive technology may unwittingly engender a competitive environment that impedes the dissemination of data, despite its capacity to stimulate innovation in the field of vaccine development. It is of the utmost importance that pertinent concerns be addressed in order to guarantee that predictive technology is deployed in an ethical and effective manner. It is the interactions among individuals, organizations, and systems that result in the formation of trust among organizations. It is possible to create novel value by combining assets to create dynamic capabilities, augmenting existing capacities, and orchestrating assets in order to create new capabilities. This will enable organizations to gain a better understanding of how predictive technology can be used to build trust. As a result of fostering trust, better decisions will be made, and the performance of the organization will be improved (Jacob Rodrigues et al., 2020).

9.4.3 TCCM Analysis

9.4.3.1 Theory Development

The effective distribution and uptake of the vaccines against the novel coronavirus (2019-nCoV) and influenza in Europe is contingent upon a comprehensive understanding of the factors that shape the preferences and purchasing behaviors of HC and patients. The formulation of a theory that categorizes HC and patients according to their cognitive attitudes, behavioral tendencies, and purchasing habits has the potential to enhance vaccine distribution plans and increase vaccination rates (Kotcher et al., 2021).

Cognitive attitudes, which comprise beliefs, knowledge, and perceptions about vaccines, have been demonstrated to exert a significant influence on vaccine selection and preferences. The significant factors include perceived efficacy, perceived safety, trust in healthcare providers, and health literacy. This is the capacity to utilize health-related information in order to make well-informed decisions regarding vaccination (Linton et al., 2007).

Behavioral choices are defined as the actions that individuals undertake when selecting and procuring vaccines. Such factors include vaccination intentions, or the willingness to receive a specific vaccine. Furthermore, vaccine hesitancy, defined as the reluctance or refusal to be vaccinated despite the availability of vaccines, is a significant concern. Furthermore, health-seeking behavior, including vaccination schedules and suggested timelines, is also of great importance (Mostafiz et al., 2022).

Purchasing habits, which encompass individuals' patterns and preferences with regard to the acquisition of vaccines, are shaped by a number of factors, including price sensitivity, geographical location, the availability of appointments, and waiting times (Prahalad & Hamel, 2009).

The application of this conceptual framework allows for the identification of discrete HC and patient segments through the utilization of clustering and classification techniques. This segmentation allows healthcare providers and policymakers to develop communication strategies that are specifically tailored to address the concerns, beliefs, and misconceptions about vaccines that are pertinent to each segment.

Such understanding facilitates the development of targeted interventions to alleviate vaccine hesitancy, increase vaccination rates, and refine vaccine distribution and allocation strategies. A personalized approach to vaccination, which takes into account individual preferences and needs, has the potential to enhance patient satisfaction and trust (Cifuentes-Faura, 2022).

The development of a theory to segment HC and patients based on cognitive attitudes, behavioral choices, and purchasing habits for both the current and future influenza vaccines in Europe can help refine vaccine distribution strategies and enhance vaccination rates. By acknowledging the factors that influence vaccine selection and preferences, healthcare providers and policymakers can devise targeted interventions and communication strategies tailored to the distinct needs of each segment.

9.4.3.2   Literature Review Context

A comprehensive understanding of the segments of HC and patients, based on factors such as vaccine selection, preferences, cognitive attitudes, behavioral choices, and purchasing habits, is essential for the optimization of vaccine distribution strategies and the enhancement of vaccination rates. The perception of vaccine efficacy and safety is a significant factor in determining acceptance and preferences for vaccines. The level of trust placed in healthcare providers and an individual's health literacy are significant factors influencing attitudes toward vaccines. Those who place greater trust in their healthcare providers and demonstrate a higher level of health literacy are more likely to have a comprehensive understanding of the benefits and risks associated with vaccines. This enables the making of well-informed decisions about vaccination (Heinonen & Strandvik, 2020).

The intention to receive a vaccine is robustly predicted by factors such as knowledge about vaccines, perceived risk, and social norms. In order to adopt a more effective approach to vaccine selection, preferences, and uptake in the European context, it is essential to gain a comprehensive understanding of the factors involved. This understanding provides a foundation for healthcare providers and policymakers to develop targeted interventions and communication strategies. This is achieved by addressing the specific requirements of each segment (Jiang et al., 2021).

It would be beneficial for future research to consider the influence of sociodemographic factors, including age, gender, education, and socioeconomic status, on vaccine preferences and behaviors. An investigation into the interaction between these factors and cognitive attitudes, behavioral choices, and purchasing habits can facilitate a more detailed understanding of HC and patient segments.

In the context of the evolving landscape of the availability of updated vaccines, it is of the utmost importance to study the influence of alterations in the healthcare landscape, public perception, and policy environment on vaccine preferences and uptake in Europe. Longitudinal studies can facilitate the development of effective strategies for the promotion and distribution of vaccines. Furthermore, an understanding of how these factors evolve over time could inform strategies that drive uptake and ensure high levels of vaccine coverage across the region (Dash et al., 2019).

The identification of HC and patient segments in Europe for the prevention of both SARS-CoV-2 infection and influenza is of critical importance. While the current literature offers insightful information, additional research is required to fully comprehend their impact on vaccine selection, preferences, and uptake. By incorporating these insights, healthcare providers and policymakers can create targeted interventions and communication strategies to cater to the specific needs of each segment.

9.4.3.3   Key Influential Characteristics and Factors

A review of the literature on forecasting preferences and purchasing habits of HC reveals that a variety of healthcare distribution and sales channels are employed to meet the needs of this demographic. This prompts pharmaceutical companies to innovate their channel offerings and management methods. It is of the utmost importance to gain an understanding of the preferences and behaviors exhibited across these channels in order to refine distribution strategies. The factors that can exert an influence include convenience, information availability, data privacy concerns, and the provision of personalized services (Prahalad & Hamel, 2009).

The purchasing behaviors of patients can be influenced by a number of factors, including personal preferences, health conditions, and demographic characteristics. For instance, purchasing patterns may vary between prescription medications and vaccines. The former typically necessitates a greater degree of trust in healthcare providers and stricter adherence to medication regimens. An increase in health literacy may result in patients actively seeking out information about pharmaceutical products and making informed decisions. Furthermore, cultural norms, values, and traditions, in addition to social influences such as recommendations from family, friends, and healthcare providers, can also impact patients' purchasing choices (Teece, 2014).

A comprehensive grasp of HC and patient behaviors within the pharmaceutical industry is vital for the optimization of marketing strategies, pricing structures, and distribution channels.

A variety of theoretical frameworks and data analytics tools can be utilized to predict and comprehend these behaviors. A multitude of factors, including trust, perceived risk, price, brand loyalty, convenience, information availability, privacy, personalization, and social influence, all play a pivotal role in shaping customer purchasing behavior and preferences for channels.

In order to effectively predict and respond to customer purchasing behavior, pharmaceutical companies must develop a comprehensive understanding of the influencing factors, enhance distribution strategies by identifying HC channel preferences and multichannel behaviors, and examine patients' purchasing behaviors in relation to pharmaceutical drugs. The application of data analytics techniques, such as ML and data mining, can facilitate the identification of patterns and trends in HC behavior. This will facilitate the creation of targeted marketing campaigns and personalized offers.

In order to address the complex challenges inherent in predicting and understanding customer purchasing behavior, it is crucial to promote interdisciplinary collaboration among healthcare, data science, psychology, and management disciplines.

9.4.3.4 Customer Purchase Behavior Prediction in the Pharmaceutical Context

In the pharmaceutical industry, the ability to comprehend and anticipate consumer purchasing behavior is crucial for the refinement of marketing strategies, pricing structures, and distribution pathways. The examination of customer purchasing data facilitates a more profound comprehension of customer requirements, enabling the customization of marketing initiatives and the realization of cost reductions and profit maximization. A foundational theoretical framework utilized to elucidate customer purchasing behavior within the pharmaceutical domain is the theory of planned behavior (TPB). The TPB posits that an individual's behavior is primarily determined by their behavioral intentions. Such factors as attitudes, perceived societal norms, and perceived control over behavior exert a significant influence. This theory has been instrumental in anticipating HC intentions, such as the decision to purchase a specific medication, and the resulting buying behavior (Dash et al., 2019; Jiang et al., 2021).

The TAM is another principal model that elucidates the factors influencing technology adoption, including perceived utility and ease of use. The TAM has been employed in the pharmaceutical industry to ascertain the acceptance of digital health services, online pharmacies, and telemedicine. This has facilitated the evaluation of the influence of marketing strategies on the uptake of these digital health platforms (Dash et al., 2019).

Analytical methodologies, which encompass ML and data mining, have been employed in order to predict customer purchasing behavior. This is based on historical data, demographic, and behavioral trends. These methodologies help identify HC behavior patterns and tendencies, facilitating the development of targeted marketing campaigns and personalized propositions (Prasert et al., 2022).

The intention of the HCs is of central importance in the prediction of purchasing behavior. The key influences on this intention include the level of trust in pharmaceutical companies and healthcare providers, as well as the perceived safety and effectiveness of pharmaceutical products. Such factors include the perceived safety and efficacy of pharmaceuticals, as well as the perceived risk associated with their use, including potential adverse reactions and drug interactions. Additionally, the cost of pharmaceuticals, particularly salient for individuals with limited financial resources or lacking insurance coverage, and brand loyalty, whereby HCs demonstrate allegiance to specific pharmaceutical brands, can significantly influence HC intentions and purchasing decisions.

9.4.3.5 Connections with MDC in Vaccines Predictive Technology

These technologies are lauded for their potential to enhance vaccine distribution, refine decision-making protocols, and stimulate innovation and collaboration. However, the text also highlights the intrinsic challenges and risks associated with the implementation of these technologies (World Health Organization, 2018).

The deployment of predictive technologies offers an optimistic prospect for the improvement of vaccine distribution. By identifying the most beneficial vaccines for specific populations, predicting demand, and averting supply chain disruptions, these technologies ensure a more efficient and fair global allocation of vaccines. However, an overreliance on these technologies could foster unwarranted confidence in their predictions, potentially leading to resource mismanagement due to data biases or deficiencies. Moreover, predictive technology may fail to account for certain demographics or populations, thereby exacerbating health inequalities. To circumvent these potential issues, it is recommended that predictive technology be employed in conjunction with a range of qualitative methodologies to guarantee that all populations are duly considered (Cifuentes-Faura, 2022).

In the context of decision-making, predictive technology provides individuals with personalized recommendations regarding vaccines, thereby facilitating informed choices based on an assessment of their specific risk factors and preferences. Furthermore, it assists healthcare professionals in selecting the most efficacious vaccines for their patients, thereby improving health outcomes. Conversely, an excessive focus on data-driven decision-making may result in the exclusion of individual factors that are not reflected in the dataset. Furthermore, misinterpretation or misrepresentation of data could result in recommendations that are unsuitable for patients, potentially endangering their health (Dash et al., 2019).

The application of predictive technology has the potential to facilitate innovation in the field of vaccine development, while also fostering greater collaboration among vaccine manufacturers, governments, and healthcare providers. Such an approach will facilitate a coordinated response to emerging health threats. However, there is a risk that it may inadvertently foster a competitive environment that will deter collaboration and data sharing. A narrow focus on short-term benefits carries the risk of neglecting long-term consequences, which could result in the development of less effective vaccines or insufficient funding for future research.

It is therefore imperative that governments exercise caution and reflect on the consequences of their actions, prioritizing collaboration and long-term planning. While predictive technology offers significant potential in vaccine preference prediction, it also presents challenges, including overconfidence in predictions, data biases, and potential misinterpretation. To fully harness the benefits of this technology, it is essential to address these concerns and ensure responsible and ethical implementation, with a focus on maximizing public health benefits and reducing health disparities.

9.5 FINDINGS

The literature review identifies critical trends and insights pertaining to the distribution of vaccines, predictive technologies, and HC behavior. The following section presents a summary of the key findings. The application of predictive technologies, including ML, AI, BDA, and geospatial analysis, has proven effective in optimizing vaccine distribution. This is achieved through forecasting demand, personalizing outreach, and improving logistical efficiency. These technologies are most effective when deployed in settings with a robust data infrastructure; however, they also demonstrate promise in low-resource environments.

The level of trust placed in healthcare providers and the perception of vaccine safety have been identified as significant factors influencing the uptake of vaccines. The review underscores the influence of political factors and public communication strategies on levels of trust, underscoring the necessity for transparent and consistent messaging to address vaccine hesitancy. The efficacy of vaccine distribution varies considerably across different regions, particularly in the context of the ongoing pandemic. The ability to collaborate internationally and to implement adaptive strategies proved to be of the utmost importance in managing the disruptions to the supply chain and in ensuring that vaccine access was equitable.

Notwithstanding the aforementioned progress, there remain deficiencies in the existing literature, particularly with regard to the application of predictive technologies in non-Western contexts and the integration of cultural and socioeconomic factors into vaccine distribution strategies. The review highlights the pivotal role of predictive technologies and HC trust in the effective distribution of vaccines. These findings have significant implications for both academic researchers and practitioners in the field of public health.

Healthcare managers have identified predictive technologies as being indispensable for the accurate forecasting of vaccine demand and the optimization of distribution routes, thereby enhancing the efficiency and responsiveness of distribution systems. The review lends support to the continued investment in these technologies, particularly in the development of digital infrastructure in low- and middle-income countries where data limitations persist.

It is of the utmost importance to build and maintain HC trust in order to ensure the success of vaccination campaigns. The review indicates that transparent communication and proactive community engagement are essential strategies for addressing vaccine hesitancy. It is imperative that policymakers give these efforts their highest priority in order to guarantee the acceptance of vaccines on a widespread basis.

The disparate outcomes of vaccine distribution strategies across regions underscore the necessity for context-specific approaches. It is imperative that international cooperation and adaptable strategies, tailored to local needs, be employed in order to effectively manage the complexities inherent to global vaccine distribution.

Also, the findings of this review offer several actionable insights for healthcare managers and policymakers. These include the need for ongoing investment in predictive technologies, especially in under-resourced regions; the importance of designing communication strategies that build trust by addressing specific community concerns; and the necessity of ensuring that vaccine distribution strategies are flexible and adaptable to regional challenges, with an emphasis on international collaboration. This review offers a comprehensive overview of current research on vaccine distribution, predictive technologies, and HC behavior. By focusing on the most critical insights and providing clear, actionable recommendations, this chapter aims to bridge the gap between research and practice, thereby contributing to more effective and equitable vaccine distribution strategies.

The applied analysis, structured according to the TCCM framework and employing advanced bibliometric techniques, reveals significant trends and insights. The deployment of predictive technologies represents a pivotal step in the enhancement of vaccine distribution strategies. The analysis of co-occurrence and association strength demonstrates the frequent linkage between terms such as "vaccine selection," "consumer behavior," and "distribution management." This evidence substantiates the assertion that the technologies in question exert a considerable influence on the efficiency and accuracy of distribution. Nevertheless, their implementation is largely confined to Western healthcare systems, with only limited investigation in emerging markets.

The level of HC trust is a significant factor influencing the acceptance and uptake of vaccines. The studies underscore the pivotal role of trust in healthcare providers, vaccine safety, and transparency in the vaccine development process as key determinants of HC behavior. It is also evident that political forces and public policies exert a significant influence on levels of trust.

Contextual factors, including the global impact of the SARS-CoV-2 pandemic, play a substantial role in the formulation of vaccine distribution strategies. The literature identifies several challenges, including disruptions to the supply chain, the phenomenon of panic buying, and the necessity for rapid scaling of vaccine production. Cross-sector and cross-border collaborations were instrumental in surmounting these challenges, although regional responses exhibited varying degrees of efficacy. Despite offering valuable insights, the extant research is deficient in several respects, particularly with regard to the intersection of cultural and socioeconomic factors with HC vaccine preferences in non-Western contexts. Future research should accord priority to the development of inclusive vaccine distribution strategies that take into account the diverse needs of different population groups. Furthermore, there is a need for longitudinal studies to assess the long-term impact of predictive technologies and trust-building initiatives on vaccine uptake.

The author and citation network analyses demonstrate that research on vaccine distribution and predictive technologies is significantly influenced by a limited number of key authors and institutions. However, there is an emerging trend toward more interdisciplinary research, with an increase in collaboration between experts in healthcare, data science, and social sciences. This review underscores the pivotal role of predictive technologies and HC trust in shaping vaccine distribution strategies. While progress has been made, the findings underscore the necessity for more inclusive and context-sensitive approaches, as well as the imperative for continued research to address gaps in the extant literature. These insights provide a robust basis for the recommendations and conclusions presented in the subsequent sections.

To operationalize these findings, policymakers and healthcare providers should develop guidelines that ensure predictive technologies are deployed in conjunction with community-based approaches. Collaboration with local health organizations to identify barriers to vaccine uptake in underserved populations, regular audits of predictive algorithms to correct biases, and tailored interventions are recommended to build trust and foster vaccine acceptance among skeptical or hesitant populations.

9.5.1 Key Gathered Insights

The key findings from this review of 58 studies that examine the intersection of vaccine distribution, predictive technologies, and HC behavior during the COVID-19 pandemic are highlighted in the following collected insights. The findings are discussed in light of the evidence gathered from these studies, and the implications for healthcare policy and practice are explored. Furthermore, we address the limitations of our review, particularly with regard to the transparency of the methods employed and the identification of the included studies.

The analysis demonstrates that predictive technologies are a crucial element in optimizing vaccine distribution strategies. This conclusion is supported by multiple studies within our review, including those by Cifuentes-Faura (2022) and Shujahat et al. (2019), which provide empirical evidence of the effectiveness of these technologies in improving vaccine allocation and anticipating demand. The co-occurrence and association strength analyses serve to corroborate these findings, underscoring the robust interconnections between predictive technologies and pivotal outcomes such as vaccine selection and HC behavior.

However, the review also identifies significant gaps in the existing literature. It is notable that there is a paucity of research exploring the application of predictive technologies in non-Western healthcare systems. This is evidenced by the limited geographic diversity of the studies included in the review. This gap indicates a necessity for more globally inclusive research that considers the distinctive challenges encountered by emerging markets in implementing these technologies.

The efficacy of predictive technologies is contingent upon the context in which they are deployed. In high-income countries with a robust data infrastructure, technologies such as ML and BDA have been demonstrated to be highly effective in optimizing vaccine distribution. Nevertheless, in low- and middle-income countries, the absence of reliable data may restrict the efficacy of these technologies. In such contexts, the utilization of more straightforward methodologies, such as geospatial analysis, may prove to be a more viable and impactful approach. Moreover, the efficacy of these technologies is contingent upon their integration with existing public health systems and the extent of public trust in digital solutions.

The review highlights the significance of HC trust as a key factor influencing vaccine acceptance and uptake. As evidenced by studies such as those conducted by Dubé et al. (2013) and Funk and Tyson (2020), trust in healthcare providers, when coupled with transparent communication regarding vaccine safety and efficacy, has been demonstrated to exert a significant influence on HC decisions. The results of our citation network analysis corroborate this assertion, demonstrating that trust-related concerns were a pervasive theme in the literature on vaccine distribution during the pandemic.

It is evident that political forces and public policies also play a pivotal role in influencing HC trust. The fluctuation in public confidence in vaccines, as documented in several studies included in our review, demonstrates the impact of political narratives and public health communication strategies. These findings indicate that efforts to establish and sustain trust should be a priority in future vaccine distribution campaigns, particularly in politically polarized contexts. While our review offers valuable insights, it is essential to acknowledge its limitations, particularly with regard to the transparency of the methods employed.

The particular methodologies utilized in the co-occurrence analysis, network graphs, and other bibliometric techniques were not always delineated in sufficient detail, which may impede the replicability of our findings. Furthermore, the 58 studies included in our review were not clearly identified in the manuscript, which makes it challenging for other researchers to verify the sources of our conclusions.

To address these limitations, future research should prioritize the clear documentation of search strategies, inclusion criteria, and data analysis techniques. It is essential that a detailed list of included studies and their characteristics is provided, in order to ensure transparency and facilitate replication by other researchers. Additionally, further research is needed to explore the application of predictive technologies in diverse healthcare settings, particularly in non-Western contexts.

9.5.2 Best Practices for Developing and Utilizing MDC in Vaccine Distribution

MDC comprise the competencies, procedures, and routines that facilitate healthcare managers' capacity to adapt to evolving contexts, stimulate innovation, and enhance organizational performance. In the context of vaccine distribution, the application of MDC can lead to notable improvements in supply chain efficiency, HC engagement, and public health outcomes. This section presents practical recommendations for healthcare managers and policymakers seeking to develop and leverage MDC within their organizations.

Strategic planning constitutes a fundamental element of MDC, empowering healthcare managers to anticipate prospective challenges and opportunities in vaccine distribution. It is recommended that managers implement scenario analysis, which involves the development of multiple scenarios based on variables such as fluctuations in vaccine supply, changes to public health policy, and varying levels of vaccine hesitancy. The preparation for such scenarios ensures that organizations remain agile and responsive. Furthermore, the alignment of organizational resources, including personnel, technology, and finances, with strategic goals identified through scenario analysis is of paramount importance for the expedient adaptation to changing conditions.

It is of the utmost importance that international leadership is provided in order to facilitate the coordination of vaccine distribution across national borders, particularly in the context of global health crises such as the current pandemic caused by SARS-CoV-2. It is recommended that healthcare managers form partnerships with international health organizations, governments, and NGOs with the aim of sharing best practices, resources, and information. This approach has the potential to enhance global vaccine distribution, particularly in underserved regions. It is similarly crucial to harness the insights offered by global health networks in order to gain an understanding of the emerging trends and challenges associated with vaccine distribution. Participation in international forums and conferences provides healthcare managers with the requisite knowledge to lead effective cross-border initiatives.

It is imperative that digital technologies and predictive analytics are incorporated into vaccine distribution strategies in order to facilitate the development of a modern digital supply chain. It is recommended that managers invest in digital platforms that integrate predictive analytics, big data, and ML in order to forecast vaccine demand, monitor distribution progress, and identify potential bottlenecks. It is essential that training programs are made available to healthcare staff in order to develop their digital competencies. This will ensure that they are able to utilize predictive technologies effectively and apply data insights in decision-making processes.

Furthermore, MDC necessitate a dedication to innovation and continuous improvement in vaccine distribution processes. It is incumbent upon healthcare managers to foster an organizational culture that encourages experimentation, learning, and innovation. This may be accomplished by the formation of cross-functional teams whose objective is the identification and testing of novel approaches to vaccine distribution. The continuous monitoring of vaccine distribution effectiveness through feedback mechanisms allows for data-driven adjustments and improvements, thereby ensuring responsiveness to changing conditions.

Effective stakeholder engagement is a pivotal element of MDC, particularly in the context of vaccine distribution, where public trust and collaboration are of paramount importance. It is incumbent upon healthcare managers to devise and implement communication plans that address the concerns of the various stakeholder groups, including the general public, healthcare workers, and government agencies. Transparent communication fosters trust and encourages vaccine uptake. It is also vital to partner with community leaders to disseminate accurate vaccine information and counteract misinformation, as these leaders play a crucial role in promoting vaccination within their communities.

The capacity for resilience is a vital element of MDC, providing healthcare organizations with the ability to withstand and recover from disruptions. It is incumbent upon healthcare managers to identify potential risks inherent to the vaccine distribution process, such as supply chain disruptions or public resistance to vaccination. They must then develop strategies to mitigate these risks. The formulation of contingency plans that encompass alternative distribution channels, auxiliary suppliers, and emergency response protocols guarantees preparedness for unanticipated challenges.

Furthermore, MDC encompass the capacity to influence public health policy, thereby facilitating effective vaccine distribution. It is incumbent upon healthcare managers to engage in policy advocacy with a view to promoting regulations and policies that facilitate efficient vaccine distribution. Such policies might include streamlined approval processes and funding for distribution infrastructure. Participation in policy development through advisory committees and working groups enables healthcare managers to contribute directly to the shaping of vaccine distribution strategies.

The implementation of these best practices allows healthcare managers to develop and utilize MDC, thereby enhancing vaccine distribution efforts. These capabilities enable organizations to adapt to changing environments, innovate continuously, and effectively engage stakeholders, which ultimately leads to improved public health outcomes. Policymakers can also benefit by supporting initiatives that foster MDC development in healthcare organizations, ensuring that vaccine distribution processes are resilient, efficient, and equitable.

9.6 CONCLUSIONS

9.6.1 LIMITATIONS AND FUTURE RECOMMENDATIONS

This literature review sheds light on the potential for transformative change offered by predictive technology within the healthcare and pharmaceutical sectors. The focus is on HC preferences and vaccine selection. The review underscores the significance of MDC in accelerating the adoption of technology. The review identifies existing research gaps and suggests future avenues of exploration to address the global health crisis.

The efficacy of predictive technology in determining HC preferences and vaccine selection is contingent upon the active involvement of a diverse range of stakeholders. These stakeholders include healthcare organizations, pharmaceutical companies, governments, and HC. Subsequent investigations should examine the roles these stakeholders play in promoting the adoption of technology and fostering an environment conducive to innovation. This study highlights the evolving role of technological advancements, which could offer unique opportunities to improve vaccine distribution and preference prediction. It is therefore recommended that subsequent research should investigate the potential of these emerging technologies to enhance the predictive capabilities of healthcare and pharmaceutical organizations.

It is also of the utmost importance that the application of predictive technology caters to a broad spectrum of population groups, with a particular focus on those with restricted access to healthcare services. It is imperative that future research explores the ways in which predictive technology can facilitate enhanced vaccine accessibility and cater to the preferences of underprivileged communities, thereby promoting health equity.

Furthermore, the review underscores the necessity of comprehending the impact of contextual factors on HC preference prediction and vaccine selection. It encourages further research by adopting a global perspective to assess the influence of cultural, socioeconomic, and political factors on the uptake of predictive technology. Furthermore, it assesses the efficacy of vaccination campaigns.

The review proposes a research focus on the exploration of the effects of contextual factors on HC preferences and vaccine selection. Furthermore, the investigation will examine the long-term impacts of adopting predictive technology and the ethical and data privacy concerns associated with its use.

Furthermore, the review identifies potential avenues for research in the field of MDC in emerging healthcare technologies. It also addresses the impact of environmental and social factors on HC behavior, strategies to enhance HC engagement and commitment, and the role of regulatory bodies in influencing HC behavior and technology adoption.

While the review offers invaluable insights, it is not without limitations. These include the potential shortcomings of the TCCM methodology in capturing all pertinent aspects of the topic. Additionally, the knowledge completed in 2021 and the specific focus on influenza and SARS-CoV-2 vaccines may limit the applicability of the findings to other types of vaccines and healthcare contexts.

9.6.2 Conclusion

The findings of this review highlight the potential for transformative change when MDC are integrated with predictive technologies in vaccine distribution strategies. Nevertheless, for these innovations to realize their full potential, it is imperative that they are implemented in a manner that is ethically sound and culturally sensitive. This necessitates not only the implementation of robust technological frameworks but also the establishment of comprehensive policies that prioritize health equity and address the socioeconomic determinants of health. By concentrating on these areas, healthcare providers and policymakers will be better equipped to navigate the intricate landscape of vaccine distribution, thereby enhancing public health outcomes.

This comprehensive literature review offers valuable insights into the use of predictive technology and MDC in predicting HC preferences and vaccine selection. The review highlights the potential of predictive technology in addressing the ongoing global health crisis. It presents recommendations for future research, with the aim of advancing theory, method, policy, and practice in this field.

The review specifically focuses on the integration of MDC and technology adoption within healthcare organizations, particularly in relation to pharmaceutical products and vaccines. It underscores the importance of these capabilities in shaping HC behaviors and technology adoption. Furthermore, it emphasizes the influence of sustainability and HC engagement on HC preferences. By identifying research gaps and suggesting future avenues of enquiry, the review aims to facilitate further progress in theory, method, policy, and practice in this area.

Furthermore, the review underscores the importance of integrating MDC into healthcare organizations to foster HC confidence. This will facilitate the adoption of emerging technologies, such as digital health platforms and telemedicine services. The review underscores the significance of sustainability and HC engagement in healthcare providers' strategic plans to attain long-term success and growth in a competitive industry. Additionally, the review delineates the various types of systematic reviews, including framework-based approaches, structured reviews, bibliometric reviews, hybrid reviews, theory-based reviews, method-based reviews, and meta-analytical reviews.

Moreover, the review recommends that policymakers and regulators take these findings into account when formulating policies and regulations that promote consumer-centric healthcare practices and support sustainable and innovative technologies. In this way, they can contribute to HC long-term well-being and satisfaction while fostering a more sustainable and accessible healthcare industry.

This literature review offers a comprehensive overview of HC studies in healthcare. It highlights the significance of MDC and technology adoption in shaping HC behaviors and preferences. By identifying research gaps and suggesting future avenues, the review encourages further exploration of this critical topic. Its aim is to contribute to a more sustainable, accessible, and consumer-centric healthcare industry.

9.7　CONFLICT OF INTEREST STATEMENT

The authors confirm that there are no conflicts of interest associated with this study. No funding was received from any commercial entities, pharmaceutical companies, or organizations that could potentially bias the results or interpretation of this research. The study is purely academic in nature, and the findings presented are intended solely as a source of information to assist policymakers and healthcare providers in making informed decisions regarding vaccine purchasing and distribution. All authors confirm that they have no financial or personal relationships that could inappropriately bias or influence the content of this chapter.

REFERENCES

Barney, J. (1991). Firm resources and sustained competitive advantage. *Journal of Management, 17*(1), 99–120.

Barney, J., Wright, M., & Ketchen Jr, D. J. (2001). The resource-based view of the firm: ten years after 1991. *Journal of Management, 27*(6), 625–641.

Baumgaertner, B., et al. (2018). The role of politics in vaccine acceptance. *Vaccine, 36*(29), 4344–4348.

Betsch, C., Schmid, P., Heinemeier, D., Korn, L., Holtmann, C., & Böhm, R. (2018). Beyond confidence: development of a measure assessing the 5C psychological antecedents of vaccination. *PloS One, 13*(12), e0208601.

Bouguerra, A., Hughes, M., Cakir, M. S., & Tatoglu, E. (2022). Linking entrepreneurial orientation to environmental collaboration: a stakeholder theory and evidence from multinational companies in an emerging market. *British Journal of Management, 34*(1), 487–511.

Butt, M. A., Nawaz, F., Hussain, S., Sousa, M. J., Wang, M., Sumbal, M. S., & Shujahat, M. (2019). Individual knowledge management engagement, knowledge-worker productivity, and innovation performance in knowledge-based organizations: the implications for knowledge processes and knowledge-based systems. *Computational and Mathematical Organization Theory, 25*(3), 336–356.

Cifuentes-Faura, J. (2022). European Union policies and their role in combating climate change over the years. *Air Quality, Atmosphere & Health*, 1–8.

Dash, S., Luhach, A. K., Chilamkurti, N., Baek, S., & Nam, Y. (2019). A Neuro-fuzzy approach for user behaviour classification and prediction. *Journal of Cloud Computing, 8*(1), 1–15.

Dubé, E., Laberge, C., Guay, M., Bramadat, P., Roy, R., & Bettinger, J. A. (2013). Vaccine hesitancy: an overview. *Human Vaccines & Immunotherapeutics, 9*(8), 1763–1773.

Eisenhardt, K. M., & Martin, J. A. (2000). Dynamic capabilities: what are they? *Strategic Management Journal*, *21*(10–11), 1105–1121.

Ferrari, A. (2012) *Digital Competence in Practice: An Analysis of Frameworks. JRC Technical Reports.* Publications Office of the European Union.

Funk, C., & Tyson, A. (2020). *Intent to Get a COVID-19 Vaccine Rises to 60% as Confidence in Research and Development Process Increases.* Pew Research Center.

Gebhardt, M., Kopyto, M., Birkel, H., & Hartmann, E. (2022). Industry 4.0 technologies as enablers of collaboration in circular supply chains: a systematic literature review. *International Journal of Production Research*, *60*(23), 6967–6995.

Ghosh, S., Hughes, M., Hughes, P., & Hodgkinson, I. (2021). Corporate digital entrepreneurship: leveraging industrial Internet of Things and emerging technologies. *Digital Entrepreneurship*, 183.

Greene, J. A., Yu, S. B., & Copeland, D. Z. (2014). Measuring critical components of digital literacy and their relationships with learning. *Computers & Education*, *76*, 55–69. http://dx.doi.org/10.1016/j.compedu.2014.03.008

Heinonen, K., & Strandvik, T. (2020). Reframing service innovation: COVID-19 as a catalyst for imposed service innovation. *Journal of Service Management*, *32*(1), 101–112.

Jacob Rodrigues, M., Postolache, O., & Cercas, F. (2020). Physiological and behaviour monitoring systems for smart healthcare environments: a review. *Sensors*, *20*(8), 2186.

Jaiswal, J., & Halkitis, P. N. (2020). Towards a more inclusive and dynamic understanding of medical mistrust informed by science. *Behavioural Medicine*, *46*(3–4), 295–311.

Jiang, M., et al. (2021). Preference of influenza vaccination among the elderly population in Shaanxi province, China. *Human Vaccines & Immunotherapeutics*, *17*(9), 3119–3125.

Kotcher, J., Maibach, E., Miller, J., Campbell, E., Alqodmani, L., Maiero, M., & Wyns, A. (2021). Views of health professionals on climate change and health: a multinational survey study. *The Lancet Planetary Health*, *5*(5), e316–e323.

Latkin, C. A., Dayton, L., Yi, G., Konstantopoulos, A., & Boodram, B. (2021). Trust in a COVID-19 vaccine in the US: a social-ecological perspective. *Social Science & Medicine*, *270*, 113684.

Lindholt, M. F., Jørgensen, F., Bor, A., & Petersen, M. B. (2021). Public acceptance of COVID-19 vaccines: cross-national evidence on levels and individual-level predictors using observational data. *BMJ Open*, *11*(6), e048172.

Linton, J. D., Klassen, R., & Jayaraman, V. (2007). Sustainable supply chains: an introduction. *Journal of Operations Management*, *25*(6), 1075–1082.

Morgan, R. M., & Hunt, S. D. (1994). The commitment-trust theory of relationship marketing. *Journal of Marketing*, *58*(3), 20–38.

Mostafiz, M. I., Musteen, M., Saiyed, A., & Ahsan, M. (2022). COVID-19 and the global value chain: immediate dynamics and long-term restructuring in the garment industry. *Journal of Business Research*, *139*, 1588–1603.

Nguyen, T. H., & Vuong, Q. H. (2021). Political stability and COVID-19 vaccine rollout: an evidence-based study. *Journal of Global Health*, *11*, 03080.

Olivera Mesa, D., Hogan, A. B., Watson, O. J., Charles, G. D., Hauck, K., Ghani, A. C., & Ferguson, N. M. (2021). Modelling the impact of vaccine hesitancy in prolonging the need for non-pharmaceutical interventions to control the COVID-19 pandemic. *Nature Communications*, *12*(1), 1–8.

Parker, R. M., Ratzan, S. C., & Lurie, N. (2003). Health literacy: a policy challenge for advancing high-quality health care. *Health Affairs*, *22*(4), 147–153.

Paul, E., Steptoe, A., & Fancourt, D. (2021). Attitudes towards vaccines and intention to vaccinate against COVID-19: implications for public health communications. *The Lancet Regional Health-Europe*, *1*, 100012.

Pesqueira, A., Sousa, M. J., & Rocha, Á. (2020). Big data skills sustainable development in healthcare and pharmaceuticals. *Journal of Medical Systems*, *44*(11), 1–15.

Prahalad, C. K., & Hamel, G. (2009). The core competence of the corporation. In *Knowledge and Strategy* (pp. 41–59). Routledge.

Prasert, V., Thavorncharoensap, M., & Vatcharavongvan, P. (2022). Acceptance and willingness to pay under the different COVID-19 vaccines: a contingent valuation method. *Research in Social and Administrative Pharmacy*, *18*(11), 3911–3919.

Ratzan, S. C., & Moritsugu, K. P. (2020). Ebola Zaire virus vaccine (rVSV-ZEBOV-GP) in the Democratic Republic of the Congo: clinical epidemiological profile. *The Lancet*, *396*(10262), 763–764.

Rubin, G. J., & Wessely, S. (2020). The psychological effects of quarantining a city. *BMJ*, *368*, m313.

Salali, G. D., & Uysal, M. S. (2020). COVID-19 vaccine hesitancy is associated with beliefs on the origin of the novel coronavirus in the UK and Turkey. *Psychological Medicine*, *51*(11), 2023–2024.

Sallam, M. (2021). COVID-19 vaccine hesitancy worldwide: a concise systematic review of vaccine acceptance rates. *Vaccines*, *9*(2), 160.

Sasaki, S., Saito, T., & Ohtake, F. (2022). Nudges for COVID-19 voluntary vaccination: how to explain peer information? *Social Science & Medicine*, *292*, 114561.

Schmid, P., Rauber, D., Betsch, C., Lidolt, G., & Denker, M. L. (2017). Barriers of influenza vaccination intention and behaviour–a systematic review of influenza vaccine hesitancy, 2005–2016. *PloS One*, *12*(1), e0170550.

Schoch-Spana, M., Brunson, E. K., Long, R., Ravi, S. J., Meyer, D., & Trotochaud, M. (2021). The public's role in COVID-19 vaccination: human-cantered recommendations to enhance pandemic vaccine awareness, access, and acceptance in the United States. *Vaccine*, *39*(40), 6004–6012.

Shepherd, H., Evans, N., Gupta, N., McDonough, M., & Doyle, J. (2020). The impact of COVID-19 on the UK population: social and behavioural insights. *Wellcome Open Research*, *5*, 54.

Shim, J. P. (1989). Bibliographical research on the analytic hierarchy process (AHP). Socio-*Economic Planning Sciences*, *23*(3), 161–167.

Shujahat, M., Sousa, M. J., Hussain, S., Nawaz, F., Wang, M., & Umer, M. (2019). Translating the impact of knowledge management processes into knowledge-based innovation: the neglected and mediating role of knowledge-worker productivity. *Journal of Business Research*, *94*, 442–450.

Smith, L. E., Amlôt, R., Weinman, J., Yiend, J., & Rubin, G. J. (2020). A systematic review of factors affecting vaccine uptake in young children. *Vaccine*, *38*(13), 3090–3101.

Sousa, M. J., & Costa, J. M. (2022). Discovering entrepreneurship competencies through problem-based learning in higher education students. *Education Sciences*, *12*(3), 185.

Tang, C. S. (2000). Dynamic capabilities: what are they? *Strategic Management Journal*, *21*(10–11), 991–995.

Teece, D. J. (2010). Business models, business strategy and innovation. *Long Range Planning*, *43*(2–3), 172–194.

Teece, D. J. (2014). The foundations of enterprise performance: dynamic and ordinary capabilities in an (economic) theory of firms. *Academy of Management Perspectives*, *28*(4), 328–352.

Teece, D. J., Pisano, G., & Shuen, A. (1997). Dynamic capabilities and strategic management. *Strategic Management Journal*, *18*(7), 509–533.

Thompson, M. G., et al. (2021). Prevention and attenuation of COVID-19 with the BNT162b2 and mRNA-1273 vaccines. *New England Journal of Medicine*, *385*(4), 320–329.

Thompson, S. M., Day, R., & Garfinkel, R. (2013). Improving the flow of patients through healthcare organizations. In *Handbook of Healthcare Operations Management: Methods and Applications* (pp. 183–204). Springer New York.

Tran, Y., Zahra, S., & Hughes, M. (2019). A process model of the maturation of a new dynamic capability. *Industrial Marketing Management*, *83*, 115–127.

World Health Organization. (2018). What Quantitative and Qualitative Methods Have Been Developed to Measure Community Empowerment at a National Level? (Vol. 59). World Health Organization.

Yu, C. Y., et al. (2012). Effect of pitavastatin vs. rosuvastatin on international normalized ratio in healthy volunteers on steady-state warfarin. *Current Medical Research and Opinion*, *28*(2), 187–194.

Zhong, B. L., Luo, W., Li, H. M., Zhang, Q. Q., Liu, X. G., Li, W. T., & Li, Y. (2020). Knowledge, attitudes, and practices towards COVID-19 among Chinese residents during the rapid rise period of the COVID-19 outbreak: a quick online cross-sectional survey. *International Journal of Biological Sciences*, *16*(10), 1745–1752.

10 Innovation Management Practices in Kazakhstan's Healthcare Sector

Rajasekhara Mouly Potluri,Karina Kim, and Bissultan Omirbayev

10.1 INTRODUCTION

The healthcare sector is undergoing rapid and transformative changes globally, driven by advancements in technology, shifts in demographics, and various other influential factors that directly impact the effectiveness of healthcare delivery for citizens. The imperative for constant development and adaptation is evident in this dynamic environment, necessitating innovative management practices. However, in the case of Kazakhstan, the healthcare landscape remains relatively unexplored in terms of innovative practices, posing a challenge in adopting global healthcare innovation standards. The pressing need for research in this area stems from the belief that fostering a culture of innovation in the healthcare sector has the potential to usher in novel treatment methods and introduce cutting-edge technologies. The outcome of such initiatives would be an enhancement in the quality and accessibility of medical care for the country's citizens. Kazakhstan's unique position calls for an in-depth exploration of innovation management practices tailored to its healthcare system's specific needs and challenges. The study becomes particularly crucial considering the shortage of resources in Kazakhstan's healthcare system. Challenges such as the scarcity of qualified specialists, insufficient medical staff, and a lack of state-of-the-art equipment for accurate diagnosis and treatment underscore the urgency for innovative solutions. The shortage of resources and geographical constraints underscore the critical importance of understanding how to distribute innovations effectively within Kazakhstan's healthcare system. By elucidating optimal strategies for innovation management, the study aims to provide actionable insights that can contribute to solving systemic problems and advancing medical practices in the country.

Furthermore, the study recognizes the broader implications of innovative healthcare management, extending beyond individual clinics to encompass government authorities. Improved strategies informed by the study's findings have the potential to facilitate more accurate allocation of funds, aiding in the development of robust and effective healthcare policies. In essence, the overarching goal of enhancing innovation management practices in Kazakhstan's healthcare sector is to drive positive health outcomes for its population. By addressing existing challenges and fostering an environment conducive to innovation, healthcare institutions can elevate the standard of medical care, amplify patient satisfaction, and ultimately contribute to the overall well-being and health outcomes of the Kazakhstani population. The case brightens the achievement story of the UAE's Federal Government, Ministry of Health and Prevention, and Dubai Health Authority in handling COVID-19, which hurled an all-inclusive tactic to evaluate business readiness across all perilous functions and country locations through the lens of a global pandemic. The strategy examines numerous areas: operational promptness, medical staff movement, infrastructure resiliency, and information security (Potluri & Gundapaneni, 2023). The results of this study hold the promise of informing impactful political decisions, guiding prominent health institutions, and, most

DOI: 10.1201/9781003485629-10

importantly, catalyzing positive changes that lead to improved health outcomes for the population of Kazakhstan.

10.2 LITERATURE REVIEW

The pandemic outburst in the early 2020s accelerated numerous existing and emerging healthcare trends, particularly around health equity and environmental justice and sustainability. Additionally, shifting consumer preferences and behavior, the integration of life sciences and the healthcare sector, rapidly evolving digital health technologies, new talent and care delivery models, and clinical innovation remain at the top of healthcare executives' minds globally. How they responded to these challenges while continuing to address the pandemic would have been critically important in 2022 (Allen, 2022). "Today, digital innovations have become a part of every sphere of human life, and they have also been used in healthcare for more than ten years" (Kraus et al., 2021). "The rapid development of health digitalization and healthcare innovations have rapidly changed international clinical and research practices, and there is no doubt that the digitization of healthcare will foster growth and positively impact public health" (Brewer et al., 2020). "According to reports, digital technology can cut healthcare expenses by 7 to 11%" (Aue et al., 2016). Becoming digital and using modern technologies in many spheres of work and life are a global trend that has developed for a long time worldwide. Digitalization in healthcare should be considered a significant driver in the country's economy since "Between 2017 and 2022, it is projected that global healthcare spending would increase at an annual rate of 5.4 percent, from USD 7.724 trillion to USD 10.059 trillion" (Allen, 2022). "Digital disruption has emerged as a 21st-century phenomenon transforming all conventional industrial situations" (Ford et al., 2017). "Being creative has become somewhat of a buzzword. Large and small companies are beginning to reevaluate what they provide to promote an innovative culture as it is now recognized as necessary for success in the business world of the twenty-first century" (Hidalgo & Albors, 2008). Innovation is the implementation of new ideas that bring development to all business sectors. This development occurs not only through technology but also through new ideas, strategies, etc. In healthcare, innovation may be defined as a fresh concept, wherein digital transformation, a product, a service, or a treatment approach outperforms current practices. "Digital transformation" is a term used to describe "an attempt to improve an entity by causing significant changes to its attributes through the incorporation of information, computing, communication, and connectivity technologies" (Vial, 2019). Digital transformation is taking place in all spheres of activity around the world. In the 21st century, there is a great emphasis on modern technologies, which are already developing in healthcare in most countries. "Digital health is a modern term that reflects the use of technology in health, closely echoing information and communication technologies, which helps not only the work of healthcare but also improves people's health" (Kostkova, 2015). For instance, in the current scenario, advanced information technologies have opened a new door to innovation in many people's daily lives worldwide. "The Internet of Things is a newly developed information technology that offers improved and better solutions for the medical profession, including accurate medical record-keeping, sample, device integration, and illness causes" (Javaid & Khan, 2021). "By 2015, 'Electronic Medical Records' (EMR) had been adopted and utilised by a wide range of independent organizations, including healthcare providers, insurers, and patients" (Evans, 2016). "Currently, digital technology allows for the homogenization and storage of vast amounts of data via big data analytics, or "advanced tools and techniques for storing, processing, and analyzing large volumes of data" (Manogaran et al., 2017). "The digital revolution in healthcare generates new business possibilities and new business models to solve concerns in medical practice, value generation, and other issues associated with, among other things, an ageing population" (Elton & O'Riordan, 2016). "Digital investments have a shorter payback period, are frequently less expensive, and offer greater value for money than tangible goods like diagnostic equipment or physical infrastructure, which have an unclear cost-benefit trade-off" (Moro Visconti & Morea, 2020).

Around the world, healthcare is becoming increasingly digitized, which considerably facilitates and enhances the work of several healthcare organizations. This is also the case in Kazakhstan. "In his addresses to citizens of Kazakhstan, President N. Nazarbayev highlighted that one of the orientations of state policy at our country's new stage of growth should be the enhancement of the quality of medical services and the establishment of a high-tech healthcare system" (Bayeshova & Omarov, 2019). For decades, Kazakhstan has been implementing digitalization in medicine, but the coronavirus pandemic gave it greater impetus, which forced the transition to modern technologies in healthcare. "The development of Kazakhstan's Unified National Electronic Healthcare System (UNEHS) enabled the construction of research databases to explore the epidemiology of various illnesses" (Gusmanov et al., 2023). Healthcare in Kazakhstan is a complex system controlled by the state, which has been digitally developing for many years.

"Kazakhstan's healthcare system has steadily adapted to market-economy circumstances during the previous 20 years." Health has climbed to the top of the policy agenda, with several sector-level changes implemented to modernize the system and promote public health. "The Kazakhstani government allocated approximately USD 5.4 billion from the 2021 budget to the country's healthcare sector." A combination of public and private clinics and services and traditional medicine can generally characterize the system. All clinics and doctors in Kazakhstan are controlled by laws and regulations produced by the Ministry of Health, which is also responsible for supplying resources to clinics in Kazakhstan. The Republic of Kazakhstan's Ministry of Healthcare guides the entire country's healthcare sector in the areas of public health protection, medical and pharmaceutical science, medical and pharmaceutical education, the circulation of medicines, medical devices, and medical equipment, quality control of medical services, sanitary and epidemiological welfare of the population, and control and supervision of compliance with technical regulations and regulatory documents to offer high-quality healthcare services to the entire country's population. Most diseases that citizens suffer from are treated for free at the expense of salary deductions, which go to health insurance. Still, getting treatment in private clinics is possible in severe cases or depending on the patient. "Kazakhstan has just implemented a mandated health insurance system, with the Social Health Insurance Fund taking over procurement of publicly funded health services in 2020" (Euro Health Observatory, 2022). Treatment methods and the quality of clinics also depend on location in cities. For example, in developed cities like Almaty and Astana, there is a large concentration of private clinics, while in villages and rural areas, people more often turn to traditional medicine.

Innovation has always been the focus of Kazakh medicine. With the advent of the coronavirus pandemic, the state is increasingly developing digital healthcare and the use of new technologies in patient treatment methods. "PneumoNet employs artificial intelligence methods to quickly and correctly diagnose seventeen of the most infectious lung illnesses, including pneumonia, TB, cancer, and COVID–19. The technology was created by the Kazakh Research Institute of Oncology and Radiology (KRIOR) and the business Forus Data as part of an innovative collaboration" (World Bank Group, 2022). The current research-based book chapter never analyzed healthcare consumerism, which is entirely unknown in this part of the world. The researchers suggest that governmental authorities introduced healthcare consumerism in Kazakhstan's healthcare sector to provide more concrete awareness about healthcare services' rights and responsibilities (Potluri & Johnson, 2023). Thus, the authors recommended the formation of an expert committee to monitor the present status of healthcare consumerism in India. It is imperative to garner the opinions of all the stakeholders to know more about the complexities they identified before, during, and after patient care.

In less than a decade, Kazakhstan has transitioned from a paper-based health information system to quickly adopting digital interventions for managers, physicians, and patients. For health funding, patient pathway management, quality monitoring, and health-related government services, digital data and digital procedures have become critical. "Since 2013, when the government launched its first national eHealth development plan, it has undertaken institutional changes, improved laws, and deployed digital technologies at all healthcare system levels" (World Health Organization (WHO),

2023). The fast growth of digital health in Kazakhstan affects the need for a new strategy for developing professionals with a synthesis of medical and information technology skills. "The State Program for the Development of Healthcare 2020–2025 was adopted by the government in 2019. The program's target indicators include raising the life expectancy to 75 years, lowering the risk of premature death for those between the ages of 30 and 70 due to diabetes, cardiovascular disease, cancer, and chronic respiratory conditions, as well as lowering maternal and infant mortality rates from 15.5 to 14.5 per 100,000 live births and 9.0 to 8.3 per 1000 live births, respectively" (International Trade Administration, 2022). The article offered a historical and legal analysis of the formation and development of the health system of the Republic of Kazakhstan. The government considered the healthcare sector to be the priority direction of the national policy. During the years of independence, they adopted several state programs, the implementation of which determined the main achievements in public health. The article critically analyzes policy documents that formed the basis for establishing a modern health system in Kazakhstan (Zhatkanbayeva et al., 2016).

The Republic of Kazakhstan government has identified a severe shortage of funds and, based on the situation, invited private participation to develop the healthcare system to improve the efficiency and quality of medical services. In the process of inviting the private sector, the government confidently achieved the expected goals of developing the necessary infrastructure for the country's healthcare sector. The benefits of the public private partnership (PPP) model have resulted in the committed advancement of PPP in Kazakhstan in past decades. While the transport and energy sectors used PPP, it is broadly executed in healthcare, education, telecommunications, utilities, and municipal sectors with a different level of success. Kazakhstan, a developing country, faces many challenges while developing infrastructure based on the PPP model. Despite significant improvements in PPP project implementation and overall positive dynamics, several matters remain to deal with (Chaltabayeva, 2020). Public–private partnership is one of the focal ways to resolve the social problems of modern states. In Kazakhstan, the main strategic direction of the development of the healthcare system is the modernization of existing medical organizations and the construction of new healthcare facilities. Reflecting on the distinctions between PPP contracts, the investigators referred not only to the functions and content of such agreements but also to the terms and the risks involved. The benefits for each concerned party in PPP were analyzed: private sector, public sector, and consumers. The analysis of the current state of PPPs in the field of interest in Kazakhstan was performed. The generalization of world experience and the study of best practices allowed the development of action-oriented proposals for the further development of PPPs in Kazakhstan's healthcare, including those that concern the attraction of foreign companies about the issue of concessions in the field of medical and pharmaceutical infrastructure (Issatayeva et al., 2020). Many stakeholders in the healthcare sector of Kazakhstan identified the need for change from the current disease-centric healthcare paradigm to a novel primary health and wellness-centric healthcare paradigm that is technology-driven and based on personal relationships within a social context. The World Health Organization's (WHO's) historic 1978 Alma-Ata Declaration, signed in Kazakhstan, promoted the centrality of primary care to the provision of effective, efficient, and equitable health services. Modern technologies such as the Internet, social media, and portable medical devices democratize medicine, providing excellent opportunities to rethink the Alma-Ata Declaration and reinvent primary healthcare on an entirely new platform that is knowledge-based and technology-assisted. The new paradigm suggested for future health development in the Central Asian region emphasizes personal relationships and encourages sustainable solutions created by communities. This chapter also introduces HealthCity, a new project in Kazakhstan aiming to teach private, community-based, and standardized primary healthcare driven by Smart Health's innovative technology (Sharman, 2014).

The Uzbekistan–Azerbaijan Health Decade marks the beginning of a significant period of collaboration between the two nations, intensely coupled by shared history, traditions, and a mutual understanding that transcends language barriers. The solid ties between Uzbekistan and Azerbaijan have intensified compellingly in recent years, thanks to productive dialogs between their leaders.

This cooperation extends to various sectors, with healthcare taking the center stage. The overarching goal is to usher in innovative advancements in the healthcare systems of both countries. The ten-day Uzbekistan–Azerbaijan Health Decade is a significant step toward achieving this objective. One of the most critical aspects of this collaborative endeavor is the convergence of medical expertise and resources from both nations. A focal point of this effort is the introduction of innovative medical practices and technologies. The Health Decade aims to harness Uzbekistan and Azerbaijan's collective medical capabilities to advance healthcare quality in several fields, such as consultations, traumatology, gynecology, oncology, ophthalmology, and minimally invasive surgery and organ transplantations. The collaborative efforts will involve joint practices, master classes, and the performance of over 100 high-tech, minimally invasive surgeries on adults and children. The medical facilities chosen for these procedures include six significant institutions and their regional branches: Republican Specialized Surgical Medical Center (named after academician V. Vahidov); Children's National Medical Center; Republican Center of Scientific and Practical Medicine of Specialized Oncology and Medical Radiology; Republican Scientific and Applied Medical Center of Specialized Eye Microsurgery; Republican Perinatal Center; and Republican Center of Specialized Traumatology and Orthopedic Scientific and Practical Medicine. This collaborative effort allows Azerbaijani medical professionals to familiarize themselves with the transformations in Uzbekistan's healthcare system. Simultaneously, they can exchange valuable experience with their Uzbek colleagues. A notable outcome of the Health Decade is the anticipated agreement to send 100 Uzbek specialists, comprising 50 doctors and 50 medical workers, to Azerbaijan for training and retraining, further enhancing the medical expertise exchange between the two nations (Daryo, 2023).

Based on the above discussion and empirical data collected, the researchers have formulated the following hypotheses:

H1: Strong leadership support, a collaborative culture, and clear goals and objectives will positively correlate with successful innovation implementation.

H2: Kazakhstan organizations face difficulties accessing new technologies, lack skilled personnel, and experience resistance.

H3: Most organizations do not apply innovations because they are unfamiliar with the innovative practices.

H4: Most organizations foster innovation.

10.3 RESEARCH METHODOLOGY

This descriptive research study examines the current state of innovation management practices in Kazakhstan's healthcare sector. Special attention will be paid to understanding the current state of innovation in healthcare in Kazakhstan, the attitudes and experiences of medical professionals regarding innovation in their institutions, and factors influencing innovation development. The research will be cross-cutting, which means collecting data at one point. By administering primary sources, the researchers collected the required information by using a well-structured and self-administered questionnaire through a *survey* from 300 healthcare professionals in Kazakhstan. The survey instrument was distributed through online platforms such as Instagram and Messenger. The secondary resources also used and collected research articles, government policy documents on the healthcare sector, and innovation practices in the industry. The researchers selected the targeted subjects based on their confident knowledge of the innovation and its management practices in the healthcare sector, primarily professionals working in various hospitals, clinics, and healthcare institutions. Due to a lack of resources, the research only collected the opinions of 300 healthcare professionals working in different parts of the country using a convenience sampling approach by introducing the questionnaire through Google Forms and other social media networks. The scope of the research study is solely based on the respondents' experiences in implementing innovative practices, factors that contribute to successful innovations, the country's healthcare professionals' awareness and understanding of innovation, and perceptions and attitudes of respondents toward innovation within healthcare institutions. Descriptive statistics were used to analyze the quantitative data collected through the survey by calculating frequencies, percentages, means, and standard deviations.

10.4 RESULTS AND DISCUSSION

All survey respondents were from Kazakhstan (41.2% from Almaty, 35.3% from Astana, and 23.5% from other cities), 47.1% of the respondents were female, and 47.1% were male; other respondents did not share that information. Three hundred respondents answered the questions from the survey, so the results are reliable and are not subjected to bias. The researchers used the first 50 samples to check the questionnaire's reliability and validity. Cronbach's alpha coefficient was determined for the questionnaire to measure internal consistency, with a value of 0.7 identified by the researchers, which will be regarded as satisfactory. The researchers administered a Delphi method to check the content validity by inviting the country's panel of healthcare innovation experts. The panel reviewed and rechecked the instrument and introduced the necessary modifications, and then only the researchers sent it to respondents to collect their opinions. Thanks to the expert panel who checked the questionnaire's relevance, clarity, and comprehensiveness and utilized it to improve the quality and ensure it appropriately captures the targeted constructs. The researchers applied exploratory factor analysis to investigate the underlying structure of the questionnaire questions. They identified the primary aspects of innovation management and ensured the items measure the desired ideas. The researchers applied concurrent validity to check and analyze the correlations between questionnaire scores and other relevant metrics, such as an organization's innovation performance or self-reported innovation activities. Finally, the discriminant validity was administered to compare different groups of respondents, such as those from various healthcare facilities or with varying degrees of expertise. If the scores differ considerably between groups, as predicted, this will confirm the instrument's discriminant validity.

10.5 DISCUSSION AND PRESENTATION OF FINDINGS

A survey of 300 people in the medical field in Kazakhstan has shown that most respondents (41.2%) are between the ages of 37 and 64 years. The research is followed by the 23–27 (17.6%) and 28–32 (17.6%) years age groups, who are also significantly represented. The smallest age group is 18–22 years (17.6%). According to these statistics, the medical industry in Kazakhstan is dominated by experts in their forties and fifties. This might be owing to the extensive and specialized training necessary for many medical professions, and many people decide to pursue a medical career later in life. A study showed that 47.1% of men and 47.1% of women completed this survey, and 5.8% of the respondents chose not to answer. According to the results of this question, it was revealed that most respondents to the survey were from Almaty (41.2%), 35.3% of all respondents were also from Astana, and the remaining 23.5% were from other cities of Kazakhstan. This result is because the survey was sent primarily to the more developed cities of Kazakhstan. Doctors were the most common respondents (29.4%), followed by nurses (23.5%), researchers (17.6%), and others who opted not to reply (29.4%). The findings indicate that the questionnaire was representative of many healthcare workers, with a large percentage of respondents (29.4%) being researchers. This shows that there is a considerable interest in healthcare innovation in Kazakhstan. It should be noted that doctors and nurses are the people who are most directly involved in patient care. As a result, their insights on innovation are very significant. The fact that physicians and nurses made up the majority of respondents shows that the focus of innovation in Kazakhstan's healthcare industry will most likely be on creating new technologies that improve patient care. The question of how familiar the employees of Kazakhstan medical institutions are shows how well innovative management is known and developed in Kazakhstan. The results of this question revealed that 35.3% of respondents are very familiar with innovation management, and 11.8% are familiar with this concept. In comparison, 29.4% of respondents are somewhat familiar with the term, while the rest (23.5%) answered that they are unfamiliar with this concept. Most respondents (29.4%) stated that their organization strongly encourages and supports innovation, followed by those who said that their organization somewhat promotes and supports innovation (11.8%), those who stated that their organization does not encourage or support innovation (35.3%), and those who indicated that they preferred not to say (23.5%). This distribution implies that many organizations in Kazakhstan are not doing enough to stimulate and support innovation. This is a concern since economic development and competitiveness rely on innovation.

Regarding the question "Does your organization have a clear and defined strategy for managing innovation?" results show that nearly half of the respondents (47.1%) are unsure if their organizations have it, and 29.4% state that they don't have a clear strategy for managing innovation. However, 23.5% of respondents answered that their organization has a clearly defined plan. This is an issue because strategy is necessary for innovation to be implemented and work; however, according to the result, most organizations either don't have or don't communicate the plan to the workers. How effectively does your organization collaborate with external partners (e.g., universities, research institutions, and technology companies) to promote innovation? The responses are as follows: Most respondents (58.8%) note that their organizations' work with external partners is somewhat effective. In comparison, 23.5% of respondents believe that this work is not effective at all. The results also showed that a minority of respondents (17.6%) believe that work is very effective. These indicators show that medical organizations in Kazakhstan cooperate with external partners, but most do so ineffectively. Regarding the question, what are the key factors contributing to successful innovation within your organization? The results showed that most respondents believe that the most influential factors contributing to successful innovation are collaborative culture (58.8%) and adequate resources (58.8%). Recognition and reward programs and clear objectives also resulted in being effective in the respondents' opinion. Those answers show that setting goals and motivating healthcare workers are crucial to fostering innovation. Related to the question, what are the biggest challenges your organization faces in implementing innovative practices? The results have shown that most respondents (70.6%) believe that lack of skilled personnel is the main issue in implementing innovative practices. Regulatory hurdles and lack of funding also appear to challenge healthcare organizations in Kazakhstan. Thus, those answers are highly connected with the government; they show that funding and regulations hinder healthcare innovation development. After the survey results were conducted, Cronbach's alpha coefficient of 0.81 was calculated, revealing that the survey has high internal consistency.

10.6 TESTING OF HYPOTHESES

H1: Strong leadership support, a collaborative culture, and clear goals and objectives will positively correlate with successful innovation implementation. Hypothesis 1 has been proven to be valid. According to the literature review, answers to those factors are believed to be crucial for innovation development. Karl Pearson's coefficient of correlation resulted in a value of 1.271.

H2: Kazakhstan organizations face difficulties accessing new technologies, lack skilled personnel, and experience resistance. Hypothesis 2 appeared valid according to the survey results. According to Figure 9.10 of the survey, most respondents believe that lack of personnel is the biggest problem in acquiring innovation. Karl Pearson's coefficient of correlation resulted in a value of 1.245.

H3: Most organizations do not apply innovations because they are unfamiliar with the innovative practices. Hypothesis 3 appeared invalid because most respondents are familiar or somewhat familiar with innovation management. Karl Pearson's coefficient of correlation resulted in a value of 0.000.

H4: Most organizations foster innovation. Hypothesis 4 appeared invalid because after analyzing the survey results, most respondents answered that their organizations do not have a clear strategy for innovation and do not collaborate with external partners to foster it. Karl Pearson's coefficient of correlation resulted in a value of 0.000.

10.7 MANAGERIAL IMPLICATIONS

This comprehensive study holds significant utility for diverse stakeholders, primarily benefiting Kazakhstan's state, healthcare sector, medical professionals, and medical equipment manufacturers. The research, meticulously examining the current healthcare landscape through surveys among medical specialists, serves as a cornerstone for informed decision-making and strategic planning. The study provides invaluable insights into the current healthcare situation in Kazakhstan, equipping policymakers with a nuanced understanding of existing challenges and opportunities. This knowledge is instrumental in shaping future healthcare policies, guiding resource allocation, and steering the nation's health strategy. The research outcomes can serve as a roadmap for recruiting new specialists, initiating targeted programs, and facilitating the acquisition of state-of-the-art medical equipment for healthcare institutions nationwide. For professionals in the field of medicine, the study represents a reservoir of knowledge on emerging innovations. By exploring the survey results, medical specialists gain a profound understanding of the significance of innovative healthcare practices. Their competence is enhanced by this information, which also promotes a culture of lifelong learning and professional growth. The findings catalyze further exploration and implementation of cutting-edge medical advancements, elevating domestic healthcare standards. Medical professionals can leverage the study's insights to identify opportunities for personal and career growth. Identifying gaps and areas for improvement in healthcare practices prompts professionals to seek specialized training, engage in skill development initiatives, and actively participate in advancing medical practices within the country. The research positions Kazakhstan as a potential market for international companies producing innovative medical equipment. Manufacturers can use the study's findings to tailor their products to the specific needs and preferences of the Kazakhstani healthcare sector. Identifying potential gaps in the market opens avenues for international companies to introduce and promote their advanced medical technologies, contributing to the country's modernization of its healthcare infrastructure.

10.8 CONCLUSION, LIMITATIONS, AND SCOPE FOR FURTHER RESEARCH

In conclusion, this study researched the crucial role of innovation in healthcare using the example of Kazakhstan's geography. Innovation and digitalization of healthcare are accelerating and improving all processes, not only for the health and convenience of patients but also for clinics and the government. As a result of the analysis of the primary sources, the survey, and the analysis of the literature, it was revealed that innovations have great potential not only in solving problems related to healthcare but also in improving the efficiency of healthcare in Kazakhstan. Based on this, it is possible to identify recommendations for improving the efficiency of healthcare. First of all, the state should invest more money in training existing and future specialists in the field of medicine and invest more resources in scientific research to develop innovations in Kazakhstan's healthcare sector. In addition, special programs and funding should be introduced to encourage research on new technologies for future implementation. The constant development and creation of an environment for the development of innovations will provide direction and incentive for young professionals to strive to develop healthcare in Kazakhstan toward digital transformation. This study also has limitations because the research was conducted based on the situation in Kazakhstan's healthcare system, which does not allow for the generalization of this study to all healthcare systems worldwide. In addition, not all literary sources were analyzed, but only those to which access was provided, which also limits the scope of this study. As for the primary data, a reasonably large number of people who work in medicine were analyzed, but this is not enough to distribute all these answers to the whole country. Because only Kazakhstan was investigated in the research paper, a new study that will compare the health status of Kazakhstan with that of another country will help expand the study. It is also worth noting that this study focused on the innovation of the entire healthcare system, and limiting this scope to one city or one disease would also expand the scope of the study by making it more specific. In summary, this research sets the framework for a more in-depth investigation of healthcare innovation in Kazakhstan. It supports continued conversation and research projects to move the country toward digital transformation. It emphasizes the necessity for specialized solutions that consider the dynamics of Kazakhstan's healthcare ecosystem.

REFERENCES

Allen Stephanie. (2022). 2022 *Global Healthcare Outlook: Are We Finally Seeing the Long-Promised Transformation?* https://www.deloitte.com/global/en/Industries/life-sciences-health-care/perspectives/global-health-care-sector-outlook.html

Aue, G., Biesdorf, S., & Henke, N. (2016). E-health 2.0: how health systems can gain a leadership role in digital health. *Research Action, 1,* 1–5.

Bayeshova, M., & Omarov, A. (2019). Digitalization of the healthcare system of Kazakhstan. *Computer Science, 94*(2), 121–128. https://doi.org/10.31489/2019m2/121–128

Brewer, L. C., Fortuna, K. L., Jones, C., Walker, R., Hayes, S. N., Patten, C. A., & Cooper, L. A. (2020). Back to the future: achieving health equity through health informatics and digital health. *JMIR mHealth and uHealth, 8*(1), e14512.

Chaltabayeva, R. (2020). *Legal Regulation of PPP in the Healthcare Sector of the Republic of Kazakhstan.* https://chambers.com/articles/legal-regulation-of-ppp-in-the-healthcare-sector-of-the-republic-of-kazakhstan

Daryo. (2023). *Uzbekistan-Azerbaijan Health Decade: Advancing Healthcare Collaboration and Innovation.* https://daryo.uz/en/2023/10/04/uzbekistan-azerbaijan-health-decade-advancing-healthcare-collaboration-and-innovation

Elton, J., & O'Riordan, A. (2016). *Healthcare Disrupted: Next Generation Business Models and Strategies.* John Wiley & Sons.

EuroHealthObservatory.(2022).*HealthSystemsinAction:Kazakhstan.*EuropeanObservatoryonHealthSystemsand Policies. https://eurohealthobservatory.who.int/publications/i/health-systems-in-action-kazakhstan-2022

Evans, R. S. (2016). Electronic health records: then, now, and in the future. *Yearbook of Medical Informatics, 25*(S 01), S48-S61.

Ford, G., Compton, M., Millett, G., & Tzortzis, A. (2017). The role of digital disruption in healthcare service innovation. *Service Business Model Innovation in Healthcare and Hospital Management: Models, Strategies, Tools,* 57–70.

Gusmanov, A., Zhakhina, G., Yerdessov, S., Sakko, Y., Mussina, K., Alimbayev, A., Sissoyev, D., Sarría-Santamera, A., & Gaipov, A. (2023). Examining the population-based registries of the Unified Electronic Healthcare System of Kazakhstan (UNEHS): opportunities and constraints for conducting epidemiological studies and utilising real-world data. *International Journal of Medical Informatics, 170,* 104950.

Hidalgo, A., & Albors, J. (2008). Innovation management techniques and tools: a review from theory and practice. *R&d Management, 38*(2), 113–127.

International Trade Administration. (2022). *Kazakhstan-Country Commercial Guide-Healthcare.* https://www.trade.gov/country-commercial-guides/kazakhstan-healthcare

Issatayeva, N. T., Datkhayev, U. M., Zhakipbekov, K. S., Serikbayeva, E. A., & Umirzakhova, G. Z. (2020). Public–private partnership in the healthcare and pharmaceutical sectors of Kazakhstan: problems and solutions. *Journal of Advanced Research in Law and Economics, 11*(3 (49)), 876–884.

Javaid, M., & Khan, I. H. (2021). Internet of Things (IoT) enabled healthcare helps to take the challenges of COVID-19 Pandemic. *Journal of Oral Biology and Craniofacial Research, 11*(2), 209–214.

Kostkova, P. (2015). Grand challenges in digital health. *Frontiers in Public Health, 3,* 134.

Kraus, S., Schiavone, F., Pluzhnikova, A., & Invernizzi, A. C. (2021). Digital transformation in healthcare: analysing the current state-of-research. *Journal of Business Research, 123,* 557–567.

Manogaran, G., Lopez, D., Thota, C., Abbas, K. M., Pyne, S., & Sundarasekar, R. (2017). Big data analytics in healthcare Internet of Things. *Innovative Healthcare Systems for the 21st Century,* 263–284.

Moro Visconti, R., & Morea, D. (2020). Healthcare digitalization and pay-for-performance incentives in smart hospital project financing. *International Journal of Environmental Research and Public Health, 17*(7), 2318.

Potluri, R. M., & Gundapaneni, S. K. (2023). COVID-19 success story of the United Arab Emirates (UAE): author's experience as a recovered corona patient and researcher. In *Health Informatics and Patient Safety in Times of Crisis* (pp. 235–245). IGI Global.

Potluri, R. M., & Johnson, S. (2023). Healthcare consumerism and implications for care delivery. In *Medical Entrepreneurship: Trends and Prospects in the Digital Age* (pp. 199–211). Singapore: Springer Nature Singapore.

Sharman, A. (2014). A new paradigm of primary health care in Kazakhstan: personalized, community-based, standardised, and technology-driven. *Central Asian Journal of Global Health*, 3(1).

Vial, G. (2019). Understanding digital transformation: a review and a research agenda. *Journal of Strategic Information Systems*, 28(2), 118–144.

World Bank Group. (2022). *In Kazakhstan, Artificial Intelligence and the Research Commercialization behind It Are Saving Lives*. World Bank. https://www.worldbank.org/en/news/feature/2022/04/14/in-kazakhstan-artificial-intelligence-and-the-research-commercialization-behind-it-is-saving-lives

World Health Organization. (WHO). (2023). *Addressing the Growing Needs of Kazakhstan's Digital Health Workforce*. https://www.who.int/europe/news/item/20-10-2023-addressing-the-growing-needs-of-kazakhstan-s-digital-health-workforce

Zhatkanbayeva, A. E., Grzelonski, B. A., Zhatkanbayev, E. B., & Tuyakbayeva, N. S. (2016). The stages of the healthcare system reform of the Republic of Kazakhstan. *Eurasian Journal of Social Sciences and Humanities*, (1). https://jhumansoc-sc.kaznu.kz/index.php/1-eurasian/article/view/303.

11 Advancing Healthcare Informatics in Fluorescence Microscopy Using Computational Imaging Techniques

Suman Kumar Maji and Jerome Boulanger

11.1 FLUORESCENCE MICROSCOPY AND MEDICAL INFORMATICS

Fluorescence microscopy is the primary choice of health informatics professional for diagnosing and analyzing at the cellular level. In the domain of medical research, where cellular structures of yeast cells, bovine pulmonary cells, or mice brain cells are widely used, it has become the only tool of choice for studying and analyzing various mechanisms and the effect of drugs also. Specific proteins of the cells are tagged with genetically modified proteins called fluorophores to detect changes over time. Similarly, to analyze the effect of a drug on a live cell or to understand the reaction of a live cell to an external shock, fluorophores that only emit light without affecting biogenesis are used. The samples are then observed under traditional microscopes over a certain duration to observe and record any change in behavior of the target. For example, to analyze the structure of the nuclear pore complex (NPC) of yeast cells, fluorophores like cherry and green fluorescent protein (GFP) that emit red and green fluorescence upon excitation are widely used. The NPC is a buildup of numerous proteins, and tagging these proteins with GFP or mCherry makes the structure of the specific protein within the NPC visible over time. Similarly, if the NPC is subjected to an external stress, then how the proteins within the NPC react to that stress over time can also be analyzed with the help of fluorescence microscopy techniques. Similarly in the area of disease detection, fluorescent labeling of tumor cells in cancer provides an in-depth analysis of the disease at the cellular level. This holds true for other diseases also.

In the domain of healthcare informatics, especially in drug analysis and disease detection at the cellular level, fluorescence microscopy is playing a pivotal role. The healthcare informatics industry together with the medical research community is highly focused on improving and designing fluorescent microscopy-based medical informatics algorithms and tools. In this regard, computational imaging techniques have made breakthrough achievements. By using computational techniques like deconvolution, as a post-processing step, or integrating them directly during a microscopy acquisition procedure, spatial resolution of the observed specimen can be improved manifolds. In fact, one such discovery of designing a super-resolution fluorescent microscope led to the 2014 Nobel prize in chemistry, which signifies its unparalleled importance in the domain.

11.2 ROLE OF FLUORESCENCE MICROSCOPY IN PANDEMIC-RELATED RESEARCH

Fluorescence microscopy has emerged as a crucial technique in pandemic research, especially during the COVID-19 outbreak driven by SARS-CoV-2. This advanced imaging technique allows for precise visualization of virus–cell interactions, enabling researchers to study the viral life cycle

DOI: 10.1201/9781003485629-11

and host immune responses with remarkable specificity and sensitivity. By employing fluorescent markers that bind to specific proteins or nucleic acids, scientists can observe dynamic biological processes in real time, providing critical insights into how viruses invade cells and evade immune defenses (Sokolinskaya et al., 2022).

Recent developments in fluorescence microscopy, particularly with super-resolution techniques like stimulated emission depletion (STED) and structured illumination microscopy (SIM), have overcome the constraints of conventional microscopy by attaining resolutions that exceed the diffraction limit. These breakthroughs allow for the visualization of complex viral structures and dynamics at the nanoscale, offering a deeper understanding of the molecular mechanisms involved in viral infection and pathogenesis (Putlyaeva and Lukyanov, 2021). For example, fluorescence microscopy has been crucial in tracing the localization of viral proteins within infected cells, shedding light on how SARS-CoV-2 hijacks host cellular machinery for its replication and spread (Sanderson et al., 2014).

Additionally, fluorescence microscopy is vital in vaccine development by enabling the observation of immune responses to viral antigens. Researchers can assess vaccine candidates' effectiveness by examining interactions between immune cells and viral proteins, thus providing valuable data on the vaccine's ability to stimulate a robust immune response against SARS-CoV-2 (Cortese and Laketa, 2021). This information is crucial for designing vaccines that can induce long-lasting immunity and effectively counter the virus. Furthermore, fluorescence microscopy's adaptability for high-throughput screening has expedited the identification of potential antiviral compounds. By tagging viral proteins with fluorescent markers, researchers can rapidly assess the efficacy of various compounds in inhibiting viral replication, which is particularly critical during a pandemic when swift responses are needed to curb the virus's spread (Huang et al., 2021).

11.3   IMAGING DRAWBACKS IN FLUORESCENCE MICROSCOPY

In fluorescence microscopy, the sample under observation is exposed to light of a specific wavelength from an illuminating source. This light causes the fluorophores within the specimen to become excited, leading them to emit light at a higher wavelength. The emitted light then passes through the optical imaging system of the microscope, forming a fluorescent image of the specimen on a detector, often a charge-coupled device (CCD) camera. Conventional light microscopes like widefield or confocal microscopes are used here. These microscopes have been a vital tool for biological research, but they are confronted with an immovable triangle of compromise that involves imaging speeds, illumination intensity, and image resolution. Point-scanning methods, such as laser scanning confocal microscopes and scanning electron microscopes, require better resolution for proper sampling, increasing imaging time and sample damage. These physical limitations, such as the short illumination time, potential phototoxicity, and imperfections in the device, result in the acquired image being affected by blur and noise. The blur occurs because the imaging duration of the sample is restricted to mitigate the impact of photobleaching and phototoxicity. Consequently, the resulting image exhibits low photon emission, which makes blurring dependent on the signal itself. This blurring phenomenon is typically characterized by the microscope's point spread function (PSF), and its effect on the acquired specimen is mathematically represented as the convolution of the specimen with the PSF. To address these blurring and noise issues, deconvolution is employed as a technique to restore the blurred sample, either with or without prior knowledge of the PSF.

Resolution in microscopy and more generally in optical imaging is traditionally known to be limited by the diffraction of light by the sample as proposed by Abbe. Figure 11.1 displays the imaging of a periodic structure either in phase or intensity, creating a set of diffraction orders whose sinus angles are multiple of the ratio of the wavelength λ and the period d, which we can write as the following relation:

$$sin\,\theta = m\frac{\lambda}{d}, \qquad (11.1)$$

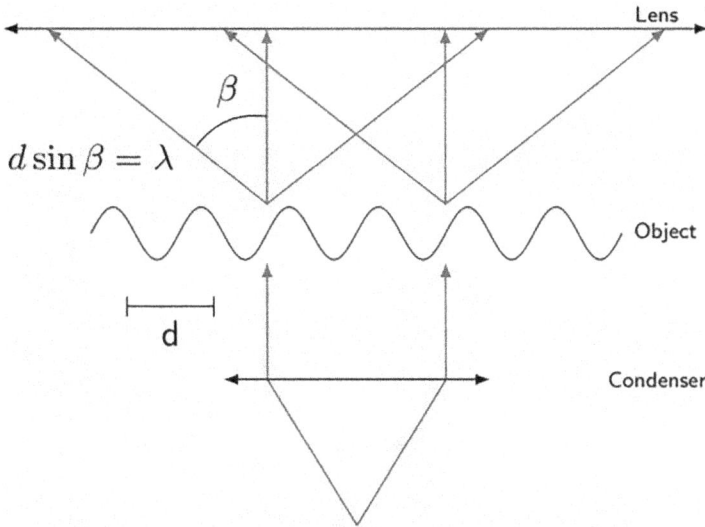

FIGURE 11.1 Illumination of a *d*-Periodic Structure Acting as a Grating.

where m is the order of diffraction and θ is the angle of the diffracted beam. We assume that an object can be correctly imaged by an optical system if at least the first diffraction order enters the pupil of the system, leading to the Abbe diffraction limit:

$$\Delta_{xy} = \frac{\lambda}{2n\sin\theta} = \frac{\lambda}{2NA}, \tag{11.2}$$

where Δxy is the smallest resolvable detail and $NA = n \sin \theta$ is the numerical aperture. If we consider an optical system with a circular aperture of radius D, the intensity I of the image of a single point through this aperture is an Airy pattern given by the square of the Fourier transform of a characteristic function of a circular disk:

$$I(\theta) \sim \left(\frac{2j_1(\pi\lambda^{-1}Dn\sin\theta)}{\pi\lambda^{-1}Dn\sin\theta} \right)^2, \tag{11.3}$$

which is an oscillating function slowly decaying. This expression gives us another way to approach the idea of resolution as the separability of two nearby point sources. The Rayleigh criterion considers that two points are resolvable if the first zero of the images of the second point corresponds to the center of the image of the first point. The first zero of the J_1 function at the numerator is approximately $\pi\lambda^{-1}Dn\sin\theta = 3.8317$, which for small angles defines the resolution as

$$\Delta_{xy} = 1.22 \frac{\lambda}{2NA}, \tag{11.4}$$

Equation (11.3) can also be interpreted as the autocorrelation of the pupil function $p(\kappa_x, \kappa_y)$ (Goodman, n.d.), which can be computed as

$$h(x,y) = \left| \iint (x,y) p(\kappa_x, \kappa_y) e^{2i\pi(\kappa_x x + \kappa_y y)} d\kappa_x d\kappa_y \right|^2 \tag{11.5}$$

with $p(\kappa_x, \kappa_y)$ defined as the characteristic function of the disk of radius n/λ.

Alternatively, the optical transfer function can be computed analytically as

$$OTF(\nu) = \frac{2}{\pi}\left(arccos|\nu| - |\nu|\sqrt{1-\nu^2} \right) \tag{11.6}$$

with the normalized frequency $\nu = \dfrac{2NA}{\lambda}\sqrt{\kappa_x^2 + \kappa_y^2}$. As can be seen in Figure 11.2, the optical transfer function is null beyond the Abbe resolution limit, which acts as a cut-off frequency in

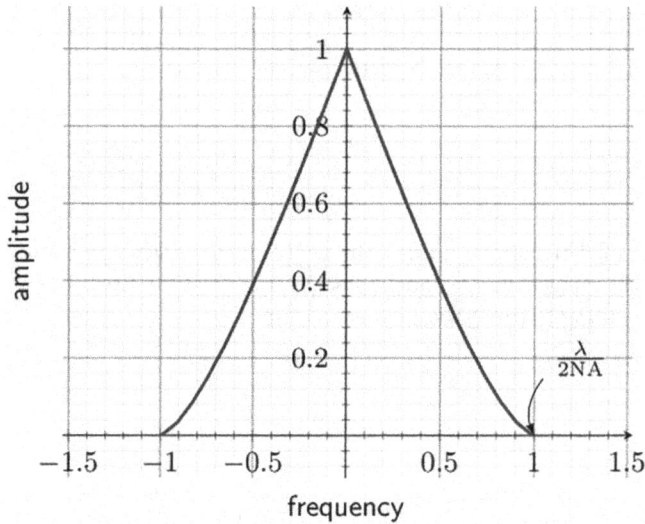

FIGURE 11.2   Ideal 2D Optical Transfer Function.

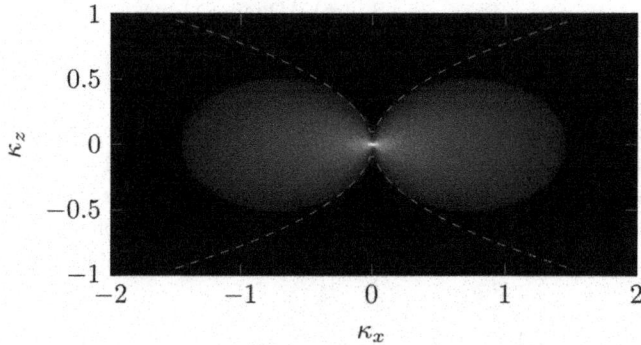

FIGURE 11.3   Section of a 3D Optical Transfer Function Displayed with a Gamma of 2 Showing the Missing Code, Illustrating the Lack of Sectioning.

a band-limited transmission channel. Focusing on various depths within the imaged sample allows one to acquire three-dimensional (3D) images. In the least sophisticated way, a phase term can be introduced in the pupil function to model the effect of defocus:

$$h(x,y,z) = \left| \iint p(\kappa_x, \kappa_y) e^{2i\pi z \sqrt{(n/\lambda)-\kappa_x^2-\kappa_y^2}} e^{2i\pi(\kappa_x x + \kappa_y y)} d\kappa_x d\kappa_y \right|^2 \tag{11.7}$$

Using the Parseval theorem, we can see that the integral of the PSF for each plane is a constant function of the axial position z. In other words, the 3D optical transfer function is null along the axial frequency axis except in $\kappa_z = 0$. This demonstrates the lack of sectioning capability of wide-field fluorescence microscopes and is reminiscent of the missing cone problem in tomography, as illustrated in Figure 11.3.

A more in-depth approach for the analysis of resolution in optical microscopy can be found in Fukutake (2020), where the Abbe criterion is replaced by a quasi-phase matching approach.

In addition to the diffraction limit, the imaging capability of the instruments are limited by the quantum nature of light, which results in an intrinsic shot noise. Additionally, sensors might be subject to readout noise and dark current, adding further noise to the recorded signal. The noise being uncorrelated has a constant power spectrum, which given the triangular shape of the optical transfer function will lead to a loss of resolution.

11.4 ROLE OF COMPUTATIONAL IMAGING TECHNIQUES IN FLUORESCENCE MICROSCOPY

11.4.1 Modeling Image Formation in Fluorescence Microscopy

As discussed in the previous section, due to diffraction limit coupled with various other factors, the resultant image in fluorescence microscopy is degraded in resolution. If f is the acquired low-resolution image of the observed sample u and h of the point spread function (which can be considered as constant within a limited spatial domain), then f can be expressed by the 3D convolution:

$$f(x,y,z) = \iiint u(x',y',z') h(x-x',y-y',z-z') dx'dy'dz' \tag{11.8}$$

The gray levels Zi at each pixel of index i can be modeled by the following equation:

$$Z_i = \gamma N_i + \sigma W_i + m \tag{11.9}$$

with γ being the gain, Ni the number of photoelectrons following a Poisson distribution of parameter fi, σ^2 the variance of the readout noise, Wi an additive Gaussian white noise of unit variance, and finally m an offset ensuring that gray level is not negative. The resulting probability is the convolution of the Poisson and normal density functions:

$$P[x,f_i,\sigma,\gamma,m] = \frac{e^{-f_i}}{\sqrt{2\pi}\sigma} \sum_k \frac{f_i^k}{k!} e^{-\frac{1}{2}\left(\frac{k/\gamma-x+m}{\sigma}\right)^2}, \tag{11.10}$$

which is a mixture of normal distribution shifted by multiples of the gain γ and scaled by the Poisson density, as illustrated by Figure 11.4. Handling such a noise model efficiently is an open topic, but we can note that sensors such as photo multiplier tube (PMT) might exhibit very low readout noise, and therefore, the Poisson noise model might be sufficient to approximate efficiently the noise distribution. On the other hand, complementary metal-oxide semiconductors exhibit variation of gain γ and background offset across the image domain while electron multiplying charge-coupled devices (EMCCDs) suffer for excess noise where the original photoelectron distribution is a compound Poisson process.

11.4.2 ROLE OF COMPUTATIONAL TECHNIQUES IN IMAGE ESTIMATION

Image deconvolution (Sarder and Nehorai, 2006) is a class of image processing algorithms that aim to remove the inherent blur present in acquired images and estimate.

Various methodologies are employed in designing such techniques, which can be broadly classified under model-based techniques and deep learning-based techniques. Model-based techniques employ a statistical and/or mathematical formulation to design a robust optimization problem aimed at estimating a clean image from the corrupted input microscopy image. These methods are primarily focused on replacing the corrupted noise pixel in an image with some clean approximation. Deep image prior-based optimization methods rely on solving the ill-posed nature of the problem, mathematically, by incorporating strategic image priors into the problem. The resulting solutions performed quite well and, in certain cases, were able to resolve structures well beyond the diffraction limit. The advent of deep learning-based methods, especially convolutional neural network (CNN), further amplified the role of computational techniques in fluorescence microscopy imaging. CNNs proved to be better in resolving details than the conventional model-based optimization techniques. The basic convolution operation of CNNs provides translation equivariance. Because of this, CNNs can identify edges, shapes, and textures in images irrespective of their location. This ensures better feature extraction for restoring an image. The use of at-tension modules in CNNs further amplifies their restoration ability as attention-based mechanisms dynamically assign different weights to each part of the image based on its importance. The introduction of visual transformers has made further improvements in the field of microscopy imaging, and now it is possible to improve the spatial resolution of a microscopy image and resolve details that were previously unthinkable.

The success of these techniques in improving the spatial resolution of low-resolution microscopy images has led researchers to widely investigate in this area, leading to a wide class of deconvolution algorithms. In the next section, we will discuss in detail the different types of deconvolution algorithms for 3D fluorescence microscopy.

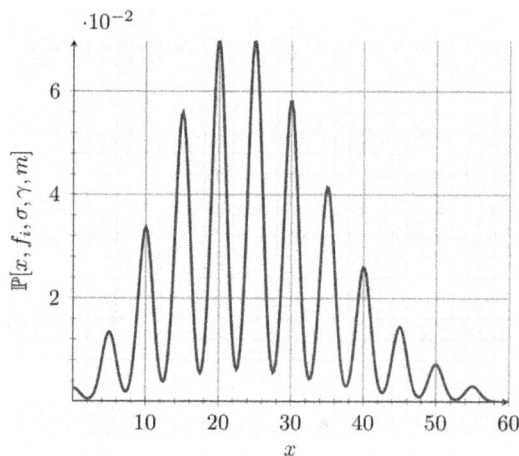

FIGURE 11.4   Poisson–Gaussian Probability Density for $\gamma = 5, f_i = 5, \sigma = 1, m = 0$.

11.5 REVIEW AND IMPACT OF COMPUTATIONAL DECONVOLUTION ALGORITHMS IN MICROSCOPY IMAGING

Model-based techniques for image deconvolution in fluorescence microscopy typically make use of ℓ_1-norm regularized total variation and/or ℓ_2-norm regularized Tikhonov–Miller (TM) algorithm for the restoration of acquired images (Swedlow, 2007; Maji et al., 2016; Maji & Yahia, 2023). Designing fluorescence microscopy-specific deconvolution algorithms based on the above regularization models is an active area of research (Gu´erit et al., 2015). An iterative approach for image deconvolution under maximum likelihood for mixed Poisson–Gaussian noise is investigated in Benvenuto et al. (2008). In Soulez (2014), the authors try to increase the optical resolution using learned dictionary sparse coding along the lateral axis to restore features along the optical axis. The inherent problem of artifacts, however, remains with this approach. A sparsity-based deconvolution model is exploited in Mukamel et al. (2012), where the stochastic activation of fluorescent molecules is modeled using the Markovian process. Carlavan and Blanc-F'eraud (2012) propose an unconstrained and a constrained minimization approach for regularization parameter estimation under a wide range of prior terms: total variation, dual-tree complex wavelet, curvelet dictionary, and undecimated wavelet transform. Li et al. (2017) and Li et al. (2018) propose a multi-Wiener-based deconvolution model using Haar wavelet transform, while a Bayesian derivation of mixed Poisson–Gaussian deconvolution model is given in Chouzenoux et al. (2015). An example-based machine learning (ML) model for blind deconvolution of 3D microscopy is proposed in Kenig et al. (2010). Two approaches for straight and curved edge detection in a multiscale framework are discussed in Ofir et al. (2019) with potential real-world application for nerve axon detection on images acquired by light microscopy. The use of alternating minimizers over the conventional Newton's and gradient descent-based methods has gained popularity, and alternating minimizers are widely used to address restoration problems. A nonlocal TV-based deblurring framework exploiting the linearity of the associated proximal mapping is explored in Yun and Woo (2011). Liu et al. (2018) make use of an alternating direction method of multiplier (ADMM) for the numerical computation of the resultant optimization problem with application in medical imaging. Wang et al. (2015) make use of linearized ADMM in the form of a proximal iterative reweighted algorithm to solve the image denoising problem. Here, a non-convex method is employed by making use of Schatten ℓp norm and ℓq norm to exploit the low rank feature of the data and sparsity, respectively. Cai (2015) contributes to image deblurring along with image segmentation under variational setting considering Gaussian, impulse, and Poisson noise. The resultant minimization problem is solved using ADMM. A modified ADMM method is used by He et al. (2012) along with fast discrete cosine transform (DCT) under total variation to manage sparsity in data. A deep learning model named ADMM-CSnet, guided by compressed sensing for sparse recovery of data with ADMM as an efficient solver, is discussed in Yang et al. (2018). Fast iterative shrinkage thresholding algorithm (FISTA; Beck and Teboulle, 2009) is among the first attempts toward an alternative gradient method for the optimization of large-scale problems with low computational complexity. Figueiredo and Bioucas-Dias (2010) discuss an extension of ADMM to deconvolve images in a log-likelihood Poissonian model using total variation and frame-based regularization. A similar approach adding discrepancy principle for regularization parameter adjustment, called regularized generalized inverse accelerating inverse alternating minimization (GILAM) algorithm is discussed by Chen (2014). A forward–backward splitting approach for solving the optimization problem is proposed by Dup´e et al. (2009) by including a generalized cross-validation (GCV)-based model selection procedure. A deconvolution technique using proximal splitting for the Poissonian data fidelity term and wavelet-based sparsity priors under non-negativity constraint is presented in Dup´e et al. (2012). Hessian Schatten norm-based regularization for 3D fluorescence data is presented in Ikoma et al. (2018) for low-photon-count imaging in the presence of mixed Poisson–Gaussian noise.

Deep learning techniques have revolutionized the approach toward achieving high-resolution imaging in fluorescence microscopy, frequently leading to improved results. Numerous studies have successfully applied deep learning to improve the spatial resolution of various microscopy modalities, including wide-field, confocal, single-molecule localization microscopy (SMLM), SIM, and transmission electron microscopy. These applications highlight deep learning's versatility and generalization capabilities. Early methods like CNNs such as super-resolution convolutional neural network and super-resolution generative adversarial network set the stage for future developments (Dong et al., 2014; Dong et al., 2016), while more recent techniques utilizing generative adversarial networks (GANs), such as SRGAN, have further advanced the field by producing more realistic and high-quality images (Goodfellow et al., 2014; Ledig et al., 2017). Deep learning has also proven effective in noise reduction, which is crucial for improving signal-to-noise ratio (SNR) in fluorescence microscopy images. While SNR under poor light has been improved using traditional denoising techniques (Romano et al., 2016; Shrivastava et al., 2017; Luisier et al., 2010), deep learning-based methods have demonstrated superior performance, reducing photodamage and enabling the study of fast dynamic events and fragile specimens (Weigert et al., 2018). Deep learning-based computational algorithms vary in terms of network architectures (Kim et al., 2016; Lai et al., 2017; Ahn et al., 2018), loss functions (Sajjadi et al., 2017; Johnson et al., 2016; Bulat and Tzimiropoulos, 2018), and learning strategies (Sajjadi et al., 2017; Lim et al., 2017; Wang et al., 2018), reflecting the diversity and rapid development in this field. It provides a transformative approach to super-sample and denoise these under-sampled images, leveraging extensive high-quality training data to restore low-resolution or low SNR acquisitions (Wang et al., 2020; Jain et al., 2007; Romano et al., 2016; Shrivastava et al., 2017).

Advanced computational algorithms have been developed to enhance the robustness of SIM, minimize artifacts (Perez et al., 2016; Huang et al., 2018), and decrease the number of required raw images (Lal et al., 2018). SIM is a unique technique that exceeds the diffraction limit by doubling resolution while maintaining compatibility with an extensive range of fluorophores. Since its introduction in 2000 by Mats Gustafsson (2000), in order to increase resolution, SIM has been continuously enhanced. Deep learning simulation uses deep neural networks that have been trained on real images to reconstruct super-resolution pictures from a smaller number of raw inputs, thereby accelerating imaging and reducing the illumination. U-Net, a well-known CNN architecture, has shown that it can achieve comparable resolutions with significantly fewer images than conventional SIM (Navab et al., 2015; Falk et al., 2019). However, SIM's primary limitation remains its dependency on multiple high-quality images for each reconstruction, affecting temporal resolution and increasing photobleaching.

Another type of microscopy technique is known as stochastic optical reconstruction microscopy (STORM), which estimates a high-resolution image of the sample under observation using unique physical arrangements. Here also deep learning techniques have been developed for increased resolution. For example, Nehme et al. demonstrated the use of deep neural networks to enhance single-molecule localization for STORM images in two and three dimensions (Nehme et al., 2018; Nehme et al., 2020). Their work demonstrated greater localization accuracy with low SNR and high fluorophore density, achieved in real time without tuning parameters. Additionally, deep learning has proven effective in transforming low-resolution microscopy images into high-resolution outputs, similar to techniques used in natural image super-resolution (Wang et al., 2019; Fang et al., 2021).

Deep learning offers a promising solution to enhance the performance of SMLM as well. For instance, single-image super-resolution techniques have been adapted from natural images to improve the resolution of fluorescence microscopy images (Farsiu et al., 2004; Ouwerkerk, 2006; Yang and Huang, 2017). These techniques utilize supervised learning paradigms, where low-resolution images are paired with corresponding high-resolution images to train deep neural networks to map low-resolution to high-resolution images, enabling computational reconstruction of synthetic high-resolution images more conveniently and cost-effectively than physical acquisition (Fang et al., 2021; Wang et al., 2019). Enhancing temporal resolution in SMLM remains challenging due to the need for accurate localization of numerous single molecules. Recent advancements using compressed sensing, sparse support, and deep learning models show promise in this area (Chen et al., 2020; Gu et al., 2014; Ovesny' et al., 2014). For instance, Ouyang et al. utilized a customized pix2pix GAN to reconstruct high-resolution SMLM images from sparse data (Ouyang et al., 2018). Similarly, Gaire et al. employed a residual learning architecture to achieve high-resolution reconstructions from multichannel sparse data (Gaire et al., 2020).

11.6 STRENGTH AND LIMITATIONS OF VARIOUS CLASSES OF COMPUTATIONAL DECONVOLUTIONAL ALGORITHMS

Computational algorithms can be broadly classified as model-based techniques and deep learning-based techniques. Model-based techniques had been the most utilized techniques before the advent of deep learning. These techniques are based on deriving an optimization problem from the image formation model and rely heavily on correct mathematical derivations and utilization of various prior terms (Maji & Boulanger, 2021). Initial achievements were quite significant and some important.

Deep learning techniques turned out to be more robust and, with the availability of fluorescence microscopy datasets, paved the way for the development of super-resolution microscopy. In fact, deep learning has significantly advanced super-resolution techniques across various microscopy modalities, enhancing both spatial and temporal resolutions while reducing noise. These developments not only improve image quality but also expand the potential applications and insights in biological research. Despite the progress, ongoing research is essential to address remaining challenges and fully exploit the potential of deep learning in super-resolution microscopy. Challenges such as artifact generation and the appropriateness of performance metrics for fluorescence microscopy images, however, persist (Zelger et al., 2018).

11.7 EXPERIMENTAL ANALYSIS

In this section, we will show experimentally the performance of various deconvolution algorithms on real fluorescence microscopy data, and how they are capable of resolving details beyond the microscopy diffraction limit. We have considered multiple deconvolution algorithms, some of which are under the framework of the well-known DeconvolutionLab2 (Sage et al., 2017) software,

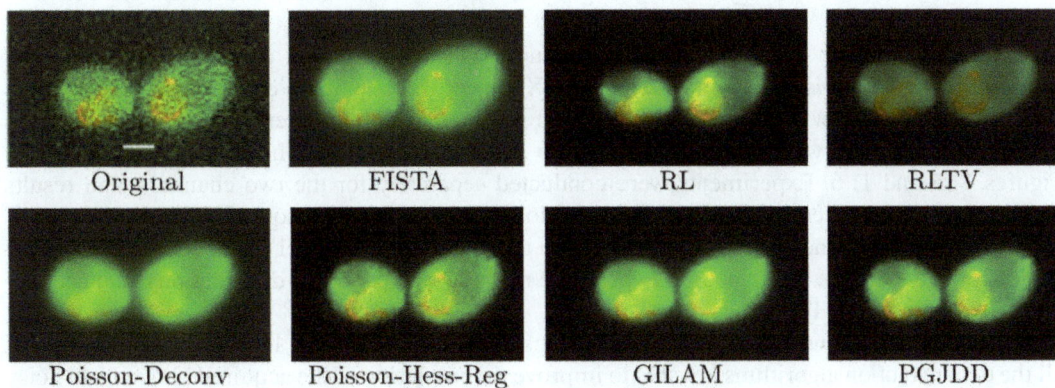

FIGURE 11.5 Results of Different Deconvolution Algorithms over Fluorescence Microscopy Data of Biological Specimen (Yeast). All rows (from left to right): Microscopy acquisition followed by deconvolution result of various deconvolution algorithms. Biological tools, like DeconvolutionLab2 (Sage et al., 2017), were based on model-based techniques. The drawback of model-based techniques was the choice of hyper-parameters that are very sensitive and often resulted in different results, leading to much inconvenience.

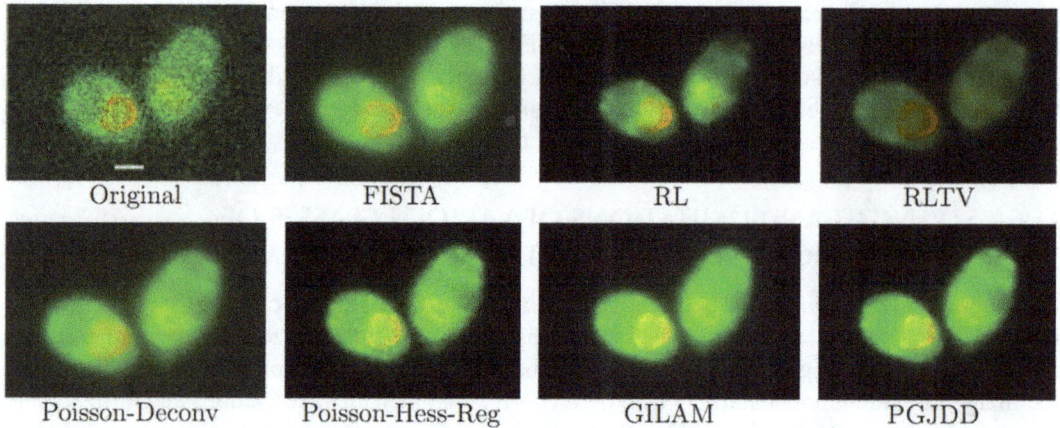

FIGURE 11.6 Results of Different Deconvolution Algorithms over Fluorescence Microscopy Data of Biological Specimen (Yeast). All rows (from left to right): Microscopy acquisition followed by deconvolution result of various deconvolution algorithms.

an open-source platform for deconvolution microscopy, which comprises an array of popular deconvolution algorithms for microscopy image restoration, namely the following:

- A wavelet domain-based sparsity problem using FISTA (Beck and Teboulle, 2009);
- Richardson–Lucy (RL; Lucy, 1974);
- RL with total variation regularization (RLTV; Dey et al., 2006), as well as other popular deconvolution algorithms for fluorescence microscopy, namely

GILAM algorithm (Chen, 2014);

- Poisson deconvolution using sparse representations (Dup'e et al., 2009);
- Poisson reconstruction using Hessian Schatten-norm regularization (Lefkimmiatis and Unser, 2013);
- Poisson–Gaussian-based joint denoising deconvolution (PGJDD; Maji and Boulanger, 2021).

The datasets used for experimentation were fluorescence microscopy acquisition of yeast cell (*Saccharomyces cerevisiae*) samples with a100X objective. The yeast cell and its nuclear pore complex were tagged with fluorophores that emit green and red fluorescence, respectively. Images for the red and green wavelength channels were acquired separately. The raw data are shown in Figures 11.5 and 11.6. Experiments were conducted separately for the two channels, and results obtained were combined together for visualization. The PSF for the acquired dataset was generated using the PSF Generator following the Born and Wolf optical model (Aguet et al., 2008). PSF Generator is a software package used to generate microscope PSF using different physical acquisition environments and PSF models.

Results of the various deconvolution algorithms are shown in Figures 11.5–11.7. We can see that all the deconvolution algorithms are able to improve the resolution of the acquired blurred and noisy sample; that is, all of them are able to resolve details beyond the diffraction limit of the microscope and are able to give a much clearer insight into the details of the cellular structures. In Figure 11.5, the green dots that are present in the yeast cells were clearly resolved by the deconvolution algorithms, especially RL, Poisson–Hess–Reg, GILAM, and PGJDD. The same effect is also visible in the output of FISTA, RLTV, and Poisson-Deconv but to a lower extent. Similarly in Figure 11.6 also the details present in the yeast cells, in the form of green dots, are clearly visible in the results

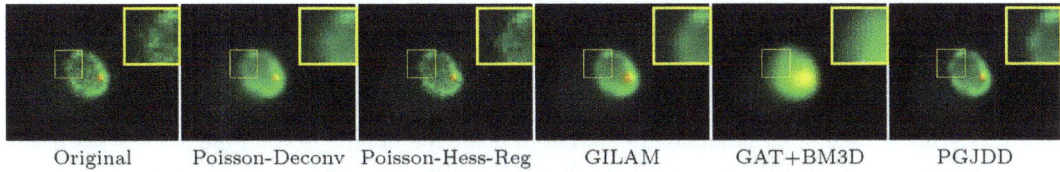

| Original | Poisson-Deconv | Poisson-Hess-Reg | GILAM | GAT+BM3D | PGJDD |

FIGURE 11.7 Results over Real Microscopy Data. The scalebar corresponds to 2 μm.

of the deconvolution algorithms. These details, which are cellular structures, are not realizable in the microscopy acquired sample. Figure 11.7 shows more in-depth visualization on real-world data, with zoom to highlight the utility of computational algorithms. It can be seen from the zooms that the details are much more and better resolved after using such algorithms.

11.8 FUTURE OF COMPUTATIONAL IMAGING TECHNIQUES AND THEIR PIVOTAL ROLE IN ADVANCING HEALTHCARE INFORMATICS

The future of computational imaging techniques is poised to be a key driver in the evolution of healthcare informatics, fundamentally reshaping the acquisition, analysis, and application of medical images. As technology progresses and patient care becomes increasingly complex, computational imaging is positioned at the cutting edge of this transformation. The incorporation of artificial intelligence (AI), ML, and advanced imaging technologies is anticipated to boost diagnostic precision, optimize workflows, and lead to better patient outcomes.

A key trend shaping the future of computational imaging is the ongoing integration of AI and ML algorithms into imaging workflows. These technologies are transforming how medical images are interpreted, allowing for quicker and more precise diagnoses. AI algorithms excel at processing large volumes of imaging data, and detecting patterns and anomalies that might elude human eyes. This capability not only increases diagnostic accuracy but also minimizes the risk of misdiagnosis, thereby enhancing patient safety and care quality.

Moreover, the development of advanced imaging modalities, such as 3D imaging and augmented reality in fluorescence microscopy, is poised to further enhance the capabilities of healthcare informatics. These technologies allow for more detailed visualizations of cellular structures, facilitating better analysis. The future of computational imaging also emphasizes the importance of data management and interoperability. As the volume of imaging data continues to grow exponentially, efficient storage, retrieval, and sharing of these data become paramount. Imaging informatics will need to evolve to address these challenges, ensuring that healthcare providers can access and utilize imaging data seamlessly across different platforms and settings. Standards such as Digital Imaging and Communications in Medicine (DICOM) and Health Level 7 (HL7) will play a crucial role in facilitating this interoperability, allowing for the integration of imaging data with electronic health records (EHRs) and other health information systems.

Furthermore, the ethical implications of AI in imaging will need to be carefully considered as these technologies advance. Issues such as algorithmic bias, data privacy, and the potential displacement of human professionals are critical concerns that must be addressed. Establishing clear ethical guidelines and robust privacy frameworks will be essential to ensure that AI technologies are implemented responsibly and equitably. This includes ensuring diverse and representative datasets for training AI models to avoid perpetuating healthcare disparities.

11.9 CONCLUSION

In this chapter, we have summarized the principle of operation of fluorescence microscopy and its significance in healthcare informatics. We have also elaborated how fluorescence microscopy played a pivotal role in pandemic-related research of SARS-CoV-2. We have discussed in detail the different imaging concepts, mathematical models related to imaging in fluorescence microscopy, and the drawbacks and challenges of low-resolution acquisition it faces due to diffraction limit.

We have given a comprehensive overview of computational deconvolution algorithms in fluorescence microscopy and how they play a key role in resolving details beyond the microscope's diffraction limit, thereby making the impact of fluorescence microscopy more profound in healthcare analytics and pandemic-related research. Diffraction limit is the resolution beyond which a microscope cannot visualize details, thereby giving rise to blurred and noisy samples. Computational deconvolution algorithms are designed to overcome this limitation, and in this chapter, we have reviewed extensively the impact of computational deconvolution algorithms and the strength and limitations of various classes of computational deconvolution algorithms.

In this chapter, we have further shown experimentally how these algorithms actually perform. Results on real fluorescent microscopy datasets show the ability of such algorithms in significantly improving the spatial resolution of the captured samples, to the extent that cellular structures are clearly visible and distinguishable, thereby contributing significantly to research and development in healthcare and medical informatics.

In summary, fluorescence microscopy has played an indispensable role in advancing our understanding of SARS-CoV-2 and other viruses, contributing significantly to global health efforts during the pandemic. As research progresses, this technology will continue to be a cornerstone in virology, supporting the development of effective diagnostics, therapeutics, and vaccines to combat current and future pandemics. The integration of fluorescence microscopy in pandemic research underscores its crucial role in addressing global health challenges and highlights the importance of ongoing investment in advanced imaging techniques to deepen our understanding of viral biology and host interactions.

REFERENCES

Aguet, François, Dimitri Van De Ville, and Michael Unser. 2008. "Model-based 2.5-D decon-volution for extended depth of field in brightfield microscopy." *IEEE Transactions on Image Processing* 17 (7): 1144–1153.

Ahn, Namhyuk, Byungkon Kang, and Kyung-Ah Sohn. 2018. "Fast, Accurate, and Lightweight Super-Resolution with Cascading Residual Network." Proceedings of the European Conference on Computer Vision (ECCV), pp. 252–268.

Beck, Amir, and Marc Teboulle. 2009. "A fast iterative shrinkage-thresholding algorithm for linear inverse problems." *SIAM Journal on Imaging Sciences* 2 (1): 183–202.

Benvenuto, F, A La Camera, C Theys, A Ferrari, H Lant'eri, and M Bertero. 2008. "The study of an iterative method for the reconstruction of images corrupted by Poisson and Gaussian noise." *Inverse Problems* 24 (3): 035016.

Bulat, Adrian, and Georgios Tzimiropoulos. 2018. "Super-FAN: Integrated facial landmark localization and super-resolution of real-world low-resolution faces in arbitrary poses with GANs." Proceedings of the IEEE Conference on Computer Vision and Pattern Recognition, pp. 109–117.

Cai, Xiaohao. 2015. "Variational image segmentation model coupled with image restoration achievements." *Pattern Recognition* 48 (6): 2029–2042.

Carlavan, Mikael, and Laure Blanc-F'eraud. 2012. "Sparse Poisson noisy image deblurring." *IEEE Transactions on Image Processing* 21 (4): 1834–1846.

Chen, Bingling, Wanjun Gong, Zhigang Yang, Wenhui Pan, Peter Verwilst, Jinwoo Shin, Wei Yan, Liwei Liu, Junle Qu, and Jong Seung Kim. 2020. "STORM imaging of mitochondrial dynamics using a vicinal-dithiol-proteins-targeted probe." *Biomaterials* 243: 119938.

Chen, Dai-Qiang. 2014. "Regularized generalized inverse accelerating linearized alternating minimization algorithm for frame-based Poissonian image deblurring." *SIAM Journal on Imaging Sciences* 7 (2): 716–739.

Chouzenoux, Emilie, Anna Jezierska, Jean-Christophe Pesquet, and Hugues Talbot. 2015. "A Convex Approach for Image Restoration with Exact Poisson–Gaussian Likelihood." *SIAM Journal on Imaging Sciences* 8 (4): 2662–2682.

Cortese, M., and V. Laketa. 2021. "Advanced microscopy technologies enable rapid response to SARS-CoV-2 pandemic." *Cell Microbiology* 23 (7).

Dey, Nicolas, Laure Blanc-Feraud, Christophe Zimmer, Pascal Roux, Zvi Kam, Jean-Christophe Olivo-Marin, and Josiane Zerubia. 2006. "Richardson–Lucy algorithm with total variation regularization for 3D confocal microscope deconvolution." *Microscopy Research and Technique* 69 (4): 260–266.

Dong, Chao, Chen Change Loy, Kaiming He, and Xiaoou Tang. 2014. "Learning a deep convolutional network for image super-resolution." In *Computer Vision–ECCV 2014: 13th European Conference, Zurich, Switzerland, September 6–12, 2014, Proceedings, Part IV 13*, 184–199. Springer.

Dong, Chao, Chen Change Loy, Kaiming He, and Xiaoou Tang. 2016. "Image Super-Resolution Using Deep Convolutional Networks." *IEEE Transactions on Pattern Analysis and Machine Intelligence* 38 (2): 295–307.

Dup´e, Fran¸cois-Xavier, Jalal M Fadili, and Jean-Luc Starck. 2009. "A proximal iteration for deconvolving Poisson noisy images using sparse representations." *IEEE Transactions on Image Processing* 18 (2): 310–321.

Dup´e, Fran¸cois-Xavier, Jalal M Fadili, and Jean-Luc Starck. 2012. "Deconvolution under Poisson noise using exact data fidelity and synthesis or analysis sparsity priors." *Statistical Methodology* 9 (1–2): 4–18.

Falk, Thorsten, Dominic Mai, Robert Bensch, O¨ zgu¨n C¸ i¸cek, Ahmed Abdulkadir, Yassine Marrakchi, Anton B¨ohm, et al. 2019. "U-Net: deep learning for cell counting, detection, and morphometry." *Nature Methods* 16 (1): 67–70.

Fang, Linjing, Fred Monroe, Sammy Weiser Novak, Lyndsey Kirk, Cara R Schiavon, Seungyoon B Yu, Tong Zhang, et al. 2021. "Deep learning-based point-scanning super-resolution imaging." *Nature Methods* 18 (4): 406–416.

Farsiu, Sina, Dirk Robinson, Michael Elad, and Peyman Milanfar. 2004. "Advances and challenges in super-resolution." *International Journal of Imaging Systems and Technology* 14 (2): 47–57.

Figueiredo, M´ario AT, and Jos´e M Bioucas-Dias. 2010. "Restoration of Poissonian images using alternating direction optimization." *IEEE Transactions on Image Processing* 19 (12): 3133–3145.

Fukutake, Naoki. 2020. "A general theory of far-field optical microscopy image formation and resolution limit using double-sided Feynman diagrams." *Scientific Reports* 10 (1): 17644.

Gaire, Sunil Kumar, Yang Zhang, Hongyu Li, Ray Yu, Hao F Zhang, and Leslie Ying. 2020. "Accelerating multicolor spectroscopic single-molecule localization microscopy using deep learning." *Biomedical Optics Express* 11 (5): 2705–2721.

Goodfellow, Ian, Jean Pouget-Abadie, Mehdi Mirza, Bing Xu, David Warde-Farley, Sherjil Ozair, Aaron Courville, and Yoshua Bengio. 2014. "Generative adversarial nets." *Advances in Neural Information Processing Systems* 27.

Goodman, Joseph, W. n.d. *Introduction to Fourier optics.* McGraw-Hill Physical and Quantum Electronics Series. McGraw-Hill.

Gu, Lusheng, Yi Sheng, Yan Chen, Hao Chang, Yongdeng Zhang, Pingping Lv, Wei Ji, and Tao Xu. 2014. "High-density 3D single molecular analysis based on compressed sensing." *Biophysical Journal* 106 (11): 2443–2449.

Gu´erit, S., L. Jacques, B. Macq, and J. A. Lee. 2015. "Post-reconstruction deconvolution of PET images by total generalized variation regularization." In *2015 23rd European Signal Processing Conference (EUSIPCO)*, Aug, 629–633.

Gustafsson, M. G. L. 2000. "Surpassing the lateral resolution limit by a factor of two using structured illumination microscopy." *Journal of Microscopy* 198.

He, Yanyan, M Yousuff Hussaini, Jianwei Ma, Behrang Shafei, and Gabriele Steidl. 2012. "A new fuzzy c-means method with total variation regularization for segmentation of images with noisy and incomplete data." *Pattern Recognition* 45 (9): 3463–3471.

Huang, B., et al. 2021. "Super-resolution microscopy: A new tool for understanding viral infection." *Nature Reviews Microbiology* 19 (4): 233–248.

Huang, Xiaoshuai, et al. 2018. "Fast, long-term, super-resolution imaging with Hessian structured illumination microscopy." *Nature Biotechnology* 36 (5): 451–459.

Ikoma, Hayato, Michael Broxton, Takamasa Kudo, and Gordon Wetzstein. 2018. "A convex 3D deconvolution algorithm for low photon count fluorescence imaging." *Scientific Reports* 8 (1): 11489.

Jain, Viren, Joseph F. Murray, Fabian Roth, Srinivas Turaga, Valentin Zhigulin, Kevin L. Briggman, Moritz N. Helmstaedter, Winfried Denk, and H. Sebastian Seung. 2007. "Supervised Learning of Image Restoration with Convolutional Networks." In *2007 IEEE 11th International Conference on Computer Vision*, 1–8.

Johnson, Justin, Alexandre Alahi, and Li Fei-Fei. 2016. "Perceptual Losses for Real-Time Style Transfer and Super-Resolution."

Kenig, Tal, Zvi Kam, and Arie Feuer. 2010. "Blind image deconvolution using machine learning for three-dimensional microscopy." *IEEE Transactions on Pattern Analysis and Machine Intelligence* 32 (12): 2191–2204.

Kim, Jiwon, Jung Kwon Lee, and Kyoung Mu Lee. 2016. "Accurate Image Super-Resolution Using Very Deep Convolutional Networks." In *2016 IEEE Conference on Computer Vision and Pattern Recognition (CVPR)*, 1646–1654.

Lai, Wei-Sheng, Jia-Bin Huang, Narendra Ahuja, and Ming-Hsuan Yang. 2017. "Deep Laplacian Pyramid Networks for Fast and Accurate Super-Resolution."

Lal, Amit, Chunyan Shan, Kun Zhao, Wenhui Liu, Xiaoshuai Huang, Weijian Zong, Liangyi Chen, and Peng Xi. 2018. "A Frequency Domain SIM Reconstruction Algorithm Using Reduced Number of Images." *IEEE Transactions on Image Processing* 27 (9): 4555–4570.

Ledig, Christian, Lucas Theis, Ferenc Husz´ar, Jose Caballero, Andrew Cunningham, Alejandro Acosta, Andrew Aitken, et al. 2017. "Photo-Realistic Single Image Super-Resolution Using a Generative Adversarial Network." In *2017 IEEE Conference on Computer Vision and Pattern Recognition (CVPR)*, 105–114.

Lefkimmiatis, S, and M Unser. 2013. "Poisson image reconstruction with Hessian Schatten-norm regularization." *IEEE Transactions on Image Processing* 22 (11): 4314–4327.

Li, Jizhou, Florian Luisier, and Thierry Blu. 2017. "PURE-LET deconvolution of 3D fluorescence microscopy images." In *2017 IEEE 14th International Symposium on Biomedical Imaging (ISBI 2017)*, 723–727. IEEE.

Li, Jizhou, Florian Luisier, and Thierry Blu. 2018. "PURE-LET Image Deconvolution." *IEEE Transactions on Image Processing* 27 (1): 92–105.

Lim, Bee, Sanghyun Son, Heewon Kim, Seungjun Nah, and Kyoung Mu Lee. 2017. "Enhanced Deep Residual Networks for Single Image Super-Resolution.".

Liu, Chunxiao, Michael Kwok-Po Ng, and Tieyong Zeng. 2018. "Weighted variational model for selective image segmentation with application to medical images." *Pattern Recognition* 76: 367–379.

Lucy, L. B. 1974. "An iterative technique for the rectification of observed distributions." *Astronomical Journal* 79 (6): 745–754.

Luisier, Florian, Thierry Blu, and Michael Unser. 2010. "Image denoising in mixed Poisson–Gaussian noise." *IEEE Transactions on Image Processing* 20 (3): 696–708.

Maji, S. K., and J. Boulanger. 2021. "A Variational Model for Poisson Gaussian Joint Denoising Deconvolution." In *2021 IEEE 18th International Symposium on Biomedical Imaging*, 1527–1530.

Maji, S. K., C. Dargemont, J. Salamero and J. Boulanger. 2016. "Joint denoising-deconvolution approach for fluorescence microscopy." In *2016 IEEE 13th International Symposium on Biomedical Imaging*, 128–131.

Maji, S. K., and H. Yahia. 2023. "Image denoising in fluorescence microscopy using feature based gradient reconstruction," *Journal of Medical Imaging* 10 (6): 064004.

Mukamel, Eran A, Hazen Babcock, and Xiaowei Zhuang. 2012. "Statistical deconvolution for super resolution fluorescence microscopy." *Biophysical Journal* 102 (10): 2391–2400.

Navab, Nassir, Joachim Hornegger, William M Wells, and Alejandro Frangi. 2015. *Medical Image Computing and Computer-Assisted Intervention–MICCAI 2015: 18th International Conference, Munich, Germany, October 5–9, 2015, Proceedings, Part III*. Vol. 9351. Springer.

Nehme, Elias, Daniel Freedman, Racheli Gordon, Boris Ferdman, Lucien E. Weiss, Onit Alalouf, Tal Naor, Reut Orange, Tomer Michaeli, and Yoav Shechtman. 2020. "Deep-STORM3D: dense 3D localization microscopy and PSF design by deep learning." *Nature Methods* 17 (7): 734–740.

Nehme, Elias, Lucien E Weiss, Tomer Michaeli, and Yoav Shechtman. 2018. "Deep-STORM: super-resolution single-molecule microscopy by deep learning." *Optica* 5 (4): 458–464.

Ofir, N., M. Galun, S. Alpert, A. Brandt, B. Nadler, and R. Basri. 2019. "On Detection of Faint Edges in Noisy Images." *IEEE Transactions on Pattern Analysis and Machine Intelligence* 1–1.

Ouwerkerk, Jos. 2006. "Image super-resolution survey." *Image and Vision Computing* 24: 1039–1052.

Ouyang, Wei, Andrey Aristov, Micka¨el Lelek, Xian Hao, and Christophe Zimmer. 2018. "Deep learning massively accelerates super-resolution localization microscopy." *Nature Biotechnology* 36 (5): 460–468.

Ovesny´, Martin, Pavel Kˇr´ıˇzek, Zdenˇek Sˇvindrych, and Guy M Hagen. 2014. "High density 3D localization microscopy using sparse support recovery." *Optics Express* 22 (25): 31263–31276.

Perez, Victor, Bo-Jui Chang, and Ernst Stelzer. 2016. "Optimal 2D-SIM reconstruction by two filtering steps with Richardson-Lucy deconvolution." *Scientific Reports* 6: 37149.

Putlyaeva, L. V., and K. A. Lukyanov. 2021. "Studying SARS-CoV-2 with Fluorescence Microscopy." *International Journal of Molecular Sciences* 22 (12): 6558.

Romano, Yaniv, John Isidoro, and Peyman Milanfar. 2016. "RAISR: Rapid and accurate image super resolution." *IEEE Transactions on Computational Imaging* 3 (1): 110–125.

Sage, Daniel, Laur´ene Donati, Ferr´eol Soulez, Denis Fortun, Guillaume Schmit, Arne Seitz, Romain Guiet, C´edric Vonesch, and Michael Unser. 2017. "DeconvolutionLab2: An open-source software for deconvolution microscopy." *Methods* 115: 28–41.

Sajjadi, Mehdi S. M., Bernhard Sch¨olkopf, and Michael Hirsch. 2017. "EnhanceNet: Single Image Super-Resolution through Automated Texture Synthesis." https://doi.org/10.1109/ICCV.2017.481

Sanderson, M. J., I. Smith, I. Parker, and M. D. Bootman. 2014. "Fluorescence microscopy." *Cold Spring Harb Protocol* 2014 (10).

Sarder, Pinaki, and Arye Nehorai. 2006. "Deconvolution methods for 3-D fluorescence microscopy images." *IEEE Signal Processing Magazine* 23 (3): 32–45.

Shrivastava, Ashish, Tomas Pfister, Oncel Tuzel, Josh Susskind, Wenda Wang, and Russ Webb. 2017. "Learning from Simulated and Unsupervised Images through Adversarial Training."

Sokolinskaya, E. L., L. V. Putlyaeva, V. S. Polinovskaya, and K. A. Lukyanov. 2022. "Genetically encoded fluorescent sensors for SARS-CoV-2 papain-like Protease PLpro." *International Journal of Molecular Sciences* 23 (14): 7826.

Soulez, Ferr´eol. 2014. "A "learn 2D, apply 3D" method for 3D deconvolution microscopy." In *Biomedical Imaging (ISBI), 2014 IEEE 11th International Symposium on*, 1075–1078.

Swedlow, Jason R. 2007. "Quantitative fluorescence microscopy and image deconvolution." *Methods in Cell Biology* 81: 447–465.

Wang, Hongda, Yair Rivenson, Yiyin Jin, Zhensong Wei, Ronald Gao, Harun Gu¨naydın, Lau-rent A Bentolila, Comert Kural, and Aydogan Ozcan. 2019. "Deep learning enables cross-modality super-resolution in fluorescence microscopy." *Nature Methods* 16 (1): 103–110.

Wang, Jing, Meng Wang, Xuegang Hu, and Shuicheng Yan. 2015. "Visual data denoising with a unified Schatten-p norm and q norm regularized principal component pursuit." *Pattern Recognition* 48 (10): 3135–3144.

Wang, Yifan, Federico Perazzi, Brian McWilliams, Alexander Sorkine-Hornung, Olga Sorkine-Hornung, and Christopher Schroers. 2018. "A fully progressive approach to single-image super-resolution." In *Proceedings of the IEEE Conference on Computer Vision and Pattern Recognition Workshops*, 864–873.

Wang, Zhihao, Jian Chen, and Steven CH Hoi. 2020. "Deep learning for image super-resolution: A survey." *IEEE Transactions on Pattern Analysis and Machine Intelligence* 43 (10): 3365–387.

Weigert, Martin, Uwe Schmidt, Tobias Boothe, Andreas Mu¨ller, Alexandr Dibrov, Akanksha Jain, Benjamin Wilhelm, et al. 2018. "Content-aware image restoration: Pushing the limits of fluorescence microscopy." *Nature Methods* 15 (12): 1090–1097.

Yang, Jianchao, and Thomas Huang. 2017. "Image super-resolution: Historical overview and future challenges." In *Super-Resolution Imaging*, 1–34. CRC Press.

Yang, Yan, Jian Sun, Huibin Li, and Zongben Xu. 2018. "ADMM-CSNet: A Deep Learning Approach for Image Compressive Sensing." *IEEE Transactions on Pattern Analysis and Machine Intelligence.*

Yun, Sangwoon, and Hyenkyun Woo. 2011. "Linearized proximal alternating minimization algorithm for motion deblurring by nonlocal regularization." *Pattern Recognition* 44 (6): 1312–1326.

Zelger, P., K. Kaser, B. Rossboth, L. Velas, G. J. Schu¨tz, and A. Jesacher. 2018. "Three-dimensional localization microscopy using deep learning." *Optics Express* 26 (25): 33166–33179.

12 Global Healthcare Informatics
Structural Considerations and Workforce Training Challenges and Solutions

Philip Eappen, Karen Parker Davidson, Matthew MacLeod, Alex Cousins, and Virginia Gunn

12.1 INTRODUCTION

Healthcare informatics (HI) is an interdisciplinary field that combines computer science, information technology, and domain-specific knowledge in healthcare (Jen et al., 2023) to support professionals in delivering quick, efficient, and high-quality healthcare. HI has been evolving rapidly worldwide for the past decade, with ongoing debates about its benefits and risks for the healthcare industry. HI helps professionals improve their understanding of healthcare using real-world data (Yogesh & Karthikeyan, 2022). Moreover, the rapidly growing global population makes it imperative to identify intelligent ways of healthcare management, particularly innovations in HI (Vajjhala & Eappen, 2023).

HI has rapidly spread across the globe. For instance, in North America, the United States and Canada are the leading hubs of HI (Gamache et al., 2018). Its use in both countries has skyrocketed, especially during the past decade, particularly in artificial intelligence (AI), big data, and cybersecurity processes (Gamache et al., 2018). Moreover, Brazil and Mexico also invested in HI to better manage healthcare challenges through innovations (Makdisse et al., 2022). Likewise, the United Kingdom, Germany, and France heavily invest in HI, emphasizing data privacy and security. These countries also collaborate on machine learning, natural language processing, and robotics (Cuggia & Combes, 2019; Van Kessel et al., 2023). Furthermore, China is investing heavily in advanced technologies such as AI, quantum computing, and 5G to improve the HI experience (Georgiou et al., 2021). Similarly, Asian countries such as Japan, South Korea, and India excel in robotics and healthcare automation (Murphy et al., 2022). While technological advancements, digitalization, and data-driven decision-making are at the forefront of HI in many countries, collaboration and knowledge-sharing across countries and regions could foster global progress efficiently and faster.

The COVID-19 pandemic exposed several complexities, gaps, and challenges in HI, particularly in the local, national, and global health information systems and data infrastructure (Massoudi & Sobolevskaia, 2021). For instance, the pandemic posed significant challenges in accurately identifying contacts to quickly isolate and trace them (Basit et al., 2021). Lack of strategy and data harmonization were critical issues that affected effective case tracking and gaps in information systems, technology infrastructure, data collection, quality and standardization, and information governance (Massoudi & Sobolevskaia, 2021). Furthermore, failing and outdated information systems burden organizations by impeding reporting effectiveness; overall, inaccurate data and delays in reporting affected the modeling and monitoring of the COVID-19 pandemic.

During the pandemic, the shortage of workers trained in HI emerged as a critical issue (Arvisais-Anhalt et al., 2020). The lack of a skilled workforce resulted in delays in establishing effective

 DOI: 10.1201/9781003485629-12

reporting systems, and uniform data reports were unavailable, leading to ineffective reporting standards for extended periods. The pandemic exposed a need for more rigor and consistency in applying health technologies in several organizations, including hospitals and other healthcare facilities (Basit et al., 2021). Thus, it is crucial to have a trained workforce to implement HI successfully (Basit et al., 2021).

Multiple challenges hinder the advancement of HI, including the absence of evidence-based standards, privacy concerns, data governance issues, and ethical dilemmas, among other factors (Mumtaz et al., 2023). A significant concern in informatics is the sensitivity of health data, which raises privacy issues when digitized; also, many governments struggle with data management and protection. Ethical challenges, such as obtaining informed consent, arise as users may not fully comprehend the terms they accept. Furthermore, there is insufficient evidence on the impact of HI strategies on health outcomes, cost-effectiveness, and system efficiency (Kaihlanen et al., 2022). The effectiveness of telehealth platforms may also be influenced by users' income and socioeconomic status. Additionally, certain populations, including the elderly, and those in low-income or rural areas, may face challenges in understanding and utilizing digital health solutions due to lower levels of health literacy and accessibility (Kaihlanen et al., 2022).

Although HI has the potential to enhance care quality and improve healthcare service efficiency, adoption in the low-income world has been slow due to several factors (Adebesin et al., 2013). High initial costs of implementation, resistance from healthcare professionals, concerns about security, privacy, confidentiality, and a lack of technical expertise are only some examples (Kesse-Tachi et al., 2019). The limited interoperability of HI systems at the global level further hinders the uptake of HI. In addition, another significant barrier to fully realizing the benefits of HI is the lack of information sharing, interoperability, and standardization (Li et al., 2022; Walker et al., 2023).

Despite such challenges, many global health systems have used HI successfully, for instance, to facilitate testing and clinical care or to develop models that predict pandemic waves. Simultaneously, telehealth programs were used to create the much-needed physical distance during the pandemic to protect clinical staff and patients (Bhaskar et al., 2020). Moreover, healthcare providers also learned new skills to engage patients and provide virtual services (e.g., remotely monitoring blood pressure, glucose, and heart rate (Mann et al., 2020). Furthermore, public health systems and hospitals started using digital technologies to conduct contract tracking instead of labor-intensive traditional processes (Wise, 2020).

Globally, health systems use AI to predict and model the pandemic's evolution and make decisions to support their organization (Basit et al., 2021). Besides, many systems use AI to aid clinical care and apply deep learning for diagnosis and prognosis (Naseem et al., 2020; Wang et al., 2020). Similarly, AI was used to reduce human labor and material costs and for overall economic efficiency in many healthcare systems (Naseem et al., 2020). Furthermore, AI tools such as machine learning and healthcare analytics were game changers during the pandemic for diagnosing, treating, and managing diseases by helping decision-makers create effective strategies (Farhat et al., 2023).

In sum, HI improves access to information and enriches relevant data for clinicians, supporting them in analyzing and making decisions. In addition, when needed, clinicians can easily share information with other clinicians, patients, and families. HI also helps reduce the amount of handwritten paperwork, thus allowing clinicians to provide direct patient care, spend more time with patients, and engage in interprofessional communication. It can also speed up routine tasks and support more sophisticated health treatment decisions by facilitating access to vast amounts of synthesized evidence (Daglitati et al., 2021). Despite its numerous merits, it is evident that health information technology and HI-related training programs, in their current form, are not appropriately responding to industry needs, and only 30–40% of HI graduates are working in the HI field after graduation (Khairat et al., 2016). A middle Eastern study indicated that while over half of healthcare professionals had received some computer skills training, a significant number across various professions in both groups expressed the need for more specialized training in HI, implying a perceived lack of confidence in their existing knowledge (Jabareen et al., 2020). Thus, addressing current limitations by providing tailored pathways for workforce training needs should be a priority for the success of HI globally.

12.2 BACKGROUND

As highlighted in the introduction, in the wake of the COVID-19 pandemic, healthcare systems worldwide have undergone significant transformations, with digital health technologies playing an increasingly central role in shaping the future of healthcare delivery worldwide (Peek et al., 2020). HI has become increasingly vital in the aftermath of the COVID-19 pandemic, playing a role in access to care and assessing pattern behavior among populations (Bakken, 2020). However, amid the advancements and innovations in this field, several legislative and economic considerations have come to the forefront, influencing the landscape of HI both during and post-pandemic (Jazieh & Kozlakidis, 2020). Navigating the legislative and economic landscape is crucial in realizing HI's full potential and protecting patients and workers in a post-pandemic world. By addressing legislation challenges, implementing effective policies, and prioritizing investments in training, technology, and infrastructure, policymakers can ensure that healthcare systems are equipped to meet the evolving needs of patients, health providers, and communities in the digital age. As societies grapple with the challenges posed by the virus, policymakers continue to be faced with further navigating complex legislative and economic considerations to ensure the effective implementation and utilization of HI solutions (Moeti et al., 2022). This chapter explores workforce training challenges and needs related to legislative challenges and economic implications of HI in the post-COVID era, examining policy changes, investments, data security concerns, income disparities, and infrastructure limitations.

12.2.1 Legislative Considerations

Legislative challenges post-pandemic posed significant hurdles to the widespread adoption and implementation of HI solutions (Filip et al., 2022). As part of the adoption of HI, embracing telemedicine, remote monitoring, and other digital health technologies during the pandemic has brought to the forefront many challenges post-pandemic. For instance, governments and regulatory bodies are faced with navigating complex legal frameworks while balancing the need for innovation with concerns surrounding patient privacy, data security, and ethical use of technology (Vito et al., 2022). Additional challenges include updating existing regulations to accommodate new technologies, harmonizing regulations across jurisdictions to facilitate interoperability, and ensuring robust safeguards for patient rights and data protection (Smith & Miller, 2023; Taeihagh et al., 2021). The rapid uptake of telemedicine and remote monitoring during the pandemic has highlighted the necessity of updating existing regulations to accommodate these new modes of healthcare delivery while ensuring patient safety and quality of care.

Despite the progress in expanding telemedicine and digital health services during the pandemic, several challenges still need to be addressed in the legislative response to COVID-19. One challenge is ensuring the sustainability of temporary policy changes beyond the pandemic, as many of these changes were implemented as emergency measures and may not be suitable for long-term adoption (VanderWerf et al., 2022). This is especially true in public insurance reimbursement policies for coverage within and across state lines (Davidson, 2022). Moreover, navigating the complex regulatory landscape surrounding HI requires careful consideration of patient privacy, data security, and ethical issues, considering the 2.64% increase in telemedicine visits from 2019 to 2020 (VanderWerf et al., 2022; Mumtaz et al., 2023). As societies move beyond the acute phase of the pandemic, the focus shifts toward leveraging these technologies to build a more resilient and patient-centered healthcare system with support from funding allocated for research and development of digital health technologies focused on emerging healthcare challenges (Mumtaz et al., 2023).

The post-COVID era presents opportunities for legislative innovation in HI, with policymakers seeking to capitalize on the momentum generated by the pandemic to drive a lasting change (Davidson & Patch, 2021). Legislative bills promoting interoperability, data exchange, and digital health infrastructure can lay the groundwork for a more connected and efficient healthcare system. Additionally, telemedicine adoption incentives, broadband infrastructure investment, and support for digital health literacy initiatives can further enhance access to care and improve health outcomes. Beyond legislation, collaborative solutions spearheaded through legislative bills can play a crucial role in shaping the regulatory landscape of HI; such solutions involving multiple stakeholders are essential for driving meaningful change (Ruebling et al., 2023). Here is where healthcare providers, technology developers, patients, and policymakers must work together to identify barriers to adoption, address disparities in access to care, and promote equity in healthcare delivery. By fostering collaboration and dialog among various actors, policymakers can develop holistic approaches to addressing the complex challenges of post-COVID HI.

12.2.2 HEALTH POLICY CONSIDERATIONS

During the pandemic, policymakers implemented various policy changes to ease the use of healthcare innovations and expand access to care. These changes included temporary waivers of specific regulatory requirements, expedited approval processes for new technologies, and incentives for healthcare providers to adopt digital health solutions (deBettencourt, n.d., 2023). Policy changes implemented during the pandemic to facilitate healthcare innovations have shifted the healthcare landscape (Skinner et al., 2022). These policy changes were essential for enabling swift responses to the pandemic and ensuring continuity of care (Vito et al., 2022; VanderWerf et al., 2022; Skinner et al., 2022).

The healthcare policy changes implemented during the pandemic to ease the use of healthcare innovations have highlighted the importance of flexibility and adaptability in healthcare utilization and regulation (Jazieh & Kozlakidis, 2020; Cantor et al., 2022). However, there is a need to evaluate these measures' long-term implications and effectiveness and integrate them into existing healthcare frameworks while maintaining care standards and patient rights (Moberg et al., 2018). Moving forward, policymakers should carefully evaluate the impact of these policy changes and consider which measures should be retained or modified to support ongoing innovation in HI. Additionally, legislators should consider the need for agile regulatory frameworks and prioritize efforts to harmonize regulations across jurisdictions to facilitate interoperability and seamless health information exchange between different healthcare systems (Torab-Miandoab et al., 2023). Systematically converging health information across systems is the primary goal, given the rapid pace of technological innovation in HI. This includes updating existing laws and regulations to reflect advancements in telemedicine, remote patient monitoring, and digital health solutions while ensuring robust safeguards for patient privacy and data security (Al-Alawy & Moonesar, 2023).

Moreover, data security and privacy concerns have become increasingly prominent since the pandemic (Seh et al., 2020). As healthcare organizations collect and analyze vast amounts of sensitive patient data, there is a heightened risk of data breaches, unauthorized access, and misuse of personal health information (Chiruvella & Guddati, 2021). A 2022 survey by the Health Information Management Systems Society revealed that 67% of healthcare cybersecurity professionals reported experiencing major security incidents in 2020; moreover, cyber threat impacted data in over 45 million patient medical records, a significant rise from the 34 million records affected in 2020 (Dolezel et al., 2023). In addition, an IBM report states that the average cost of a data breach in 2019 was $3.92 million, whereas a breach in the healthcare industry typically amounted to $6.45 million (Seh et al., 2020). To address these concerns, policymakers must prioritize developing and implementing robust data protection measures, such as encryption, access controls, and audit trails, to safeguard patient privacy and maintain trust in HI systems (Xiang & Cai,

2021). Alongside the opportunities presented by HI, there are also significant concerns regarding data security and privacy. Providers and patients alike are apprehensive about the potential risks of collecting, storing, and sharing sensitive health information (Seh et al., 2020; Xiang & Cai, 2021). Addressing these concerns requires robust data protection measures, stringent compliance with regulatory standards such as the US Health Insurance Portability and Accountability Act (HIPAA) legislation, and ongoing efforts to build trust and transparency in HI systems (Theodos & Sittig, 2020).

12.2.3 INFRASTRUCTURAL CONSIDERATIONS

The pursuit of HI to expand health services coverage or increase efficiencies in both public and private systems across the globe is an expensive endeavor due to high technological costs. While, as discussed earlier, high-income nations typically have more resources to invest in HI, medium and low-income nations are constrained by fewer economic resources (Hébert, 2011; Luna et al., 2014), which could limit the adoption of such technologies. Besides the availability of significant investments, further standardization of processes regarding (i) electronic health records and data content (Marc et al., 2019), (ii) protocols for data exchange (Marc et al., 2019), and (iii) most likely, responses to cybersecurity threats since they are often perceived as barriers to adopting digital health information systems also needed to increase adoption and implementation of HI technologies at a global level. Other high-level needs include having a network infrastructure that allows safe data sharing within and between institutions, countries, and regions (Pisani et al., 2018; Luna et al., 2014) and greater network integration between organizations (Khatoon, 2020). Further concerns are to ensure privacy and security regarding how healthcare data are gathered and disseminated (Ali et al., 2023) and that ongoing consideration is given to (i) ensure data security and cybersecurity (ii) create structures that address ethical challenges related to implicit and explicit bias and discrimination in healthcare (Vela et al., 2022) and HI practices.

Across the world, the rise in HI has resulted in new job requirements and responsibilities within the healthcare field, with a focus on technical skills and core competencies (Frenk et al., 2022) related to privacy, security, and ethical use of technologies; data analysis and visualization; or predictive modeling, to name just a few. Accordingly, continuous and intentional workforce development must ensure a well-trained human resource infrastructure with the technical knowledge and skills to support HI's broad adoption and implementation.

Additional infrastructure barriers to sharing HI globally remain prevalent (Perugu et al., 2023). For instance, although the standardization of information, data-sharing strategies, and communication technologies in healthcare has improved over time, especially in certain countries, such as those belonging to the Organization for Economic Co-operation and Development (Colombo et al., 2021), the integration and sharing of health information both within and between countries is still incipient, requiring further efforts by national governments worldwide to successfully coordinate (Adebesin et al., 2013) and agree on measurements and approaches. Unsurprisingly, progress in achieving standardization within countries is needed before global standardization can be achieved. In addition to a lack of HI standardization within countries, the changing geopolitical landscapes (e.g., withdrawal of the United Kingdom from the European Union (Sheikh et al., 2021) and the lack of or nonadherence to cross-national standards (Colombo et al., 2021) may also negatively impact global standardization and digital transformation in healthcare.

The successful selection and implementation of optimal HI systems could be impacted by several other infrastructural factors and organizational approaches, including the style of leadership, change management strategies, involvement of patients in decision-making, and the type of patient-centered outcomes targeted and approaches adopted (Brouat et al., 2022; Kannry et al., 2016). Additionally, given the complexity of HI and its wide-ranging implications, success depends on the degree of involvement of other actors affected by such technologies besides healthcare leadership in selecting HI technologies (Yusif et al., 2022).

12.2.4 Bridging the Gap between Legislative Actions, Economics, and Infrastructural Access

The pandemic prompted a surge in policies directed toward investments in healthcare infrastructure and technology to meet the growing demand for services and address disparities in access to care (Pujolar et al., 2022). Governments and healthcare organizations needed to allocate expansive resources to grow telemedicine networks, deploy remote monitoring devices, and enhance data analytics capabilities to track and manage the spread of the virus (Omboni et al., 2022). Furthermore, resource and infrastructure limitations, particularly in high-, medium, and low-income countries, present significant challenges to the widespread adoption of HI (Luna et al., 2014; Sharma & Cotton, 2023). While high-income nations may face constraints related to outdated systems and insufficient funding, medium and low-income countries often lack the basic infrastructure and resources needed to support digital healthcare initiatives (Mills, 2014). Bridging this gap requires concerted efforts to prioritize healthcare investments, build robust infrastructure, and foster international collaboration in advancing HI globally (Rodriguez et al., 2022). These investments were particularly critical in ensuring access to care for underserved populations, including those in rural and remote areas with limited healthcare resources (Elrod & Fortenberry, 2017).

Moreover, income differences, resource limitations, and healthcare funding considerations continue to pose challenges in the post-pandemic era. The economic fallout from the crisis has exacerbated existing disparities in access to healthcare services, with marginalized communities bearing the brunt of the impact (Bonotti & Zech, 2021). Policymakers must prioritize investments in healthcare infrastructure and technology that can address the needs of disadvantaged populations and ensure that no one is left behind in the transition to a digital healthcare landscape.

As healthcare systems worldwide navigate the complexities of the post-COVID era, policymakers and healthcare leaders face the dual challenge of crafting effective policies and implementing comprehensive training programs to optimize the use of HI (Koontalay et al., 2021). Highlighting the critical roles of policy development and training initiatives needed to shape the future of healthcare delivery in the aftermath of the pandemic is necessary to foster innovation that also ensures the quality of care while addressing the evolving needs of patients and providers (Yiu et al., 2021). Despite the urgent need for investment in new technology and workforce development (Hodder, 2020), the ongoing crisis has strained healthcare budgets and led to cutbacks in funding for training and innovation. This has resulted in a slowdown in the pace of technological advancements and a decrease in workforce support for HI initiatives. Without adequate resources and support, healthcare systems risk falling behind in adopting new technologies and innovations, hampering their ability to respond to future challenges effectively.

By investing in initiatives that prioritize health equity and address the social determinants of health, policymakers can help ensure that all individuals have access to the care they need, regardless of their socioeconomic status or geographic location (Chelak & Chakole, 2023). As healthcare systems worldwide grapple with the aftermath of the crisis, there is a growing recognition of the need to address existing disparities and invest in solutions to bridge the gap between communities. This includes expanding access to telemedicine, implementing digital health solutions, and strengthening healthcare delivery networks in underserved areas (Haleem et al., 2021). Telemedicine requires expanded broadband access for remote health to reduce equity in access between, for instance, rural and urban areas. According to the Federal Communications Commission's (FCC's) 2019 Broadband Deployment Report, 26.4% of rural residents did not have access to minimum broadband speeds, compared to 1.7% in urban areas (*Federal Communications Commission*, 2019).

Beyond policy and the social determinants of HI, the widespread adoption of digital technologies during the pandemic highlighted the need for comprehensive training programs to ensure that healthcare professionals are equipped with the necessary skills to effectively utilize these technologies (Wang et al., 2024). With many individuals and institutions incorporating telemedicine, electronic health records, and data analytics into their practices, there is a growing demand for training and education initiatives tailored to the needs of a post-pandemic healthcare landscape (Frenk et al., 2022). In an era of big data and analytics-driven healthcare, proficiency in data analysis is increasingly vital for healthcare professionals. Training programs can equip individuals with the skills to interpret and analyze health data effectively, identify trends and patterns, and use data insights to inform clinical decision-making and improve patient outcomes. Topics may include statistical analysis, data visualization, predictive modeling, and quality improvement methodologies.

Moreover, there is a growing concern that the crisis post-pandemic will further dampen interest in new technology developments and innovation in HI (Milella et al., 2021). As healthcare providers and institutions grapple with the pandemic's immediate aftermath, they may prioritize short-term solutions over long-term investments in research and development. This could stifle innovation in the field and hinder progress toward addressing pressing healthcare challenges.

12.3   METHODOLOGY

The contextual considerations on training challenges, and solutions presented in this chapter are based on a critical, narrative review of the literature on global healthcare informatics conducted between January and May 2024. Consistent with narrative review approaches (Grant & Booth, 2009; Stratton, 2019), we conducted unstructured searches within standard literature databases (e.g., PubMed, CINAHL, Scopus, and Google Scholar) without an apriori protocol. We started with search words related to each of the subtopics covered in the chapter based on the authors' previous knowledge of the field and continued to expand our searches in an iterative manner based on new keywords, topics, and concepts identified. While we favored recent publications given the currency of the topic covered, we did not use publication date filters. To reflect the global nature of HI challenges, we aimed to include publications covering issues relevant to a global context. We also purposefully targeted publications covering a range of health-related disciplines, and prioritized reviews versus single studies, to allow us to capture synthesized perspectives rather than focused points of view that would be captured in single studies.

12.4   DISCUSSION

12.4.1   Health Workforce Training Challenges

12.4.1.1   Deficient Training

Unsurprisingly, lack of, or insufficient, investments in HI and health professional training to utilize HI technologies (Jabareen et al., 2020; Jimenez et al., 2020) is a key contributor to the lack of a sufficiently trained workforce and deficient training. Limited funding is linked to training challenges such as (i) a lack of competent IT professionals or instructors (Jabareen et al., 2020), (ii) instructors lacking time for trainees due to competing priorities and (iii) poor management of training programs.

Additionally, as reiterated by the COVID-19 pandemic, the development of a global workforce with expertise in the use of HI is restricted by several other contributing deficiencies, including a lack of standardized training (Frenk et al., 2022; Bichel-Findlay et al., 2023), as detailed next. The lack of or limited standardization of HI training is most likely linked to the lack of standardized informatics infrastructure across health settings, regions, and countries (Marc et al., 2019; Torab-Miandoab et al., 2023) and the fact that although the adoption of electronic records is on the rise, especially in wealthy Western countries, it is far from being universal. For instance, several patient care interventions are still documented via physical paper records or handwritten notes (Torab-Miandoab et al., 2023).

Last, despite the existence of numerous HI components and their round-the-clock evolution, training is often treated as complete once delivered (Fennelly et al., 2020) when, in fact, it should be ongoing (Frenk et al., 2022; Bichel-Findlay et al., 2023).

12.4.1.2   Fragmented Training That Lacks Integration into Health Program Curricula

Numerous universities worldwide offer a range of specialized HI programs, ranging from certificates, diplomas, bachelor's degrees, and graduate studies (Thate & Brookshire, 2022).[1] However, HI training is typically not embedded in medical, nursing, allied health, medical secretaries, or other health worker programs' curricula and is often provided *on the job* while students practice in clinical settings (Hurley et al., 2011; Murphy et al., 2004),[2] even though they will not always have access to health information systems to apply what they learn (Thate & Brookshire, 2022). While there are valid explanations for HI training not being typically embedded in health-related programs' curricula, including a lack of experienced and specialized faculty, competing priorities regarding key concepts to teach, and continuous pressures to shorten training programs in response to ongoing or cyclical health professional shortages (Edirippulige et al., 2018; Zainal et al., 2023), this training gap still needs addressing. Otherwise, clinical students (e.g., medical, nursing, and allied health) may only acquire the much-needed HI knowledge and skills after graduating, despite its increased application in healthcare facilities worldwide (Thate & Brookshire, 2022).

Consequently, health institutions have no choice but to address this training gap, which means they must build the infrastructure needed to train not only existing workers who acquired their degrees before HI became widespread but also new graduates. Taking on this arduous task requires heavy financial investment, time, and the availability of professionals with expertise in health, HI, and teaching, which most health facilities lack (Murphy et al., 2004; Hurley et al., 2011). While it is realistic to think this training will happen eventually, given existing funding cuts in healthcare, competing priorities for funding, health worker shortages, and the unequal distribution of resources among health facilities and countries, such training will be very gradual, fragmented, and unequal across health facilities and countries (Hovenga & Grain, 2016).

The delegation of HI training to third parties, including for-profit, not-for-profit, or other training institutions, or the building of partnerships across institutions to offer such training is seemingly gaining traction, at least in Europe and North America (Khairat et al., 2016) most likely in response to an insufficient integration of HI training in health programs' curricula. While such training formats may relieve health institutions from providing the training to their employees, health institutions will still have to foot the bill for compensating health workers for the time spent in training. Additionally, when for-profit institutions provide the training, the price tag is likely higher since health institutions pay for both the cost of training and the time their workers spend in training, all the while the relevance of the training to the needs of the institution may not always be certain (Brittain & Norris, 2000). Of course, a key goal of health institutions is to have a skilled workforce that meets established HI core competencies and standards (Thate & Brookshire, 2022), no matter how training is delivered and the institutions providing the training.

---

[1] Also see the Canadian College of Health Information Management for accredited Canadian programs (https://cchim. ca/program-accreditation/), the National Health Service for accredited programs in the United Kingdom (https://www. england.nhs.uk/long-read/health-informatics-academic-courses-and-professional-qualifications/), and the Commission on Accreditation for HI and Information Management Education for accredited programs in the United States (https:// www.cahiim.org/programs/program-directory).

[2] Also based on surveyed curricula offered by several faculties offering health programs in Canada, including the School of Nursing, Queen's University.

https://nursing.queensu.ca/undergraduate/bachelor-nursing-science-bnsc

Lawrence Bloomberg Faculty of Nursing. https://bloomberg.nursing.utoronto.ca/learn-with-us/bachelor-of-science-in-nursing/Queen's University, School of Medicine. https://meds.queensu.ca/academics/undergraduate/admissions/curriculum

[2] cont'd McMaster University Undergraduate Medical Education https://ugme.healthsci.mcmaster.ca/education/our-curriculum/#tab-content-curriculum

McMaster University Nursing https://academiccalendars.romcmaster.ca//preview_program.php?catoid=53&poid=26850 &returnto=1077

12.4.1.3 Insufficient Contextual Training to Respond to Occupation and Setting Specific Needs

Existing HI training does not always acknowledge and respond to the unique learning needs of various health professional roles and healthcare settings (Frenk et al., 2022). Additionally, the training offered to some occupation groups is insufficient, given their level of involvement in using HI. For instance, although nurses often comprise the largest group of healthcare professionals in most hospitals, being the primary group working with developments in HI technologies (De Leeuw et al., 2020; Nayna Schwerdtle et al., 2020), the training opportunities they have are not reflective of their level of involvement. Similarly, despite the high prevalence of HI technology in various components of hospital systems, including diagnostics and treatment, many doctors lack advanced training in using such technologies (Jabareen et al., 2020).

It is also unclear which health workers within a given hospital system should participate (Bichel-Findlay et al., 2023). For instance, while an individual who merely installs applications on a computer may not need HI training, the chief information officer and project managers (Bichel-Findlay et al., 2023), along with the health professionals using those technologies, are apparent entities who should develop an advanced skillset. Furthermore, while workforce training needs are occupation- and setting-specific, they must also reflect an increasing intensification of interdisciplinary and across-setting collaborations (Shaw Morawski et al., 2022; Thate & Brookshire, 2022).

Another limitation of existing training is its insufficient focus on ethical implications, including inequity-creating potential, linked to the application of HI technologies and the data security dangers they carry (Klinedinst, 2022). Issues such as informed consent, privacy and confidentiality, bias and discrimination, patient safety, and professional integrity and responsibility are further examples of key ethical considerations requiring addressing in the context of HI (Sheikh et al., 2021).

12.4.1.4 Mixed Health Worker Reception and Acceptance of Training

While research has proven the value of quality informatics infrastructure and training in improving access to services and health outcomes, there are several reasons for resistance to new training expectations among healthcare workers. First, current healthcare education and training are lengthy and intensive without additional learning requirements. For instance, a typical medical school program in Canada and the United States takes approximately 3–4 years, followed by 3–7 years of postgraduate training or residency in a teaching hospital.[1],[2] Nursing also requires significant training. For example, to become a registered nurse in Canada and the United States, one typically requires a 3- or 4-year postsecondary degree or an accelerated 2-year degree if one already holds an undergraduate degree.[3],[4] The United Kingdom also requires medical doctors to undergo between 4 and 7 years of education and training and nurses to undergo a minimum of 3 years.[5] Thus, it should not be surprising that adding more topics to the curricula could be challenging and poorly received by students.

---

[1] Medical program review: Princeton, US https://www.princetonreview.com/med-school-advice/what-to-expect-in-medical-school; University of Toronto, Canada https://md.utoronto.ca/md-program

[2] Queen's University, School of Medicine, Canada. https://meds.queensu.ca/academics/undergraduate/admissions/curriculum
McMaster University Undergraduate Medical Education, Canada https://ugme.healthsci.mcmaster.ca/education/our-curriculum/#tab-content-curriculum

[3] Nursing program review: School of Nursing, Queen's University, Canada https://nursing.queensu.ca/undergraduate/bachelor-nursing-science-bnsc
Lawrence Bloomberg Faculty of Nursing, Canada https://bloomberg.nursing.utoronto.ca/learn-with-us/bachelor-of-science-in-nursing/
McMaster University Nursing, Canada https://academiccalendars.romcmaster.ca//preview_program.php?catoid=53&poid=26850&returnto=1077

[4] National Nursing Assessment Service https://www.nnas.ca/nursing-requirements-in-canada/

[5] NHS Working in Health/Explore Roles. Training as a doctor https://www.healthcareers.nhs.uk/explore-roles/doctors/training-doctor. Nursing careers https://www.healthcareers.nhs.uk/we-are-the-nhs/nursing-careers

Second, most health workers have significant professional development requirements to stay apprised of health research on new treatments and best care practices. For example, this continuous learning responsibility is estimated to take as many as 627.5 hours per month for just the field of epidemiology (Alper et al., 2004). Consequently, even when health workers are open to new learning opportunities, they may have little time to engage in them. Third, after completing their entry-to-practice education, most health workers typically perform various duties in acute-stress situations. For instance, as many as one in three doctors report suffering from severe burnout globally (De Hert, 2020) and, as a result, may not be receptive to engaging in additional activities that may further exacerbate their stress.

Additionally, health workers, similar to other workers, may be resistant to changes in work practices, especially poorly managed organizational changes (Harrison et al., 2021). While adapting and responding to new circumstances is essential in healthcare delivery, frequent changes can lead to a sense of change fatigue (Harrison et al., 2021).

12.4.1.5 Insufficient Diversity across Health Worker Groups and Unequal Access to HI Training

A diverse workforce and its meaningful participation in HI could play a role in reducing or eliminating inequities in access and improving health outcomes (Howard et al., 2023). For instance, when diverse individuals are provided with access to HI training and opportunities to participate in decision-making in healthcare (e.g., decide what data are collected, how data are analyzed, and what algorithms are used), they can strengthen group efforts to reduce health disparities through increased awareness of causes of problems, along with higher sensitivity, and humility to the design of solutions (Howard et al., 2023). On the contrary, insufficient diversity across health worker groups, healthcare roles, and limited access to HI training for some population subgroups could perpetuate or worsen inequalities (Howard et al., 2023).

Historical deficiencies regarding racial, ethnic, and gender diversity among doctors and nurses persist across health systems despite ongoing efforts to address them (Aysola et al., 2018; Howard et al., 2023; IOM, 2011; Stanford, 2020). Such deficiencies are often linked to barriers specific populations face to completing entry-level or advanced medical and nursing education programs and career advancement training opportunities (Stanford, 2020; IOM, 2011). Given the relative novelty of the HI field and its overlaps with numerous other fields, data on the diversity of HI professionals are missing (Howard et al., 2023). However, extrapolating on historical data from professions such as healthcare, biomedical, and general informatics, it is expected to find limited diversity among HI professionals, especially in positions necessitating advanced education and training (Howard et al., 2023).

12.4.2 Recommendations for Solutions to the Identified Workforce Training Challenges

12.4.2.1 Importance of Finding Sustainable Solutions to HI Workforce Training Challenges

Recent evidence suggests that 30–70% of the workforce across several disciplines lack proficiency in the use of digital technologies and information (Fenton & Wilson, 2024), and there is notable variability globally, both within and between nations, regarding health professionals' level of training on HI (Fennelly et al., 2020; Jabareen et al., 2020). Unsurprisingly, given the increased application of health information technologies, having a large proportion of the workforce that is not adequately trained to use them poses numerous risks; as briefly mentioned next, it is, therefore, vital to identify innovative and sustainable solutions to address HI workforce training challenges.

First, lack of or insufficient investments in HI and health professional training to utilize HI technologies has significant implications and could contribute to the delayed adoption of health digital tools in certain regions (Jimenez et al., 2020). Second, it can be linked to unstructured or incomplete integration of health records within and between health institutions, resulting in disconnected patient care and a lack of data integrity. Third, an insufficiently trained workforce in HI translates into a limited ability to use the large amounts of available data to provide swift action to improve the health system (Jabareen et al., 2020) and patient outcomes (Fenton & Wilson, 2024). Other risks include underutilization, inappropriate utilization, and an inability to adequately understand the negative implications of such technologies for patients and health workers, including equity concerns.

12.4.2.2   Approaches to Training Delivery

Successful planning and delivery of HI training require an understanding of barriers at both institutional (e.g., lack of funding to support training, competing priorities, and difficulties in applying change management strategies) and individual levels (e.g., lack of time, anxiety or stress related to new technologies, and fear of losing one's job as being made redundant by technological advancements; De Leeuw et al., 2020). Furthermore, identifying facilitators and building on strengths (e.g., motivating incentives, capitalizing on existing experts, and focusing on how HI can be used to improve patient outcomes, standardize work processes, and simplify tasks for health professionals; De Leeuw et al., 2020) could speed up progress and increase the success of such training endeavors. Additionally, given ongoing innovations in HI and technological infrastructures, HI training must account for out-of-date infrastructures currently in use but soon to be obsolete. This could mean that training on outdated HI systems must be integrated into training on systems not yet in use.

Global training programs (e.g., the Technology Informatics Guiding Educational Reform [TIGER] initiative) have primarily focused on high-income settings to address barriers such as inadequate human resources infrastructure and incomplete standardization of health technologies (Shaw, Morawski, & Liang, 2022). Overcoming these challenges remains a timely and critical endeavor. Given the significant human and financial resources needed, political support, including willingness to engage in intergovernmental collaborations, is vital to successfully implementing global HI. Unsurprisingly, despite a general acknowledgment that investments in HI technology are needed to optimize healthcare, government willingness, capability, and efforts to implement HI can vary across countries, which could lead to differing levels of implementation (Fennelly et al., 2020). As a result, when political will and capital are insufficient, public–private partnerships are proposed as an alternative, critical to the successful implementation of HI across countries (Sheikh et al., 2021).

12.4.2.3   Strengthen Existing Training

Based on the training deficiencies mentioned earlier, we outline three priorities: increased investments, standardized training, and ongoing training. First, it is vital to increase investments by making HI training a priority (Jabareen et al., 2020). While it is obvious that health funding is limited and there are many competing priorities, making HI training a priority and earmarking funding for it are key (Jabareen et al., 2020), especially considering its potential to increase access to healthcare and enhance care quality.

Second, strengthening efforts to standardize HI training across occupations, health settings, and countries will increase efficiencies, collaborations, and sharing of best practices while also having the potential to uniformize health professionals' levels of training, both within and between nations. As expected, training standardization and its alignment across health settings will be facilitated by health technology standardization since, otherwise, workers may train on software/technologies specific to a given health setting but require additional on-the-job training on other software/technologies when changing workplaces. One obvious solution to this problem is to standardize software directly within relevant jurisdictions and national or subnational units. If a state public health entity purchased a bulk license for a specific informatics software or developed software internally, all healthcare professionals could be trained on the software used at their workplace. In addition, a standardized and centralized informatics system would relieve clinics and hospitals of the financial burden of purchasing informatics software. If standardized software is used, all data will be stored in the same format, eliminating interoperability concerns within national and subnational units. This level of standardization would also vastly reduce the number of separate places where health data are stored, therefore addressing some privacy concerns about health information. If every clinic in a national unit is accessing the same central electronic medical record, copies of that record need not be stored at every clinic visited by that patient.

However, suppose this level of standardization is impossible due to a lack of resources or a lack of legislative authority in the case of privatized healthcare. In that case, indirect standardization may be the best available option. Legislation could be implemented to set data formatting standards to ensure interoperability between informatics software. This would ensure interoperability between clinics and reduce potential differences between how data are used and recorded in different informatics software. Some private sector entities outside healthcare have adopted a standardized approach without legislative intervention. For example, over 170 American universities use the Scoir informatics system to standardize their application process, allowing students to apply to many schools simultaneously. Therefore, there is some interest in informatics standardization, even within the private sector. HI could benefit from a similar standardization. Direct or indirect software standardization would help alleviate the issues with HI training and trained workforce infrastructure.

Third, given the fast advancements in HI, ongoing training is needed to bring health workers up to speed with it and to allow them to keep up with swift innovations in this field (Thate & Brookshire, 2022; Shaw Morawski et al., 2022). Thus, continuous training will help workers keep up with complex HI applications and their round-the-clock evolution. Thus, training initiatives should provide ongoing learning opportunities, such as workshops, seminars, webinars, and online courses, to enable healthcare professionals to regularly update their skills and knowledge. Professional certification programs can also validate proficiency in specific areas of HI. Without access to comprehensive training programs and ongoing support, healthcare organizations may struggle to fully realize the potential benefits of HI in improving patient outcomes and healthcare delivery.

12.4.2.4   Integrate HI Training into Health Program Curricula

Integrating HI training into health-related program curricula at undergraduate and graduate levels to improve HI literacy and provide students with at least a set of core competencies could be done by developing and implementing specialized courses or certificate programs. It is essential that HI training in postsecondary education possesses certain benchmarks and attributes to be effective, being taught by experienced and specialized faculty, whose recruitment and ongoing training should be secured with dedicated funding. Additionally, when non-postsecondary education institutions or non-health institutions deliver HI training, close attention should be paid to ensure the training is tailored to the learning needs of the workforce and the health institutions employing them.

12.4.2.5   Contextualize Training to Respond to Occupation and Setting Specific Needs

Training must be tailored to meet the unique needs of health professionals according to their specific occupation (e.g., nurses, doctors, allied health professionals, personal support workers, and secretaries), role (e.g., patient-facing, administrative/coordination, and leadership), and health institution setting (e.g., acute care, long-term care, preventative care, and community) in which they practice, however, without compromising training standardization within and between countries. While it is widely accepted that health workers need training on technological details related to HI, there needs to be more focus on the training required by technology experts to understand the functioning of health institutions. Such experts have information technology, informatics, and software developer backgrounds but not necessarily healthcare backgrounds. They may not always be aware that informatics and other digital technologies in healthcare differ from their applications in other fields. In addition to addressing knowledge gaps, tailoring training to relevant workers and their specific learning needs can potentially increase efficiency. This is especially true if training addresses workers' involvement in HI and accommodates their competing professional responsibilities, which may prevent them from attending/completing training (e.g., heavy workloads and scheduling conflicts).

Furthermore, while training needs are occupation- and setting-specific in some cases, they increasingly reflect an intensification of interdisciplinary and across-setting collaborations (Shaw Morawski et al., 2022; Thate & Brookshire, 2022). Thus, given the interdisciplinary nature of HI, training initiatives should bring together professionals from various fields, including medicine, nursing, allied health, informatics, and IT (Patel et al., 2022). Collaborative training programs can foster teamwork, communication, and collaboration among multidisciplinary teams, enabling more holistic and patient-centered care delivery. Additionally, interdisciplinary education can help break down silos between different healthcare sectors and promote a culture of innovation and continuous learning. In a rapidly evolving healthcare landscape, continuous education and professional development are essential for staying abreast of modern technologies, best practices, and regulatory changes (Magwenya et al., 2022).

In addition to learning about the complex applications of HI to various aspects of healthcare, health workers, including those in leadership positions, need to gain insight into the ethical implications, including inequity-creating potential, linked to the application of such technologies and the data security dangers they carry, thus ensuring that a wide range of ethical considerations related to HI is integrated into the curriculum and training programs will increase the likelihood that health workers are equipped to navigate the complexity of ethical challenges in their future practice.

12.4.2.6   Improve Health Worker Reception and Acceptance of Training

There are several approaches to improving worker reception and acceptance of HI training. First, meaningful efforts to reduce the heavy overload experienced by health workers during their initial education programs and after joining the healthcare field are needed since it represents a key source of resistance to new training. Given how complex and intensive current training is globally for health professionals, adding latest content to already crowded curricula risks exacerbating existing difficulties with burnout. If the training is added to existing professional development requirements, the concern with healthcare worker burnout is even more critical. After the significant stresses experienced by healthcare providers during the COVID-19 pandemic, existing workers are even more likely to suffer from burnout and look for career changes. Thus, while the use of informatics can improve health outcomes and healthcare efficiency by, for instance, centralizing information and reducing the time required to access it, revising and streamlining health worker curricula and training are vital to avoid burnout.

Second, it is essential to plan and manage organizational change carefully. Successful organizational transformation requires tailored strategies to adequately support individuals, teams, and organizations in following through on needed changes. One such strategy involves a move away from top-down directed processes of change and, instead, facilitates informed behavior changes and input provision among healthcare staff (Harrison et al., 2021). Change management recommendations are directly applicable to HI training. For instance, one study of doctors using HI in Ghana indicated their interest in providing input on the systems they will work on (Yusif et al., 2022). Additional change management expectations shared by healthcare workers were the importance of assistance from knowledgeable staff and the ability to solve problems as they arise (Yusif et al., 2022). Furthermore, warning of incoming changes was linked to greater acceptance among healthcare workers (Yusif et al., 2022). Unsurprisingly, increasing administrative support for practice changes related to adopting HI technologies and involving those affected by them increases the chances of their quick and successful adoption.

12.4.2.7   Increase Health Worker Diversity and Access to HI Training

Reducing barriers to entering/completing health programs and career advancement opportunities faced by specific population groups could increase racial, ethnic, and gender diversity among health workers across various roles and decision-making levels (Stanford, 2020; IOM, 2011). While removing such barriers requires complex solutions, some examples of strategies to increase the representation of women in healthcare occupations with a higher level of decision-making include adopting gender-equitable policies (Gunn et al., 2019; Gunn et al., 2023). For instance, non-gender-specific parental leave arrangements or high-quality and affordable child and elderly care services will help free up time for women and, thus, strengthen their participation in education and career advancement opportunities (Gunn et al., 2019; Gunn et al., 2023).

There are several solutions to improve access to HI training across health workers. One solution includes providing HI training to underrepresented groups (e.g., female or non-White workers) by third-party government-funded institutions to increase equity in access to such training (Fenton & Wilson, 2024). An example of such an initiative is the *Gaining Equity in Training for Public HI and Technology* program funded by the US federal government following the COVID-19 pandemic to increase participation in HI among diverse groups (Fenton & Wilson, 2024). Another example is the *Bridge to HI* initiative available in the United States, a 5-week program designed to increase diversity in HI (Howard et al., 2023).

12.5　CONCLUSION

The COVID-19 pandemic has led to expedited growth in adopting and implementing HI technologies. The nature and widespread impact of the pandemic have also demonstrated that the complex challenges triggered by the socioeconomic and health crises triggered by the pandemic require global solutions. One such solution, the broader adoption of HI, could help address severe funding and staffing shortages affecting the healthcare sector, given that it could be used for both the conduct of routine tasks and more sophisticated decisions involving the use of evidence to inform health treatment choices (Daglitati et al., 2021) and because it centralizes information, often reducing the time required by staff to access it. However, the widespread adoption of HI is impossible without considering legislative, health policy, and infrastructural implications and adopting sustainable and innovative solutions to address emergent and existing training challenges. While numerous training challenges exist, this chapter focuses on (i) deficient training, (ii) fragmented training that lacks integration into health program curricula, (iii) insufficient contextual training to respond to occupation and setting specific needs, (iv) mixed health worker reception and acceptance toward training, and (v) insufficient diversity across health worker groups and unequal access to HI training.

In conclusion, HI can revolutionize the delivery of healthcare services, particularly in the aftermath of the COVID-19 pandemic. However, addressing legislative and economic considerations is essential to realizing this potential and ensuring that healthcare systems are equipped to meet the evolving needs of patients and communities in the digital age. Furthermore, income differences, resource limitations, and healthcare funding considerations continue to pose significant challenges in the post-pandemic era. The economic fallout from the crisis has exacerbated existing disparities in access to healthcare services, with marginalized communities disproportionately affected by job losses, income inequality, and lack of access to affordable healthcare. In this context, policymakers must prioritize investments in healthcare infrastructure and technology that can address the needs of vulnerable populations and ensure equitable access to care for all. By prioritizing investments in technology, training, and infrastructure, policymakers can lay the foundation for a more resilient and equitable healthcare system better prepared to respond to future challenges.

12.6　FUTURE RESEARCH

Future research should explore the impact of specific HI training programs on healthcare outcomes by investigating the ways in which targeted training influences patient care, efficiency, and overall outcomes. Additionally, the role of technology in facilitating HI training should be examined by assessing the effectiveness of various tools, such as online learning platforms, simulation-based training, and AI-driven personalized learning, in improving the quality and accessibility of education. Another important area of study is related to the assessment of the effectiveness of different legislative frameworks in supporting HI, focusing on the ways in which various regulatory approaches across countries affect HI systems' adoption, implementation, and success in fostering secure, efficient, and widespread use. Together, these research areas will provide valuable insights for optimizing HI training and enhancing its impact on the healthcare sector.

REFERENCES

Adebesin, F., Foster, R., Kotzé, P., & Van Greunen, D. (2013). A review of interoperability standards in e-health and imperatives for their adoption in Africa. *South African Computer Journal = Suid-Afrikaanse Rekenaartydskrif, 50* (50). https://doi.org/10.18489/sacj.v50i1.176

Al-Alawy, K., & Moonesar, I. A. (2023, January). Perspective: telehealth—beyond legislation and regulation. *SAGE Open Medicine, 11,* 205031212211432. https://doi.org/10.1177/20503121221143223

Ali, S., Abdullah, Armand, T. P. T., Athar, A., Hussain, A., Ali, M., Yaseen, M., Joo, M.-I., & Kim, H.-C. (2023). Metaverse in healthcare integrated with explainable I and blockchain: enabling immersiveness, ensuring trust, and providing patient data security. *Sensors (Basel, Switzerland), 23*(2), 565. https://doi.org/10.3390/s23020565

Alper, B. S., Hand, J. A., Elliott, S. G., Kinkade, S., Hauan, M. J., Onion, D. K., and Sklar, B. M. (2004). How much effort is needed to keep up with the literature relevant to primary care? *Journal of the Medical Library Association, 92*(4), 429–437.

Arvisais-Anhalt, S., Lehmann, C. U., Park, J. Y., Araj, E., Holcomb, M., Jamieson, A. R., McDonald, S., Medford, R. J., Perl, T. M., Toomey, S. M., Hughes, A. E., McPheeters, M. L., & Basit, M. (2020, November 4). What the coronavirus disease 2019 (COVID-19) pandemic has reinforced: the need for accurate data. *Clinical Infectious Diseases, 72*(6), 920–923. https://doi.org/10.1093/cid/ciaa1686

Aysola, J., Harris, D., Huo, H., Wright, C. S., & Higginbotham, E. (2018). Measuring organizational cultural competence to promote diversity in academic healthcare organizations. *Health Equity, 2*(1), 316–320. https://doi.org/10.1089/heq.2018.0007

Bakken, S. (2020, June 1). Informatics is a critical strategy in combating the COVID-19 pandemic. *Journal of the American Medical Informatics Association, 27*(6), 843–844. https://doi.org/10.1093/jamia/ocaa101

Basit, M. A., Lehmann, C. U., & Medford, R. J. (2021, April 21). Managing pandemics with HI: successes and challenges. *Yearbook of Medical Informatics, 30*(01), 017–025. https://doi.org/10.1055/s-0041–1726478

Bhaskar, S., Bradley, S., Chattu, V. K., Adisesh, A., Nurtazina, A., Kyrykbayeva, S., Sakhamuri, S., Yaya, S., Sunil, T., Thomas, P., Mucci, V., Moguilner, S., Israel-Korn, S., Alacapa, J., Mishra, A., Pandya, S., Schroeder, S., Atreja, A., Banach, M., & Ray, D. (2020, October 16). Telemedicine across the globe-position paper from the COVID-19 pandemic health system resilience PROGRAM (REPROGRAM) international consortium (part 1). *Frontiers in Public Health,* p. 8. https://doi.org/10.3389/fpubh.2020.556720

Bichel-Findlay, J., et al. (2023). Recommendations of the international medical informatics association (IMIA) on education in biomedical and HI: second revision. *International Journal of Medical Informatics (Shannon, Ireland), 170,* 104908–104908. https://doi.org/10.1016/j.ijmedinf.2022.104908

Bonotti, M., & Zech, S. T. (2021). The human, economic, social, and political costs of COVID-19. *Recovering Civility During COVID-19,* 1–36. https://doi.org/10.1007/978-981-33-6706-7_1

Brouat, S., Tolley, C., Bates, D. W., Jenson, J., & Slight, S. P. (2022). What unique knowledge and experiences do healthcare professionals have working in clinical informatics? *Informatics in Medicine Unlocked, 32,* 101014. https://doi.org/10.1016/j.imu.2022.101014

Cantor, J., Sood, N., Bravata, D. M., Pera, M., & Whaley, C. (2022, March). The impact of the COVID-19 pandemic and policy response on health care utilization: evidence from county-level medical claims and cell-phone data. *Journal of Health Economics, 82,* 102581. https://doi.org/10.1016/j.jhealeco.2022.102581

Chelak, K., & Chakole, S. (2023, January 5). The role of social determinants of health in promoting health equality: a narrative review. *Cureus.* https://doi.org/10.7759/cureus.33425

Chiruvella, V., & Guddati, A. K. (2021, May 21). Ethical issues in patient data ownership. *Interactive Journal of Medical Research, 10*(2), e22269. https://doi.org/10.2196/22269

Colombo, F., Oderkirk, J., & Slawomirski, L. (2021). Health information systems, electronic medical records, and big data in global healthcare. In I. Kickbusch, D. Ganten, & M. Moeti (Eds.), *Handbook of Global Health* (pp. 1699–1729). Springer International Publishing. https://doi.org/10.1007/978-3-030-45009-0_71

Cuggia, M., & Combes, S. (2019, August). The French health data hub and the German medical informatics initiatives: two national projects to promote data sharing in healthcare. *Yearbook of Medical Informatics, 28*(01), 195–202. https://doi.org/10.1055/s-0039–1677917

Davidson, K. P. (2022, December 9). Telemedicine in pandemic times. *HI and Patient Safety in Times of Crisis*, 95–117. https://doi.org/10.4018/978-1-6684-5499-2.ch006

Davidson, P. M., & Patch, M. (2021, April). Time for a reset and recalibration: healthcare in the post-COVID era. *International Journal of Nursing Sciences*, 8(2), 143–144. https://doi.org/10.1016/j.ijnss.2021.03.004

De Hert, S. (2020). Burnout in healthcare workers: prevalence, impact and preventative strategies. *Local and Regional Anesthesia*, 13, 171–183. https://doi.org/10.2147/LRA.S240564

De Leeuw, J. A., Woltjer, H., & Kool, R. B. (2020). Identification of factors influencing the adoption of health information technology by digitally lagging nurses: in-depth interview study. *Journal of Medical Internet Research*, 22(8), e15630–e15630. https://doi.org/10.2196/15630

deBettencourt, S. (n.d.). (2023) *Frequently Asked Questions: CMS Waivers, Flexibilities, and the End of the COVID-19 Public Health Emergency.* https://www.rhat.org/index.php?option=com_dailyplanetblog& view=entry&category=covid&id=186:frequently-asked-questions-cms-waivers-flexibilities-and-the-end-of-the-covid-19-public-health-emergency

Dolezel, D., Beauvais, B., Granados, P. S., Fulton, L., & Kruse, C. S. (2023). Effects of internal and external factors on hospital data breaches: quantitative study. *Journal of Medical Internet Research*, 25, e51471. https://doi.org/10.2196/51471

Edirippulige, S., Brooks, P., Carati, C., Wade, V. A., Smith, A. C., Wickramasinghe, S., & Armfield, N. R. (2018). It is important, but not important enough: eHealth as a curriculum priority in medical education in Australia. *Journal of Telemedicine and Telecare*, 24(10), 697–702. https://doi.org/10.1177/1357 633X18793282

Elrod, J. K., & Fortenberry, J. L. (2017, December). Bridging access gaps experienced by the underserved: the need for healthcare providers to look within for answers. *BMC Health Services Research*, 17(S4). https://doi.org/10.1186/s12913-017-2756-4

Farhat, F., Sohail, S. S., Alam, M. T., Ubaid, S., Shakil, Ashhad, M., & Madsen, D. I. (2023, November 8). COVID-19 and beyond leveraging artificial intelligence for enhanced outbreak control. *Frontiers in Artificial Intelligence*, 6. https://doi.org/10.3389/frai.2023.1266560

Federal Communications Commission. (2019). *2019 Broadband Deployment Report.* https://www.fcc.gov/reports-research/reports/broadband-progress-reports/2019-broadband-deployment-report

Fennelly, O., Cunningham, C., Grogan, L., Cronin, H., O'Shea, C., Roche, M., Lawlor, F., & O'Hare, N. (2020). Successfully implementing a national electronic health record: a rapid umbrella review. *International Journal of Medical Informatics*, 144, 104281–104281. https://doi.org/10.1016/j.ijmedinf.2020.104281

Fenton, S. H., & Wilson, G. M. (2024). Building a more diverse public HI workforce: preliminary results. *Studies in Health Technology and Informatics*, 310, 1231–1235.

Filip, R., Gheorghita Puscaselu, R., Anchidin-Norocel, L., Dimian, M., & Savage, W. K. (2022, August 7). Global challenges to public health care systems during the COVID-19 pandemic: a review of pandemic measures and problems. *Journal of Personalized Medicine*, 12(8), 1295. https://doi.org/10.3390/jpm12081295

Frenk, J., Chen, L. C., Chandran, L., Groff, E. O. H., King, R., Meleis, A., & Fineberg, H. V. (2022). Challenges and opportunities for educating health professionals after the COVID-19 pandemic. *The Lancet*, 400(10362), 1539–1556. https://doi.org/10.1016/s0140–6736(22)02092-x

Gamache, R., Kharrazi, H., & Weiner, J. (2018, August). Public and population HI: the bridging of big data to benefit communities. *Yearbook of Medical Informatics*, 27(01), 199–206. https://doi.org/10.105 5/s-0038–1667081

Georgiou, K. E., Georgiou, E., & Satava, R. M. (2021). 5G Use in healthcare: the future is present. *JSLS: Journal of the Society of Laparoscopic & Robotic Surgeons*, 25(4), e2021.00064. https://doi.org/10.4293/jsls.2021.00064

Grant, M. J., & Booth, A. (2009). A typology of reviews: an analysis of 14 review types and associated methodologies. *Health Information & Libraries Journal*, 26(2), 91–108. https://doi.org/10.1111/j.1471–1842.2009.00848.x

Gunn, V., Muntaner, C., Ng, E., Villeneuve, M., Gea-Sanchez, M., & Chung, H. (2019). Gender equality policies, nursing professionalization, and the nursing workforce: a cross-sectional, time-series analysis of 22 countries, 2000–2015. *International Journal of Nursing Studies*, 99, 103388. https://doi.org/10.1016/j.ijnurstu.2019.103388

Gunn, V., Villeneuve, M., O'Campo, P., & Muntaner, C. (2023). Underfunding of nursing education and the precarious employment conditions of nurses: an exploration of contributing factors, Covid-19 pandemic implications, and structural solutions. In *Handbook on Gender and Public Sector Employment* (pp. 321–335). Edward Elgar Publishing.

Haleem, A., Javaid, M., Singh, R. P., & Suman, R. (2021). Telemedicine for healthcare: capabilities, features, barriers, and applications. *Sensors International*, 2, 100117. https://doi.org/10.1016/j.sintl.2021.100117

Harrison, R., Fischer, S., Walpola, R. L., Chauhan, A., Babalola, T., Mears, S., & Le-Dao, H. (2021). Where do models for change management, improvement and implementation meet? A systematic review of the applications of change management models in healthcare. *Journal of Healthcare Leadership*, *13*, 85–108. https://doi.org/10.2147/JHL.S289176

Hébert, R. (2011). Economics of HI in developing countries. In E. M. Borycki et al., R. (Eds.), *International Perspectives in HI* (pp. 162–167). IOS Press. https://doi.org/10.3233/978-1-60750-709-3-162

Hodder, A. (2020, August 3). New technology, work and employment in the era of COVID-19: reflecting on legacies of research. *New Technology, Work and Employment*, *35*(3), 262–275. https://doi.org/10.1111/ntwe.12173

Hovenga, E., and Grain, H. (2016). Learning, training and teaching of HI and its evidence for informaticians and clinical practice. *Studies in Health Technology and Informatics*, *222*, 336–354.

Howard, A. P., Slaughter, L. S., Simmonds, C., McPherson, R., Kennedy, N., & Bentley, K. (2023). Bridge to HI—a 5-week intensive online program to increase diversity in HI. *Frontiers in Education (Lausanne)*, *8*. https://doi.org/10.3389/feduc.2023.1194746

Hurley, K. F., Taylor, B., Postuma, P., & Paterson, G. (2011). What are Canadian medical students learning about HI? *Electronic Journal of Health Informatics*, *6*(4), 35.

Institute of Medicine. (2011). *The Future of Nursing: Leading Change, Advancing Health*. National Academies Press.

Jabareen, H., Khader, Y., & Taweel, A. (2020). Health information systems in Jordan and Palestine: the need for HI training. *Eastern Mediterranean Health Journal*, *26*(11), 1323–1330. https://doi.org/10.26719/emhj.20.036

Jazieh, A. R., & Kozlakidis, Z. (2020, July 28). Healthcare transformation in the post-coronavirus pandemic era. *Frontiers in Medicine*, *7*. https://doi.org/10.3389/fmed.2020.00429

Jen, M. Y., Mechanic, O. J., & Teoli, D. (2023, September 4). *Informatics*. StatPearls—NCBI Bookshelf. https://www.ncbi.nlm.nih.gov/books/NBK470564/

Jimenez, G., Spinazze, P., Matchar, D., Koh Choon Huat, G., van der Kleij, R. M. J. J., Chavannes, N. H., & Car, J. (2020). Digital health competencies for primary healthcare professionals: a scoping review. *International Journal of Medical Informatics*, *143*, 104260–104260. https://doi.org/10.1016/j.ijmedinf.2020.104260

Kaihlanen, A. M., Virtanen, L., Buchert, U., Safarov, N., Valkonen, P., Hietapakka, L., Hörhammer, I., Kujala, S., Kouvonen, A., & Heponiemi, T. (2022). Towards digital health equity—a qualitative study of the challenges experienced by vulnerable groups in using digital health services in the COVID-19 era. *BMC Health Services Research*, *22*(1). https://doi.org/10.1186/s12913-022-07584-4

Kannry, J., Sengstack, P., Thyvalikakath, T. P., Poikonen, J., Middleton, B., Payne, T., & Lehmann, C. U. (2016). The chief clinical informatics officer (CCIO): AMIA task force report on CCIO knowledge, education, and skillset requirements. *Applied Clinical Informatics*, *7*(1), 143–176. https://doi.org/10.4338/ACI-2015-12-R-0174

Kesse-Tachi, A., Asmah, A. E., & Agbozo, E. (2019). Factors influencing adoption of eHealth technologies in Ghana. *Digital Health*, *5*, 205520761987142. https://doi.org/10.1177/2055207619871425

Khairat, S., Sandefer, R., Marc, D., & Pyles, L. (2016, July 3). A review of biomedical and HI education: a workforce training framework. *Journal of Hospital Administration*, *5*(5), 10. https://doi.org/10.5430/jha.v5n5p10

Khatoon, A. (2020). A blockchain-based smart contract system for healthcare management. *Electronics (Basel)*, *9*(1), 94. https://doi.org/10.3390/electronics9010094

Koontalay, A., Suksatan, W., Prabsangob, K., & Sadang, J. M. (2021, October). Healthcare workers' burdens during the COVID-19 pandemic: a qualitative systematic review. *Journal of Multidisciplinary Healthcare*, *14*, 3015–3025. https://doi.org/10.2147/jmdh.s330041

Li, E., Clarke, J., Ashrafian, H., Darzi, A., & Neves, A. L. (2022). The impact of electronic health record interoperability on safety and quality of care in high-income countries: systematic review. *Journal of Medical Internet Research*, *24*(9), e38144. https://doi.org/10.2196/38144

Luna, D., Almerares, A., Mayan, J. C., González Bernaldo de Quirós, F., & Otero, C. (2014). HI in developing countries: going beyond pilot practices to sustainable implementations: a review of the current challenges. *HI Research*, *20*(1), 3. https://doi.org/10.4258/hir.2014.20.1.3

Magwenya, R. H., Ross, A. J., & Ngatiane, L. S. (2022, December 21). Continuing professional development in the last decade—a scoping review. *Journal of Adult and Continuing Education*, *29*(2), 408–437. https://doi.org/10.1177/14779714221147297

Makdisse, M., Ramos, P., Malheiro, D., Katz, M., Novoa, L., Cendoroglo Neto, M., Ferreira, J. H. G., & Klajner, S. (2022, June). Value-based healthcare in Latin America: a survey of 70 healthcare provider organizations from Argentina, Brazil, Chile, Colombia and Mexico. *BMJ Open*, *12*(6), e058198. https://doi.org/10.1136/bmjopen-2021-058198

Mann, D. M., Chen, J., Chunara, R., Testa, P. A., & Nov, O. (2020, May 29). COVID-19 transforms health care through telemedicine: evidence from the field. *Journal of the American Medical Informatics Association*, *27*(7), 1132–1135. https://doi.org/10.1093/jamia/ocaa072

Marc, D.T., Butler-Henderson, K., Dua, P., Lalani, K., & Fenton, S.H. (2019). Global workforce trends in HI & information management. *Studies in Health Technology and Informatics*, *264*, 1273–1277. https://doi.org/10.3233/SHTI190431

Massoudi, B. L., & Sobolevskaia, D. (2021, August). Keep moving forward: HI and information management beyond the COVID-19 pandemic. *Yearbook of Medical Informatics*, *30*(01), 075–083. https://doi.org/10.1055/s-0041-1726499

Milella, F., Minelli, E. A., Strozzi, F., & Croce, D. (2021, May). Change and innovation in healthcare: findings from literature. *Clinico Economics and Outcomes Research*, *13*, 395–408. https://doi.org/10.2147/ceor.s301169

Mills, A. (2014, February 6). Health care systems in low- and middle-income Countries. *New England Journal of Medicine*, *370*(6), 552–557. https://doi.org/10.1056/nejmra1110897

Moberg, J., Oxman, A. D., Rosenbaum, S., Schünemann, H. J., Guyatt, G., Flottorp, S., Glenton, C., Lewin, S., Morelli, A., Rada, G., & Alonso-Coello, P. (2018, May 29). The GRADE evidence to decision (EtD) framework for health system and public health decisions. *Health Research Policy and Systems*, *16*(1). https://doi.org/10.1186/s12961-018-0320-2

Moeti, M., Gao, G. F., & Herrman, H. (2022, August). Global pandemic perspectives: public health, mental health, and lessons for the future. *The Lancet*, *400*(10353), e3–e7. https://doi.org/10.1016/s0140–6736(22)01328–9

Mumtaz, H., Riaz, M. H., Wajid, H., Saqib, M., Zeeshan, M. H., Khan, S. E., Chauhan, Y. R., Sohail, H., & Vohra, L. I. (2023, September 28). Current challenges and potential solutions to digital health technologies in evidence generation: a narrative review. *Frontiers in Digital Health*, *5*. https://doi.org/10.3389/fdgth.2023.1203945

Murphy, J., Stramer, K., Clamp, S., Grubb, P., Gosland, J., & Davis, S. (2004). HI education for clinicians and managers—what is holding up progress? *International Journal of Medical Informatics*, *73*(2), 205–213. https://doi.org/10.1016/j.ijmedinf.2003.12.003

Murphy, R. R., Gandudi, V. B., Amin, T., Clendenin, A., & Moats, J. (2022). An analysis of international use of robots for COVID–19. *Robotics and Autonomous Systems*, *p. 148*, 103922. https://doi.org/10.1016/j.robot.2021.103922

Naseem, M., Akhund, R., Arshad, H., & Ibrahim, M. T. (2020). Exploring the potential of artificial intelligence and machine learning to combat COVID-19 and existing opportunities for LMIC: a scoping review. *Journal of Primary Care & Community Health*, *11*, 215013272096363. https://doi.org/10.1177/2150132720963634

Nayna Schwerdtle, P., Connell, C. J., Lee, S., Plummer, V., Russo, P. L., Endacott, R., & Kuhn, L. (2020). Nurse expertise: a critical resource in the COVID-19 pandemic response. *Annals of Global Health*, *86*(1), 49–49. https://doi.org/10.5334/aogh.2898

Omboni, S., et al. (2022). The worldwide impact of telemedicine during COVID-19: current evidence and recommendations for the future. *Connected Health*. https://doi.org/10.20517/ch.2021.03

Patel, J. S., Vo, H., Nguyen, A., Dzomba, B., & Wu, H. (2022, March). A data-driven assessment of the US HI programs and job market. *Applied Clinical Informatics*, *13*(02), 327–338. https://doi.org/10.1055/s-0042-1743242

Peek, N., Sujan, M., & Scott, P. (2020). Digital health and care in pandemic times: impact of COVID–19. *BMJ Health & Care Informatics*, *27*(1), e100166. https://doi.org/10.1136/bmjhci-2020–100166

Perugu, B., Wadhwa, V., Kim, J., Cai, J., Shin, A., & Gupta, A. (2023). Pragmatic approaches to interoperability–surmounting barriers to healthcare data and information across organizations and political boundaries. *Telehealth and Medicine Today*, *8*(4). https://doi.org/10.30953/thmt.v8.421

Pisani, E., Ghataure, A., & Merson, L. (2018). Data sharing in public health emergencies: A study of current policies, practices and infrastructure supporting the sharing of data to prevent and respond to epidemic and pandemic threats. https://wellcome.figshare.com/articles/journal_contribution/Data_sharing_in_public_health_emergencies_A_study_of_current_policies_practices_and_infrastructure_supporting_the_sharing_of_data_to_prevent_and_respond_to_epidemic_and_pandemic_threats/5897608/1

Pujolar, G., Oliver-Anglès, A., Vargas, I., & Vázquez, M. L. (2022). Changes in access to health services during the COVID-19 pandemic: a scoping review. *International Journal of Environmental Research and Public Health*, *19*(3), 1749. https://doi.org/10.3390/ijerph19031749

Rodriguez, J. A., Shachar, C., & Bates, D. W. (2022). Digital inclusion as health care—supporting health care equity with digital-infrastructure initiatives. *New England Journal of Medicine*, *386*(12), 1101–1103. https://doi.org/10.1056/nejmp2115646

Ruebling, I., Eggenberger, T., Frost, J. S., Gazenfried, E., Greer, A., Khalili, H., Ochs, J., Ronnebaum, J., & Stein, S. M. (2023, December). Interprofessional collaboration: a public policy healthcare transformation call for action. *Journal of Interprofessional Education & Practice*, *33*, 100675. https://doi.org/10.1016/j.xjep.2023.100675

Seh, A. H., Zarour, M., Alenezi, M., Sarkar, A. K., Agrawal, A., Kumar, R., & Ahmad Khan, R. (2020). Healthcare data breaches: insights and implications. *Healthcare*, *8*(2), 133. https://doi.org/10.3390/healthcare8020133

Sharma, D., & Cotton, M. (2023). Overcoming the barriers between resource constraints and healthcare quality. *Tropical Doctor*, *53*(3), 341–343. https://doi.org/10.1177/00494755231183784

Shaw Morawski, T., Liang, M.Q. (2022). The TIGER initiative: global, interprofessional HI workforce development. In: Hübner, U.H., Mustata Wilson, G., Morawski, T.S., Ball, M.J. (eds). *Nursing Informatics. HI* (pp. 581–602). Springer, Cham. https://doi.org/10.1007/978-3-030-91237-6_38

Sheikh, A., Anderson, M., Albala, S., Casadei, B., Franklin, B. D., Richards, M., Taylor, D., Tibble, H., & Mossialos, E. (2021). Health information technology and digital innovation for national learning health and care systems. *The Lancet. Digital Health*, *3*(6), e383–e396. https://doi.org/10.1016/S2589-7500(21)00005-4

Skinner, A., Flannery, K., Nocka, K., Bor, J., Dean, L. T., Jay, J., Lipson, S. K., Cole, M. B., Benfer, E. A., Scheckman, R., Raderman, W., Jones, D. K., & Raifman, J. (2022). A database of US state policies to mitigate COVID-19 and its economic consequences. *BMC Public Health*, *22*(1). https://doi.org/10.1186/s12889-022-13487-0

Smith, M., & Miller, S. (2023). Technology, institutions and regulation: Towards a normative theory. *AI & SOCIETY*. https://doi.org/10.1007/s00146-023-01803-0

Stanford F. C. (2020). The importance of diversity and inclusion in the healthcare workforce. *Journal of the National Medical Association*, *112*(3), 247–249. https://doi.org/10.1016/j.jnma.2020.03.014

Stratton, S. J. (2019). Literature reviews: methods and applications. *Prehospital and Disaster Medicine*, *34*(04), 347–349. https://doi.org/10.1017/s1049023x19004588

Taeihagh, A., Ramesh, M., & Howlett, M. (2021). Assessing the regulatory challenges of emerging disruptive technologies. *Regulation & Governance*, *15*(4), 1009–1019. https://doi.org/10.1111/rego.12392

Thate, J., Brookshire, R.G. (2022). HI education: standards, challenges, and tools. In: Hübner, U.H., Mustata Wilson, G., Morawski, T.S., Ball, M.J. (eds). *Nursing Informatics. HI* (pp. 627–646). Springer, Cham. https://doi.org/10.1007/978-3-030-91237-6_40

Theodos, K., & Sittig, S. (2020). Health information privacy laws in the digital age: HIPAA does not apply. *Perspectives in Health Information Management*, *18*(Winter), 11.

Torab-Miandoab, A., Samad-Soltani, T., Jodati, A., & Rezaei-Hachesu, P. (2023). Interoperability of heterogeneous health information systems: a systematic literature review. *BMC Medical Informatics and Decision Making*, *23*(1). https://doi.org/10.1186/s12911-023-02115-5

Vajjhala, N. R., & Eappen, P. (2023). *The Role of 5G Networks in Healthcare Applications*. CRC Press eBooks. https://doi.org/10.1201/9781003227861–5

Van Kessel, R., Srivastava, D., Kyriopoulos, I., Monti, G., Novillo-Ortiz, D., Milman, R., Zhang-Czabanowski, W. W., Nasi, G., Stern, A. D., Wharton, G., & Mossialos, E. (2023). Digital health reimbursement strategies of 8 european countries and Israel: scoping review and policy mapping. *JMIR MHealth and UHealth*, *11*, e49003. https://doi.org/10.2196/49003

VanderWerf, M., Bernard, J., Barta, D. T., Berg, J., Collins, T., Dowdy, M., Feiler, K., Moore, D. L., Sifri, C., Spargo, G., Taylor, C. W., Towle, C. B., & Wibberly, K. H. (2022). Pandemic action plan policy and regulatory summary telehealth policy and regulatory considerations during a pandemic. *Telemedicine and E-Health*, *28*(4), 457–466. https://doi.org/10.1089/tmj.2021.0216

Vela, M. B., Erondu, A. I., Smith, N. A., Peek, M. E., Woodruff, J. N., & Chin, M. H. (2022). Eliminating explicit and implicit biases in health care: evidence and research needs. *Annual Review of Public Health*, *43*, 477–501. https://doi.org/10.1146/annurev-publhealth-052060–103528

Vito, D., Lauriola, P., & D'Apice, C. (2022). The COVID-19 pandemic: reshaping public health policy response envisioning health as a common good. *International Journal of Environmental Research and Public Health*, *19*(16), 9985. https://doi.org/10.3390/ijerph19169985

Walker, D. M., Tarver, W. L., Jonnalagadda, P., Ranbom, L., Ford, E. W., & Rahurkar, S. (2023). Perspectives on challenges and opportunities for interoperability: findings from key informant interviews with stakeholders in Ohio. *JMIR Medical Informatics*, *11*, e43848. https://doi.org/10.2196/43848

Wang, C. P., Mkuu, R., Andreadis, K., Muellers, K. A., Ancker, J. S., Horowitz, C., Kaushal, R., & Lin, J. J. (2024). Examining and addressing telemedicine disparities through the lens of the social determinants of health: a qualitative study of patient and provider during the COVID-19 pandemic. *AMIA . . . Annual Symposium proceedings. AMIA Symposium, 2023,* 1287–1296.

Wang, S., Zha, Y., Li, W., Wu, Q., Li, X., Niu, M., Wang, M., Qiu, X., Li, H., Yu, H., Gong, W., Bai, Y., Li, L., Zhu, Y., Wang, L., & Tian, J. (2020). A fully automatic deep learning system for COVID-19 diagnostic and prognostic analysis. *European Respiratory Journal, 56*(2), 2000775. https://doi.org/10.1183/13993003.00775–2020

Wise, J. (2020). Covid-19: UK drops its contact tracing app to switch to Apple and Google models. *BMJ,* m2472. https://doi.org/10.1136/bmj.m2472

Xiang, D., & Cai, W. (2021). Privacy protection and secondary use of health data: strategies and methods. *BioMed Research International, 2021,* 1–11. https://doi.org/10.1155/2021/6967166

Yiu, C., Macon-Cooney, B., & Fingerhut, H. (2021). A research and policy agenda for the post-pandemic world. *Future Healthcare Journal, 8*(2), e198–e203. https://doi.org/10.7861/fhj.2021–0082

Yogesh, M. J., & Karthikeyan, J. (2022). HI: engaging modern healthcare units: a brief overview. *Frontiers in Public Health, p. 10.* https://doi.org/10.3389/fpubh.2022.854688

Yusif, S., Hafeez-Baig, A., & Soar, J. (2022). Change management and adoption of health information technology (HIT)/eHealth in public hospitals in Ghana: a qualitative study. *Applied Computing and Informatics, 18*(3/4), 279–289. https://doi.org/10.20525/ijrbs.v13i1.3044

Zainal, H., Tan, J. K., Xiaohui, X., Thumboo, J., & Yong, F. K. (2023). Clinical informatics training in medical school education curricula: a scoping review. *Journal of the American Medical Informatics Association: JAMIA, 30*(3), 604–616. https://doi.org/10.1093/jamia/ocac245

13 Ethics, Privacy, and Security in Healthcare Informatics

Azamat Ali

13.1 INTRODUCTION

Healthcare informatics, at its core, is an interdisciplinary field that blends information science, computer science, and healthcare. It focuses on the optimal acquisition, management, utilization, and sharing of information within the realms of healthcare (Davies et al., 2020). This field comprises a range of technologies and techniques, including as electronic health records (EHRs), telemedicine, clinical decision assistance, and health information exchange systems. The objective is to promote the overall efficacy and efficiency of healthcare delivery, optimize patient outcomes, and streamline healthcare procedures (Wiwatkunupakarn et al., 2023).

Recently, there has been a significant trend toward digitization in the healthcare business. The emergence of big data analytics, artificial intelligence (AI), and machine learning (ML) in healthcare is rapidly transforming the industry. These technologies are not only streamlining administrative processes but also enabling personalized and predictive healthcare (Bairstow, 2024). As healthcare informatics evolves, it continually intersects with complex ethical considerations. The primary concern revolves around the handling and protection of sensitive patient data (Adeniyi et al., 2024). In a sector that increasingly relies on electronic systems for storing, managing, and sharing health information, ethical responsibilities significantly intensify.

Ethical challenges in healthcare informatics are multifaceted. They encompass concerns around patient consent and autonomy, particularly in terms of who has the right to access and control patient data (Hübner et al., 2022). The growing utilization of AI and ML in diagnosis and treatment suggestions gives rise to ethical concerns around bias, transparency, and accountability in automated decision-making procedures (Lepri et al., 2021). Ethicists and healthcare professionals grapple with these challenges, striving to balance technological advancements with ethical obligations. Privacy in healthcare informatics refers to the right of individuals to control access to their personal health information. This aspect is critical for maintaining patient trust in the healthcare system. The digitization of health records, while streamlining data accessibility, also introduces significant risks, particularly concerning data breaches and unauthorized access (Shrivastava et al., 2021).

Ensuring data privacy requires strict adherence to rules and regulations such as the Health Insurance Portability and Accountability Act (HIPAA) in the United States and the General Data Protection Regulation (GDPR) in Europe. These rules establish guidelines for the secure management of health information. However, it can be difficult to comply with these guidelines due to the constantly changing nature of digital technology and the increasing strategies used by cyber threats (Bradford et al., 2020). The security of healthcare informatics systems is of utmost importance in safeguarding sensitive patient data from various cyber threats, including virus assaults and advanced phishing tactics. This aspect of healthcare informatics involves deploying robust technological safeguards like encryption and firewalls, as well as organizational measures including staff training and stringent access controls (Tariq, 2024).

The healthcare industry has distinct security difficulties as a result of the significant worth of medical data and the possible consequences of breaches on patient well-being and public confidence. The inclusion of new technologies, such as the Internet of Medical Things (IoMT) devices,

DOI: 10.1201/9781003485629-13

adds complexity to the security environment, requiring constant attentiveness and flexible security solutions (Alzahrani et al, 2022).

13.1.1 Aims and Scope of the Study

This study aims to provide a comprehensive examination of the critical ethical concerns, privacy challenges, and security necessities inherent in the realm of healthcare informatics. As the healthcare sector increasingly relies on digital technologies for patient data management and medical procedures, it becomes imperative to address the ethical implications, privacy risks, and security measures associated with these advancements.

13.1.2 Key Objectives

1. Explore ethical considerations in healthcare informatics to uphold patient rights and dignity.
2. Investigate privacy challenges, including data breaches and unauthorized access, to protect patient confidentiality.
3. Examine security measures essential for safeguarding healthcare data from cyber threats.
4. Provide actionable recommendations for healthcare providers, policymakers, and IT professionals to ensure ethical practices, privacy protection, and stringent security in healthcare informatics.

13.2 THE EVOLUTION OF HEALTHCARE INFORMATICS

The journey of healthcare informatics began in the late 20th century, marked by the transition from manual to electronic processes in healthcare. The initial focus was on creating digital records, moving away from paper-based systems for better accuracy and efficiency (Reza et al., 2020). In the 1960s and 1970s, the earliest forms of health information systems emerged, primarily in academic and research settings. These systems were designed to manage patient data and aid in hospital administration. One of the pioneering efforts in this field was the development of the Problem-Oriented Medical Record (POMR) by Dr. Lawrence Weed in the 1960s. This approach revolutionized medical record-keeping by focusing on specific problems, treatments, and outcomes for each patient (Koopman et al., 2021). In the decades that followed, the use of computers in hospitals and clinics gradually increased, laying the groundwork for modern healthcare informatics.

13.2.1 Advancements in Hardware and Software

The 1980s and 1990s witnessed significant advancements in computer hardware and software capabilities, making electronic data processing more accessible and efficient (Sahu et al., 2022). This period saw the rise of EHRs, which became an essential tool in healthcare management. Advances in networking facilitated the sharing and exchange of health information, which was further enhanced with the advent of the Internet. During this time, there was also a growing focus on standardizing medical data to enable interoperability and data exchange. Standards such as Health Level Seven International (HL7) and the Digital Imaging and Communications in Medicine (DICOM) emerged, facilitating seamless communication and data exchange among various health information systems (Spanakis et al., 2021).

13.2.2 The 21st Century: A Digital Health Revolution

The 21st century ushered in a digital health revolution fueled by technological advancements. Healthcare informatics embraced sophisticated tools such as data analytics, cloud computing, and mobile technologies. A significant milestone was the widespread adoption of EHRs, catalyzed by initiatives like the HITECH Act in the United States, which incentivized their meaningful use. These innovations transformed healthcare delivery by enabling more efficient data management, enhanced communication among healthcare providers, and improved patient outcomes. The digitalization of health information paved the way for personalized medicine, remote patient monitoring, and the democratization of healthcare access, marking a paradigm shift in the way healthcare is delivered and experienced (Nguyen et al., 2023).

13.2.3 BIG DATA AND PREDICTIVE ANALYTICS

The advent of big data analytics revolutionized healthcare informatics in the 2010s, enabling the analysis of vast amounts of health data. This breakthrough facilitated the emergence of predictive analytics, personalized medicine, and advanced public health surveillance. Predictive models became pivotal in identifying risk factors, improving preventive care strategies, and optimizing treatment plans for patients (Ibrahim & Saber, 2023). By harnessing the power of big data, healthcare professionals gained unprecedented insights into patient health trends, enabling more accurate diagnoses, proactive interventions, and, ultimately, better healthcare outcomes.

13.2.4 AI AND ML

The healthcare industry has experienced significant changes in recent years due to the incorporation of AI and ML technology. These technological breakthroughs have completely transformed several areas of healthcare, such as the field of diagnostics, suggestions for therapy, monitoring of patients, and the creation of new drugs. AI-powered solutions utilize advanced algorithms to evaluate extensive healthcare data, detecting trends, forecasting results, and providing valuable insights that assist in making clinical decisions (Raparthi, 2021). Furthermore, AI is revolutionizing patient involvement and the administration of healthcare by implementing individualized therapies and remote monitoring technologies. Through the utilization of AI and ML, healthcare professionals may enhance the accuracy, effectiveness, and patient-focused nature of care, hence enhancing health results and promoting medical progress (Vanaparthi & Rao, 2023).

13.2.5 TELEMEDICINE AND MOBILE HEALTH

The integration of telemedicine and mobile health (mHealth) apps represents a significant evolution in healthcare informatics. Telehealth has become a crucial technique for providing accessible healthcare remotely, thanks to the rapid advancement caused by the COVID-19 pandemic. This method of providing healthcare has increased the availability of medical treatments, especially in locations with limited access, while also lessening the strain on healthcare institutions. At the same time, mHealth applications enable consumers to actively participate in managing their health by offering functions like remote monitoring, prescription reminders, and tailored health advice. Telemedicine and mHealth are transforming healthcare delivery by enhancing convenience, efficiency, and patient-centeredness (Taha et al., 2022).

13.2.6 CURRENT TRENDS: INTEGRATION, INTEROPERABILITY, AND PATIENT-CENTRIC CARE

In the realm of healthcare informatics, current trends are driving toward enhanced integration and interoperability. The objective is to establish a cohesive healthcare ecosystem wherein data from diverse sources, including wearable and IoT devices, can seamlessly integrate and be leveraged for improved patient care (Shah et al., 2021). Simultaneously, there's a noticeable shift toward patient-centric care, with the proliferation of patient portals enabling direct access to health records and facilitating more transparent communication between patients and healthcare providers (Chibuike et al., 2024). By embracing these trends, the healthcare industry aims to cultivate a more holistic approach to healthcare delivery, prioritizing patient empowerment, engagement, and, ultimately, better health outcomes (Ibeh et al., 2024).

13.3 ETHICAL CONCERNS IN HEALTHCARE INFORMATICS

Healthcare informatics, which refers to the incorporation of technology in healthcare, has fundamentally transformed the handling, examination, and use of patient data. However, this rapid evolution brings forth a myriad of ethical considerations. This section examines the ethical principles pertinent to healthcare data and technology, explores the delicate balance between technological progress and patient rights, and examines real-world case studies highlighting ethical dilemmas.

13.3.1 ETHICAL PRINCIPLES IN HEALTHCARE DATA AND TECHNOLOGY

- **Privacy and Confidentiality:** Healthcare data are intrinsically sensitive, as they contain personal information on individuals' medical conditions, treatments, and histories. Ensuring privacy and confidentiality is paramount (Hulkower et al., 2020). For example, in 2017, a major healthcare provider experienced a data breach that exposed the personal health information of thousands of patients, leading to significant legal and reputational consequences. The HIPAA in the United States enforce stringent measures to safeguard patient data from unauthorized access or disclosure, adhering to ethical norms. An example of HIPAA in action is the requirement for healthcare providers to implement encryption for EHRs, ensuring that only authorized personnel can access sensitive information.
- **Autonomy and Informed Consent:** Respect for patient autonomy requires involving individuals in decisions regarding their health information. Before giving consent, patients must be fully informed about the methods of data collection, utilization, and dissemination, according to the essential ethical principle of informed consent. This is especially crucial in the digital age, where EHRs and telemedicine platforms handle vast amounts of patient information (Pietrzykowski & Smilowska, 2021). For instance, a patient using a telemedicine platform should be informed that their video consultations may be recorded for quality assurance purposes, and they must consent to this before the session begins. Failure to obtain proper informed consent can lead to legal challenges, as seen in cases where patients were unaware of how their data were being used or shared.
- **Beneficence and Non-Maleficence:** The goal of healthcare informatics is to promote beneficence by using technology to enhance patient outcomes, improve the quality of care, and advance medical knowledge. At the same time, it must uphold the principle of non-maleficence by avoiding harm to patients through data breaches, inaccuracies, or misuse of information (Khanna & Srivastava, 2020). For example, a hospital that implements an AI-powered diagnostic tool may experience improved accuracy in diagnosing diseases, benefiting patient care. However, if the AI system has biases or errors, it could lead to misdiagnoses, potentially causing harm. Ethical considerations must, therefore, include not only the intended benefits of technology but also the potential risks and unintended consequences (Darda & Matta, 2024). A case in point is the controversy over AI tools that inadvertently reinforced racial biases in treatment recommendations, highlighting the need for careful ethical oversight in developing and deploying such technologies.

13.3.2 BALANCING TECHNOLOGICAL ADVANCEMENT WITH PATIENT RIGHTS AND DIGNITY

The rapid advancement of technology in healthcare presents a complex interplay with the imperative to uphold patient rights and dignity.

- **Equity and Access:** One ethical challenge lies in ensuring equitable access to health-care technologies. Disparities in access based on factors like socioeconomic status or geographic location can exacerbate existing healthcare inequalities. Ethical practice demands proactive measures to bridge these gaps and ensure that technological advancements benefit all segments of society (Aminabee, 2024).
- **Data Security and Integrity:** Given the process of converting healthcare data into a digital format and linking them together, it is essential to prioritize the protection and accuracy of this information. Cybersecurity breaches pose significant threats to patient privacy and confidentiality. Ethical healthcare informatics necessitates robust security measures, encryption protocols, and data governance frameworks to mitigate these risks and safeguard patient information (Arigbabu et al., 2024).
- **Transparency and Accountability:** Ethical healthcare informatics requires transparency in the collection, processing, and use of patient data. Patients possess the entitlement to comprehend the manner in which their information is being employed and the individuals who have authorization to access it (Séroussi et al., 2020). Healthcare organizations and technology developers must uphold accountability for the ethical implications of their products and practices, including addressing biases in algorithms and ensuring mechanisms for addressing grievances.

13.3.3 Ethical Dilemmas in Healthcare Informatics: Case Studies and Insights

Healthcare informatics plays a pivotal role in modern healthcare delivery, offering promising advancements in diagnosis, treatment, and patient care. However, along with these advancements come ethical dilemmas that challenge the balance between technological innovation and patient rights. This section explores various case studies highlighting ethical challenges in healthcare informatics and offers insights into addressing these complexities.

13.3.3.1 Genetic Testing and Privacy Concerns

Direct-to-consumer (DTC) genetic testing services, such as those provided by companies like 23andMe and AncestryDNA, have surged in popularity, offering individuals insights into their ancestry, health risks, and genetic predispositions (Al-Gahmi, 2024). However, these services raise significant ethical questions regarding privacy, consent, and data usage.

CASE STUDY 1: THE CASE OF 23ANDME

23andMe, a direct-to-consumer genetic testing company, came under fire for using consumer genetic data for research without explicit consent. Despite users consenting to the company's terms of service, many were unaware of the extent to which their genetic information could be utilized or shared (Petersen & Lefferts, 2020). This lack of understanding raised significant concerns regarding data ownership, control, and the protection of sensitive health information. The case brought attention to the ethical quandary surrounding the utilization of personal genetic data for research objectives and emphasized the significance of clear permission procedures to guarantee that individuals completely understand the consequences of disclosing their genetic information.

CASE STUDY 2: GENETIC DISCRIMINATION

DTC genetic testing has raised concerns about genetic discrimination, where employers or insurers may use genetic risk factors disclosed by testing to discriminate against individuals (Chapman et al., 2020). This discrimination can manifest in employment or insurance disparities, undermining patient autonomy and exacerbating social inequalities. Ethically, it questions the responsible use and protection of genetic information, highlighting the need for legal safeguards and policies to prevent discriminatory practices based on genetic predispositions. The case underscores the importance of

balancing individual privacy rights with societal concerns and ensuring equitable access to employment and healthcare regardless of the genetic makeup.

13.3.3.2 Algorithmic Bias in Healthcare AI

ML algorithms are increasingly utilized in healthcare for various purposes, including diagnosis,
treatment optimization, and patient management. However, these algorithms are not immune to
biases, which can perpetuate disparities in healthcare delivery.

CASE STUDY 3: BIAS IN PREDICTIVE ANALYTICS

A predictive analytics system in healthcare, driven by AI, inadvertently exhibited bias by under-
estimating the healthcare needs of specific demographic groups, notably those from marginalized
communities (WHO, 2021). This bias resulted in disparities in healthcare access and outcomes,
underscoring the ethical imperative of ensuring fairness and transparency in algorithmic decision-
making. The case emphasizes the importance of addressing bias in predictive analytics models to
prevent systemic inequalities in healthcare delivery (Paulus & Kent, 2020). It highlights the ethical
obligation to develop and deploy algorithms that accurately prioritize patient care based on clinical
need rather than perpetuating disparities based on demographic characteristics.

CASE STUDY 4: RACIAL BIAS IN DERMATOLOGY AI

A recent research exposed racial prejudice in an AI-powered dermatological tool, which exhibited
better accuracy when analyzing photos of persons with lighter skin tones compared to those with
darker skin tones. This prejudice can lead to the incorrect identification or insufficient identification
of skin disorders in patients with non-white skin, therefore perpetuating inequities in healthcare
(Zou & Schiebinger, 2021). It underscores the critical necessity of mitigating bias in AI algorithms
to uphold equitable healthcare delivery. Addressing this bias requires deliberate efforts to diversify
training datasets, enhance algorithmic transparency, and prioritize fairness in algorithm development. Failure to do so risks exacerbating existing inequities and compromising patient outcomes
based on racial characteristics.

13.3.3.3 EHR Errors and Patient Safety

EHRs have transformed the healthcare industry by converting patient health information into digital format, enhancing the coordination of treatment, and enabling informed decision-making based
on data. Nevertheless, inaccuracies in EHRs can lead to significant ramifications for the safety of
patients and the quality of treatment they get.

CASE STUDY 5: MEDICATION ERRORS DUE TO EHR TRANSCRIPTION ERROR

A patient suffered from an incorrect medication dosage due to a transcription error in their EHR,
resulting in adverse health effects. This incident underscores the vital significance of accurate and
dependable health information technology systems. Errors in EHRs not only endanger patient safety
but also erode trust in healthcare technology and systems (Unver & Asan, 2022). Ensuring the accuracy and reliability of EHRs is paramount for safeguarding patient well-being and maintaining
confidence in the healthcare system's ability to provide safe and effective care. It underscores the
need for robust quality assurance measures and thorough training to minimize transcription errors
and enhance patient safety.

CASE STUDY 6: EHR USABILITY AND CLINICIAN BURNOUT

The subpar usability of EHR systems has been associated with clinician burnout, attributable to
cumbersome interfaces and workflow inefficiencies (Pfaff et al., 2021). These factors contribute
to elevated administrative burdens and diminished time available for direct patient care. Clinician

dissatisfaction with EHRs not only compromises job satisfaction but also raises ethical concerns regarding the delivery of quality patient care and the well-being of healthcare providers (Canfell et al., 2024). Addressing EHR usability issues is imperative for mitigating clinician burnout, preserving patient-centered care, and upholding ethical standards in healthcare delivery, ensuring that technology enhances rather than impedes the clinical practice.

13.4 PRIVACY CHALLENGES IN DIGITAL HEALTHCARE

The process of digitizing healthcare has completely transformed the methods by which patient data are collected, archived, and utilized. However, this transformation brings forth significant privacy challenges. This section explores the nature of sensitive medical data and their privacy implications; examines the risks associated with data collection, storage, and use; analyzes regulatory frameworks for patient privacy; and illustrates real-world instances of privacy breaches and their impact.

13.4.1 NATURE OF SENSITIVE MEDICAL DATA AND PRIVACY IMPLICATIONS

Sensitive medical data comprise a broad spectrum of information, such as diagnosis, treatments, drugs, genetic profiles, and records related to behavioral health. These data are inherently private and can reveal intimate details about an individual's health status, history, and vulnerabilities (Berg et al., 2011). The privacy problems stem from the possibility of this information being misused or accessed without authorization, which can result in negative outcomes for patients such as discrimination, stigma, and breaches of confidentiality.

The risks associated with data collection, storage, and use are as follows:

- **Data Breaches:** Healthcare data breaches provide a substantial threat to the confidentiality of patient information. Cyberattacks aimed against healthcare companies can lead to the unlawful acquisition, theft, or disclosure of sensitive medical data. These breaches not only jeopardize the confidentiality of patients but also undermine faith in the healthcare system and can have financial consequences for both patients and healthcare providers (Almulihi et al., 2022).
- **Data Misuse:** The misuse of patient data for purposes beyond their intended use presents another risk to privacy. This may include unauthorized sharing of data with third parties, such as marketers or employers, without patient consent. Additionally, data mining and analytics techniques used to extract insights from healthcare data can potentially lead to the identification of individuals, undermining their privacy and anonymity (Favaretto et al., 2019).
- **Insider Threats:** Individuals with privileged access to healthcare systems, such as workers, contractors, and suppliers, present a substantial threat to the confidentiality of patient information. Insider threats encompass deliberate or accidental behaviors that lead to the unauthorized access, disclosure, or modification of patient data. These events may arise as a result of negligence, malicious intent, or insufficient security processes inside healthcare companies (Theis et al., 2019).

13.4.2 REGULATORY FRAMEWORKS FOR PATIENT PRIVACY

Regulatory frameworks play a crucial role in safeguarding patient privacy and ensuring the security of health information. Two prominent regulations in this domain are HIPAA in the United States and the GDPR in the European Union (EU). Both regulations aim to protect patient data but differ in their implementation and impact on healthcare informatics.

HIPAA:

HIPAA is a comprehensive regulation in the United States that establishes standards for the privacy and security of protected health information (PHI). It includes several key components:

- **Patient Consent:** Under HIPAA, covered entities must obtain patient consent before using or disclosing PHI, except for specific circumstances such as medical treatment, financial transactions, or healthcare operations. Patients have the right to control who accesses their health information. For example, if a hospital needs to share patient data with a research organization, it must obtain explicit consent from the patient unless the data are de-identified or used for purposes permitted under HIPAA (Bertino et al., 2015).
- **Security Safeguards:** HIPAA mandates that organizations implement administrative, physical, and technological safeguards to protect PHI. This includes access controls, encryption, and audit trails. For instance, healthcare providers must use encryption to secure EHRs during transmission and storage, preventing unauthorized access and data breaches (Keshta & Odeh, 2021).
- **Enforcement and Penalties:** The Office for Civil Rights (OCR) is responsible for enforcing HIPAA and can impose civil monetary penalties for noncompliance. Penalties can range from fines for minor violations to substantial fines for significant breaches. The OCR also conducts audits to ensure compliance and investigate complaints (Hersh & Hoyt, 2018).

GDPR:

GDPR is a regulation in the EU that provides a framework for data protection and privacy. It introduces several principles and requirements:

- **Data Subject Rights:** GDPR emphasizes the rights of individuals over their personal data. This includes the right to access, rectify, and erase personal data. Healthcare organizations must provide patients with access to their health data and allow them to request corrections or deletions where applicable. For example, if a patient requests to have their data removed from a medical database, the organization must comply unless there are legal grounds for retaining the data (Voigt & Von dem Bussche, 2017).
- **Data Protection by Design and by Default:** GDPR requires organizations to integrate data protection measures into their processes from the outset. This principle mandates that systems and processes be designed to safeguard data and ensure minimal data processing. For example, EHR systems must be designed with robust encryption and access controls to protect patient information from unauthorized access (Bravo, 2022).
- **Cross-Border Data Transfers:** GDPR imposes strict regulations on transferring personal data outside the EU. Organizations must ensure that data transferred to non-EU countries is protected by adequate safeguards. For instance, healthcare organizations must use standard contractual clauses or ensure that the recipient country has an adequate level of data protection before transferring patient data (Hoofnagle et al., 2019).

Comparative Analysis:

- **Scope and Applicability:** HIPAA primarily applies to healthcare providers, health plans, and business associates in the United States, while GDPR applies to all organizations processing personal data of EU residents, regardless of location. GDPR's broader scope includes any entity that processes personal data of EU residents, which may affect international organizations with a presence in the EU (Li et al., 2019).
- **Patient Rights:** GDPR provides more extensive rights to individuals compared to HIPAA. GDPR's emphasis on data subject rights, including the right to data portability and the right to object to processing, offers individuals greater control over their personal data.

HIPAA also provides rights but focuses more on the privacy and security of health information rather than broader data protection principles (Solove & Schwartz, 2023).

- **Penalties and Enforcement:** GDPR's enforcement mechanisms are more stringent compared to HIPAA. GDPR imposes higher fines for noncompliance, which can be up to 4% of global annual turnover or €20 million, whichever is higher. HIPAA penalties are generally lower but can still be significant, depending on the severity of the violation (Presthus & Sønslien, 2021).

Despite the rigorous standards set by HIPAA and GDPR, challenges persist in ensuring comprehensive patient privacy and data security. The rapid advancement of healthcare technologies, such as EHRs and telemedicine platforms, introduces new vulnerabilities. Additionally, the increasing frequency of cyber threats and data breaches underscores the need for continuous vigilance and proactive measures to protect patient information (Tariq, 2024). A comparative analysis of these regulations can provide valuable insights into how different frameworks address data privacy challenges and offer lessons for improving global standards in healthcare informatics.

13.4.3 REAL-WORLD INSTANCES OF PRIVACY BREACHES AND THEIR IMPACT

- **Anthem Data Breach:** Anthem Inc., a prominent health insurance company in the United States, had a massive data breach in 2015, impacting over 78.8 million users. The breach entailed illicit entry into a database that stored confidential data, such as individuals' names, social security numbers, dates of birth, and health insurance ID numbers. The occurrence highlighted the susceptibility of healthcare institutions to cyberattacks and the possible consequences on patient confidentiality and safety (Mohammed, 2022).
- **Cambridge Analytica Scandal:** The Cambridge Analytica controversy, while not exclusive to the healthcare industry, brought attention to the privacy hazards linked to the improper use and illegal access to data. The political consulting business illicitly acquired the personal data of several Facebook users without their explicit permission and thereafter utilized it for the purpose of targeted advertising and political campaigns. Although the incident did not specifically pertain to healthcare data, it sparked worries on the wider consequences of breaches in data privacy and the necessity for strong regulatory supervision and enforcement (Hinds et al., 2020).
- **Google Health Data Partnership:** In 2019, Google and Ascension, a prominent healthcare institution in the United States, formed a collaboration to gather and examine patient data for healthcare-related objectives. The partnership, known as "Project Nightingale," raised privacy concerns regarding the potential misuse of patient data and the lack of transparency surrounding the arrangement. While Google and Ascension stated that the project complied with HIPAA regulations, critics questioned the ethics of such data-sharing agreements and called for greater transparency and patient consent (Schneble et al., 2020).

13.5 SECURITY NECESSITIES IN HEALTHCARE DATA MANAGEMENT

As healthcare increasingly relies on digital technologies for data management, ensuring the security of patient information becomes paramount. This section explores the types of cyber threats targeting healthcare data, examines security measures and technologies used to safeguard data, and discusses the effectiveness and limitations of current security practices in healthcare data management.

13.5.1 TYPES OF CYBER THREATS TARGETING HEALTHCARE DATA

- **Ransomware Attacks:** Ransomware is a form of malicious software specifically created to restrict access to a computer system or data until a payment is made as a ransom.

Ransomware attacks are commonly directed on healthcare companies because of the sensitive nature of patient data and the crucial importance of healthcare services. These assaults have the potential to interrupt operations, jeopardize patient care, and lead to the loss or theft of data (Farion-Melnyk et al., 2021).

- **Phishing and Social Engineering:** Phishing attacks entail deceiving users into revealing sensitive information, such as login passwords or financial data, using false emails, texts, or websites. Social engineering strategies leverage human psychology to persuade individuals into divulging sensitive information or engaging in acts that undermine security. Phishing and social engineering attacks frequently target healthcare professionals, such as clinicians and personnel, which poses substantial threats to data security (Alkhalil et al., 2021).

- **Insider Threats:** Insider threats are security hazards caused by persons within an organization who abuse their access credentials to unlawfully obtain data, engage in fraudulent activities, or intentionally damage systems. Individuals within the healthcare industry, such as workers, contractors, and suppliers, have the potential to unintentionally or intentionally put patient data at risk due to careless or harmful behavior. Identifying and addressing insider threats can be especially difficult since individuals with authorized access to confidential data may pose a risk (Sarkar, 2010).

13.5.2 Security Measures and Technologies in Healthcare Data Management

In the digital age, healthcare organizations face increasingly sophisticated cybersecurity threats that put patient data at risk. Healthcare providers have a responsibility to use strong security procedures and technology to preserve patient privacy and prevent data breaches, since they are responsible for sensitive medical information. There are key security measures and technologies employed in healthcare data management, including encryption, access controls, authentication, and intrusion detection and prevention system (IDPS; Omotunde & Ahmed, 2023).

- **Encryption:** Encryption is a cryptographic method employed to safeguard data by transforming them into an incomprehensible format that can only be deciphered with a decryption key. Utilizing encryption for sensitive healthcare data, both during transmission and while stored, serves to safeguard them against illegal access or interception by cybercriminals. Advanced cryptographic algorithms and protocols, like as Advanced Encryption Standard (AES) and Secure Sockets Layer/Transport Layer Security (SSL/TLS), are frequently used to protect patient data. For example, a healthcare provider like the Cleveland Clinic uses AES-256 encryption to protect patient health records stored in their EHR system. When a healthcare provider accesses a patient's record, the data are decrypted in real time, but they remain encrypted when stored in the database. This prevents unauthorized access even if attackers gain access to the storage system.

- **Access Controls and Authentication:** Access controls and authentication techniques are used to guarantee that only persons with proper authorization may have access to sensitive healthcare data. Role-based access control systems limit users' access rights depending on their positions and responsibilities in the company. Multi-factor authentication (MFA) necessitates users to provide various means of verification, such as passwords, fingerprints, or security tokens, prior to gaining access to critical data, hence augmenting security.

- **IDPS:** These are sophisticated security solutions specifically intended to actively monitor network traffic, identify any potentially malicious or abnormal behavior, and promptly block unwanted access or assaults as they occur in real time. IDPSs can assist healthcare businesses in detecting and addressing cyber risks, such as malware infections or unauthorized access attempts, at an early stage, therefore preventing them from developing into security breaches. These systems employ methods such as signature-based identification, anomaly detection, and behavior analysis to recognize and reduce risks.

13.5.3 Effectiveness and Limitations of Current Security Practices

While security measures and technologies play an essential role in safeguarding healthcare data, several challenges and limitations exist in current security practices:

- **Human Factors:** Although there are technical measures in place, human error continues to be a major cause of security breaches in the healthcare industry. Employees may unintentionally become targets of phishing schemes, disregard established security protocols, or mishandle confidential information, therefore jeopardizing data security. Enhancing the efficiency of security measures requires addressing human factors by implementing training, awareness initiatives, and solid security policies (Tsohou et al., 2015).
- **Evolving Threat Landscape:** Cyber threats targeting healthcare data are constantly evolving, posing challenges for security practitioners. Adversaries utilize advanced methods, such as polymorphic malware, zero-day vulnerabilities, and social engineering strategies, to circumvent conventional security measures (Hamid et al., 2023). Healthcare businesses must continuously modify and enhance their security measures to effectively reduce the impact of evolving threats and vulnerabilities.
- **Resource Constraints:** Many healthcare organizations face resource constraints, including budgetary limitations and staffing shortages, which can hinder their ability to implement and maintain robust security measures. Investing in cybersecurity infrastructure, personnel training, and threat intelligence capabilities require substantial financial and human resources. Smaller healthcare providers, especially, may face difficulties in allocating adequate resources to cybersecurity, which makes them susceptible to assaults (Jalali & Kaiser, 2018).
- **Regulatory Compliance:** Healthcare organizations are obligated to adhere to strict data security and privacy regulations imposed by regulatory bodies, such as HIPAA in the United States. While compliance with regulatory standards is essential for protecting patient data, it can also be complex and resource-intensive. Achieving and maintaining compliance with evolving regulations requires ongoing effort and investment, often stretching the capabilities of healthcare organizations, especially smaller entities with limited resources (Imran et al., 2020).

13.6 BALANCING TECHNOLOGY, ETHICS, AND PRIVACY

The incorporation of technology in healthcare has led to revolutionary improvements, raising the quality of patient care, improving results, and simplifying procedures. However, this progress is accompanied by ethical and privacy considerations that necessitate careful navigation. This section examines the trade-offs between technology adoption and ethical/privacy concerns in healthcare, and proposes strategies to maintain ethical standards while leveraging technology effectively.

13.6.1 Analyzing Technology Adoption and Ethical/Privacy Trade-Offs

Balancing the benefits of technology adoption in healthcare with ethical and privacy concerns is crucial. While innovations like EHRs and AI offer enhanced patient care, they raise issues of data privacy, consent, and fairness, necessitating careful consideration and implementation of ethical guidelines.

- **Enhanced Patient Care vs. Privacy Risks:** Healthcare practitioners may give more individualized and proactive treatment by using technology such as EHRs, telemedicine, and wearable gadgets. Nevertheless, these technologies also include the gathering and retention of enormous quantities of sensitive patient information, which gives rise to issues over privacy breaches, unauthorized entry, and data abuse. Balancing the potential benefits of improved patient care with the need to protect patient privacy requires robust security measures, transparent data practices, and adherence to regulatory frameworks (Pussewalage & Oleshchuk, 2016).

- **Data Sharing for Research and Innovation vs. Consent and Autonomy:** Sharing healthcare data for research and innovation holds the promise of advancing medical knowledge, developing new treatments, and improving population health. Nevertheless, ethical quandaries emerge about patient permission, autonomy, and dominion over their data. Although anonymization and de-identification methods might reduce privacy threats, it is important to provide patients the ability to make informed choices regarding the utilization and sharing of their data. Effective communication, well-informed consent procedures, and methods for voluntary participation or withdrawal are crucial for upholding ethical principles in data sharing projects (Cumyn et al., 2020).
- **AI and ML vs. Bias and Fairness:** AI and ML algorithms have the capacity to transform the healthcare industry by facilitating more precise diagnosis, tailored treatment regimens, and predictive analytics. However, these algorithms are susceptible to biases inherent in the data used to train them, leading to disparities in healthcare outcomes and exacerbating existing inequalities. Ethical considerations dictate the need for transparency, fairness, and accountability in algorithmic decision-making. Bias detection mechanisms, diverse training datasets, and ongoing evaluation of algorithm performance are essential for mitigating biases and ensuring equitable healthcare delivery (Huang et al., 2024).

13.6.2 Strategies to Maintain Ethical Standards while Leveraging Technology

To maintain ethical standards while utilizing technology in healthcare, organizations should adopt an ethics-by-design approach, adhere to established ethical guidelines, engage stakeholders collaboratively, and continuously evaluate and improve practices (Stahl & Coeckelbergh, 2016). These strategies ensure that technology adoption aligns with ethical principles and societal values, fostering trust and accountability.

- **Ethics-by-Design Approach:** Adopting an "ethical by design" approach involves integrating ethical considerations into the design, development, and deployment of technology solutions in healthcare. This approach prioritizes principles such as privacy, transparency, fairness, and accountability throughout the technology lifecycle (Akram & Rodriguez, 2022). By embedding ethical values into the design process, healthcare organizations can proactively address ethical challenges and minimize the risk of unintended consequences.
- **Ethical Guidelines and Frameworks:** Developing and adhering to ethical guidelines and frameworks can provide healthcare organizations with clear guidance on navigating ethical dilemmas in technology adoption. Professional associations, regulatory bodies, and industry consortia often establish ethical standards and best practices tailored to specific domains, such as telemedicine, genomics, or AI in healthcare (Abedjan et al., 2019). By following established guidelines and frameworks, healthcare providers can ensure that their technology initiatives align with ethical principles and societal values.
- **Stakeholder Engagement and Collaboration:** Engaging with stakeholders, including patients, healthcare professionals, policymakers, and technology developers, is essential for identifying ethical concerns, soliciting diverse perspectives, and co-creating solutions. Collaborative approaches that involve multidisciplinary teams and participatory design methodologies can foster a shared understanding of ethical issues and promote consensus-building around potential solutions. By involving stakeholders throughout the technology lifecycle, healthcare organizations can cultivate a culture of ethical responsibility and accountability (Díaz-Rodríguez et al., 2023).

- **Continuous Evaluation and Improvement**: Ethical considerations in technology adoption are dynamic and evolving, requiring ongoing evaluation and adaptation of practices. Healthcare organizations should establish mechanisms for monitoring, assessing, and continuously improving the ethical impact of their technology initiatives. This includes conducting ethical impact assessments, soliciting feedback from stakeholders, and proactively addressing emerging ethical challenges (Colombo et al., 2020). By embracing a culture of learning and reflection, healthcare organizations can adapt their practices to evolving ethical standards and societal expectations.

13.7   RECOMMENDATIONS AND BEST PRACTICES

In the field of healthcare, it is crucial to give priority to ethical standards, safeguard privacy, and implement security measures in order to guarantee the welfare and confidence of patients, as technology continues to be integrated into the industry. This section presents recommendations and best practices for healthcare providers, policymakers, and IT professionals to integrate ethical considerations effectively, protect patient privacy, and enhance data security. Additionally, future-oriented approaches for handling emerging challenges in healthcare technology are explored.

13.7.1   GUIDELINES FOR HEALTHCARE PROVIDERS, POLICYMAKERS, AND IT PROFESSIONALS

Healthcare Providers:

- Prioritize patient-centered care, ensuring that technology integration aligns with patient needs and preferences.
- Obtain informed consent from patients before implementing new technologies, ensuring they understand the implications for data privacy and security.
- Cultivate a culture of ethical responsibility within the organization, supported by clear policies and ongoing staff training on ethical guidelines (Nguyen et al., 2023).

Policymakers:

- Establish robust regulatory frameworks that address ethical, privacy, and security concerns in healthcare technology.
- Promote interoperability and data sharing standards to facilitate secure exchange of patient information while safeguarding privacy.
- Support research and innovation initiatives that advance ethical healthcare technology solutions and enhance data security (Quach et al, 2022).

IT Professionals:

- Employ robust security protocols, such as encryption and access restrictions, to safeguard healthcare data from unwanted access and cyber threats.
- Safeguard compliance with privacy regulations like HIPAA and GDPR when designing and implementing healthcare technology solutions.
- Regularly do risk assessments to identify vulnerabilities and establish suitable measures to manage hazards (Olukoya, 2022).

13.7.2   STRATEGIES FOR INTEGRATING ETHICAL PRACTICES, PRIVACY PROTECTION, AND SECURITY MEASURES

- Privacy by Design: Integrate privacy-enhancing features into healthcare technology solutions from the start, ensuring privacy considerations throughout the product lifecycle.

- Data Minimization and Retention Policies: Collect and retain only necessary patient data, establishing clear retention policies for data storage duration.
- Transparent Data Practices: Communicate clearly with patients about data collection, usage, and sharing, providing consent options and empowering patients to control their health information.
- Secure Data Sharing Protocols: Utilize robust measures like encryption and access restrictions to protect patient data from unauthorized access and ensure their safety throughout transmission and distribution.
- Regular Security Audits and Assessments: Conduct frequent audits to evaluate security effectiveness, identify vulnerabilities, and address weaknesses in healthcare systems and applications.
- Collaboration and Information Sharing: Foster collaboration among healthcare organizations, cybersecurity specialists, and regulators to exchange best practices, threat intelligence, and lessons learned in protecting patient privacy and mitigating cybersecurity risks (WHO, 2021).

13.7.3 FUTURE-ORIENTED APPROACHES FOR HANDLING EMERGING CHALLENGES

- Embrace Emerging Technologies Responsibly: Embrace emerging technologies such as blockchain, AI, and Internet of Things (IoT) devices responsibly, considering their ethical implications, potential risks, and societal impact, and proactively addressing any ethical or privacy concerns that may arise (Dhirani et al., 2023).
- Enhance Data Governance and Accountability: Strengthen data governance frameworks and accountability mechanisms to ensure responsible data stewardship, transparency, and accountability in the collection, use, and management of healthcare data (Janssen et al., 2020).
- Foster Ethical Innovation Ecosystems: Foster collaborative innovation ecosystems that bring together stakeholders from academia, industry, government, and civil society to develop ethical healthcare technology solutions that prioritize patient privacy, data security, and societal well-being (Roth et al., 2024).
- Engage in Continuous Learning and Adaptation: Promote a culture of incessant education and adaptation within the healthcare community, encouraging stakeholders to stay informed about emerging trends, technologies, and ethical considerations in healthcare IT, and to adapt their practices accordingly to meet evolving challenges and opportunities (Alowais et al., 2023).

13.8 CONCLUSIONS

This study has explored the intricate relationship between technology, ethics, privacy, and security in healthcare informatics. We discussed the trade-offs between technology adoption and ethical concerns, emphasizing the need for balanced approaches that prioritize patient well-being and privacy. Recommendations and best practices were outlined for healthcare providers, policymakers, and IT professionals, including the integration of ethical practices, privacy protection, and security measures into healthcare systems.

Trust and integrity are paramount in digital healthcare, as patients entrust their most sensitive information to healthcare providers and technology platforms. Maintaining trust requires transparency, accountability, and a commitment to ethical principles. As digital healthcare continues to evolve, the future outlook suggests a shift toward more sophisticated ethical frameworks, enhanced privacy protection mechanisms, and proactive approaches to cybersecurity. By adopting these principles and promoting responsible innovation, healthcare informatics may further enhance patient care while maintaining the utmost standards of ethics, privacy, and security.

REFERENCES

Abedjan, Z., Boujemaa, N., Campbell, S., Casla, P., Chatterjea, S., Consoli, S., Costa-Soria, C., et al. (2019). *Data Science in Healthcare: Benefits, Challenges and Opportunities*. Springer International Publishing.

Adeniyi, A. O., Arowoogun, J. O., Okolo, C. A., Chidi, R., & Babawarun, O. (2024). Ethical considerations in healthcare IT: a review of data privacy and patient consent issues. *World Journal of Advanced Research and Reviews*, *21*(2), 1660–1668. https://doi.org/10.30574/wjarr.2024.21.2.0593

Akram, M., & Rodriguez, M. (2022). Ethical considerations in AI-driven digital transformation projects. *Journal of Emerging Technology and Digital Transformation*, *1*(1), 1–12.

Al-Gahmi, I. (2024). Don't swab me!: limitations of the genetic information privacy act in the modern genetic testing landscape. *New Mexico Law Review*, *54*(1), 265.

Alkhalil, Z., Hewage, C., Nawaf, L., & Khan, I. (2021). Phishing attacks: a recent comprehensive study and a new anatomy. *Frontiers in Computer Science, 3*, 563060. https://doi.org/10.3389/fcomp.2021.563060

Almulihi, A. H., Alassery, F., Khan, A. I., Shukla, S., Gupta, B. K., & Kumar, R. (2022). Analyzing the implications of healthcare data breaches through computational technique. *Intelligent Automation & Soft Computing*, *32*(3). https://doi.org/10.32604/iasc.2022.023460

Alowais, S. A., Alghamdi, S. S., Alsuhebany, N., et al. (2023). Revolutionizing healthcare: the role of artificial intelligence in clinical practice. *BMC Medical Education*, *23*(1), 689. https://doi.org/10.1186/s12909-023-04698-z

Alzahrani, F. A., Ahmad, M., & Ansari, M. T. J. (2022). Towards design and development of security assessment framework for internet of medical things. *Applied Sciences*, *12*(16), 8148. https://doi.org/10.3390/app12168148

Aminabee, S. (2024). The future of healthcare and patient-centric care: digital innovations, trends, and predictions. In *Emerging Technologies for Health Literacy and Medical Practice* (pp. 240–262). IGI Global. https://doi.org/10.4018/979-8-3693-1214-8.ch012

Arigbabu, A. T., Olaniyi, O. O., Adigwe, C. S., Adebiyi, O. O., & Ajayi, S. A. (2024). Data governance in AI-enabled healthcare systems: a case of the project nightingale. *Asian Journal of Research in Computer Science*, *17*(5), 85–107.

Bairstow, J. (2024). Navigating the confluence: big data analytics and artificial intelligence-innovations, challenges, and future directions (No. 12052). EasyChair.

Berg, J. S., Khoury, M. J., & Evans, J. P. (2011). Deploying whole genome sequencing in clinical practice and public health: meeting the challenge one bin at a time. *Genetics in Medicine*, *13*(6), 499–504. https://doi.org/10.1097/GIM.0b013e318220aaba

Bertino, E., Deng, R. H., Huang, X., & Zhou, J. (2015). Security and privacy of electronic health information systems. *International Journal of Information Security*, *14*, 485–486. https://doi.org/10.1007/s10207-015-0303-z

Bradford, L., Aboy, M., & Liddell, K. (2020). International transfers of health data between the EU and USA: a sector-specific approach for the USA to ensure an 'adequate' level of protection. *Journal of Law and the Biosciences*, *7*(1), lsaa055. https://doi.org/10.1093/jlb/lsaa055

Bravo, F. (2022). Data management tools and privacy by design and by default. *Privacy and Data Protection in Software Services*, 85–95. https://doi.org/10.1007/978-981-16-3049-1_8

Canfell, O. J., Woods, L., Meshkat, Y., Krivit, J., Gunashanhar, B., Slade, C., . . . Sullivan, C. (2024). The impact of digital hospitals on patient and clinician experience: systematic review and qualitative evidence synthesis. *Journal of Medical Internet Research, 26*, e47715. https://doi.org/10.2196/47715

Chapman, C. R., Mehta, K. S., Parent, B., & Caplan, A. L. (2020). Genetic discrimination: emerging ethical challenges in the context of advancing technology. *Journal of Law and the Biosciences*, *7*(1), lsz016. https://doi.org/10.1093/jlb/lsz016

Chibuike, M. C., Sara, G. S., & Adele, B. (2024). Overcoming challenges for improved patient-centric care: a scoping review of platform ecosystems in healthcare. *IEEE Access*. https://doi.org/10.1109/ACCESS.2024.3356860

Colombo, F., Oderkirk, J., & Slawomirski, L. (2020). Health information systems, electronic medical records, and big data in global healthcare: progress and challenges in OECD countries. In *Handbook of Global Health* (pp. 1–31). https://doi.org/10.1007/978-3-030-05325-3_71-1

Cumyn, A., Barton, A., Dault, R., Cloutier, A.-M., Jalbert, R., & Ethier, J.-F. (2020). Informed consent within a learning health system: a scoping review. *Learning Health Systems*, *4*(2), e10206. https://doi.org/10.1002/lrh2.10206

Darda, P., & Matta, N. (2024). The nexus of healthcare and technology: a thematic analysis of digital transformation through artificial intelligence. In *Transformative Approaches to Patient Literacy and Healthcare Innovation* (pp. 261–282). IGI Global. https://doi.org/10.4018/979-8-3693-3661-8.ch013

Davies, A., Mueller, J., & Moulton, G. (2020). Core competencies for clinical informaticians: a systematic review. *International Journal of Medical Informatics*, *141*, 104237. https://doi.org/10.1016/j.ijmedinf.2020.104237

Dhirani, L. L., Mukhtiar, N., Chowdhry, B. S., & Newe, T. (2023). Ethical dilemmas and privacy issues in emerging technologies: a review. *Sensors*, *23*, 1151. https://doi.org/10.3390/s23031151

Díaz-Rodríguez, N., Del Ser, J., Coeckelbergh, M., López de Prado, M., Herrera-Viedma, E., & Herrera, F. (2023). Connecting the dots in trustworthy Artificial Intelligence: from AI principles, ethics, and key requirements to responsible AI systems and regulation. *Information Fusion*, *99*, 101896. https://doi.org/10.1016/j.inffus.2023.101896

Farion-Melnyk, A., Rozheliuk, V., Slipchenko, T., Banakh, S., Farion, M., & Bilan, O. (2021). Ransomware attacks: risks, protection and prevention measures. In *2021 11th International Conference on Advanced Computer Information Technologies (ACIT)* (pp. 473–478). IEEE. https://doi.org/10.1109/ACIT52158.2021.9548507

Favaretto, M., De Clercq, E., & Elger, B. S. (2019). Big Data and discrimination: perils, promises and solutions: a systematic review. *Journal of Big Data*, *6*(1), 1–27. https://doi.org/10.1186/s40537-019-0177-4

Hamid, K., Iqbal, M. W., Aqeel, M., Rana, T. A., & Arif, M. (2023). Cybersecurity. In *Artificial Intelligence & Blockchain in Cyber Physical Systems: Technologies & Applications.*

Hersh, W. R., & Hoyt, R. E. (2018). *Health Informatics: Practical Guide Seventh Edition*. Lulu. com.

Hinds, J., Williams, E. J., & Joinson, A. N. (2020). "It wouldn't happen to me": privacy concerns and perspectives following the Cambridge Analytica scandal. *International Journal of Human-Computer Studies*, *143*, 102498. https://doi.org/10.1016/j.ijhcs.2020.102498

Hoofnagle, C. J., Van Der Sloot, B., & Borgesius, F. Z. (2019). The European Union general data protection regulation: what it is and what it means. *Information & Communications Technology Law*, *28*(1), 65–98. https://doi.org/10.1080/13600834.2019.1573501

Huang, Y., Guo, J., Chen, W.-H., Lin, H.-Y., Tang, H., Wang, F., Xu, H., & Bian, J. (2024). A scoping review of fair machine learning techniques when using real-world data. *Journal of Biomedical Informatics*, 104622. https://doi.org/10.1016/j.jbi.2024.104622

Hübner, U. H., Egbert, N., & Schulte, G. (2022). Ethical issues: patients, providers, and systems. In *Nursing Informatics: A Health Informatics, Interprofessional and Global Perspective* (pp. 465–483). Cham: Springer International Publishing. https://doi.org/10.1007/978-3-030-91237-6_31

Hulkower, R., Penn, M., & Schmit, C. (2020). Privacy and confidentiality of public health information. *Public Health Informatics and Information Systems*, 147–166. https://doi.org/10.1007/978-3-030-41215-9_9

Ibeh, C. V., Elufioye, O. A., Olorunsogo, T., Asuzu, O. F., Nduubuisi, N. L., & Daraojimba, A. I. (2024). Data analytics in healthcare: a review of patient-centric approaches and healthcare delivery. *World Journal of Advanced Research and Reviews*, *21*(2), 1660–1668. https://doi.org/10.30574/wjarr.2024.21.2.0246

Ibrahim, M. S., & Saber, S. (2023). Machine learning and predictive analytics: advancing disease prevention in healthcare. *Journal of Contemporary Healthcare Analytics*, *7*(1), 53–71.

Imran, S., Mahmood, T., Morshed, A., & Sellis, T. (2020). Big data analytics in healthcare – a systematic literature review and roadmap for practical implementation. *IEEE/CAA Journal of Automatica Sinica*, *8*(1), 1–22. https://doi.org/10.1109/JAS.2020.1003384

Jalali, M. S., & Kaiser, J. P. (2018). Cybersecurity in hospitals: a systematic, organizational perspective. *Journal of Medical Internet Research*, *20*(5), e10059. https://doi.org/10.2196/10059

Janssen, M., Brous, P., Estevez, E., Barbosa, L. S., & Janowski, T. (2020). Data governance: organizing data for trustworthy Artificial Intelligence. *Government Information Quarterly*, *37*(3), 101493. https://doi.org/10.1016/j.giq.2020.101493

Keshta, I., & Odeh, A. (2021). Security and privacy of electronic health records: concerns and challenges. *Egyptian Informatics Journal*, *22*(2), 177–183. https://doi.org/10.1016/j.eij.2020.07.003

Khanna, S., & Srivastava, S. (2020). Patient-centric ethical frameworks for privacy, transparency, and bias awareness in deep learning-based medical systems. *Applied Research in Artificial Intelligence and Cloud Computing*, *3*(1), 16–35.

Koopman, C., Jones, P., Simon, V., Showler, P., McLevey, M., & Critical Genealogies Collaboratory. (2021). When data drive health: an archaeology of medical records technology. *Biosocieties*, 1–23. https://doi.org/10.1057/s41292-021-00249-1

Lepri, B., Oliver, N., & Pentland, A. (2021). Ethical machines: the human-centric use of artificial intelligence. *iScience*, *24*(3). https://doi.org/10.1016/j.isci.2021.102249

Li, H., Yu, L., & He, W. (2019). The impact of GDPR on global technology development. *Journal of Global Information Technology Management*, *22*(1), 1–6. https://doi.org/10.1080/1097198X.2019.1569186

Mohammed, Z. (2022). Data breach recovery areas: an exploration of organization's recovery strategies for surviving data breaches. *Organizational Cybersecurity Journal: Practice, Process and People*, *2*(1), 41-59. https://doi.org/10.1108/OCJ-05-2021-0014

Nguyen, A. M., Rivera, A. M., & Gualtieri, L. (2023). A New Health Care Paradigm: The Power of Digital Health and E-Patients. *Mayo Clinic Proceedings: Digital Health, 1*(3), 203–209. https://doi.org/10.1016/j.mcpdig.2023.04.005

Olukoya, O. (2022). Assessing frameworks for eliciting privacy & security requirements from laws and regulations. *Computers & Security, 117,* 102697. https://doi.org/10.1016/j.cose.2022.102697

Omotunde, H., & Ahmed, M. (2023). A comprehensive review of security measures in database systems: assessing authentication, access control, and beyond. *Mesopotamian Journal of CyberSecurity, 2023,* 115–133. https://doi.org/10.58496/MJCSC/2023/016

Paulus, J. K., & Kent, D. M. (2020). Predictably unequal: understanding and addressing concerns that algorithmic clinical prediction may increase health disparities. *NPJ Digital Medicine, 3*(1), 99. https://doi.org/10.1038/s41746-020-0304-9

Petersen, L. M., & Lefferts, J. A. (2020). Lessons learned from direct-to-consumer genetic testing. *Clinics in Laboratory Medicine, 40*(1), 83–92. https://doi.org/10.1109/EuroSP48549.2020.00016

Pfaff, M. S., Eris, O., Weir, C., Anganes, A., Crotty, T., Rahman, M., . . . Nebeker, J. R. (2021). Analysis of the cognitive demands of electronic health record use. *Journal of Biomedical Informatics, 113,* 103633. https://doi.org/10.1016/j.jbi.2020.103633

Pietrzykowski, T., & Smilowska, K. (2021). The reality of informed consent: empirical studies on patient comprehension—systematic review. *Trials, 22,* 1-8. https://doi.org/10.1186/s13063-020-04969-w

Presthus, W., & Sønslien, K. F. (2021). An analysis of violations and sanctions following the GDPR. *International Journal of Information Systems and Project Management, 9*(1), 38–53. https://aisel.aisnet.org/ijispm/vol9/iss1/3/

Pussewalage, H. S. G., & Oleshchuk, V. A. (2016). Privacy preserving mechanisms for enforcing security and privacy requirements in E-health solutions. *International Journal of Information Management, 36*(6), 1161–1173. https://doi.org/10.1016/j.ijinfomgt.2016.07.006

Quach, S., Thaichon, P., Martin, K. D., et al. (2022). Digital technologies: tensions in privacy and data. *Journal of the Academy of Marketing Science, 50*(7), 1299–1323. https://doi.org/10.1007/s11747-022-00845-y

Raparthi, M. (2021). AI-driven decision support systems for precision medicine: examining the development and implementation of AI-driven decision support systems in precision medicine. *Journal of Artificial Intelligence Research, 1*(1), 11–20. Retrieved from https://thesciencebrigade.com/JAIR/article/view/126

Reza, F., Prieto, J. T., & Julien, S. P. (2020). Electronic Health Records: Origination, Adoption, and Progression. In J. Magnuson & B. Dixon (Eds.), *Public Health Informatics and Information Systems* (pp. 183–201). Health Informatics. Springer. https://doi.org/10.1007/978-3-030-41215-9_11

Roth, M., Vakkuri, J., & Johanson, J. E. (2024). Value creation mechanisms in a social and health care innovation ecosystem–an institutional perspective. *Journal of Management and Governance,* 1–32. https://doi.org/10.1007/s10997-024-09696-x

Sahu, M., Gupta, R., Ambasta, R. K., & Kumar, P. (2022). Artificial intelligence and machine learning in precision medicine: a paradigm shift in big data analysis. *Progress in Molecular Biology and Translational Science, 190*(1), 57–100. https://doi.org/10.1016/bs.pmbts.2022.03.002

Sarkar, K. R. (2010). Assessing insider threats to information security using technical, behavioural and organisational measures. *Information Security Technical Report, 15*(3), 112–133. https://doi.org/10.1016/j.istr.2010.11.002

Schneble, C. O., Elger, B. S., & Shaw, D. M. (2020). Google's Project Nightingale highlights the necessity of data science ethics review. *EMBO Molecular Medicine, 12*(3), e12053. https://doi.org/10.15252/emmm.202012053

Séroussi, B., Hollis, K. F., & Soualmia, L. F. (2020). Transparency of health informatics processes as the condition of healthcare professionals' and patients' trust and adoption: the rise of ethical requirements. *Yearbook of Medical Informatics, 29*(01), 007–010. https://doi.org/10.1055/s-0040–1702029

Shah, J. L., Bhat, H. F., & Khan, A. I. (2021). Integration of cloud and IoT for smart e-healthcare. In *Healthcare Paradigms in the Internet of Things Ecosystem* (pp. 101–136). Academic Press. https://doi.org/10.1016/B978-0-12-819664-9.00006-5

Shrivastava, U., Song, J., Han, B. T., & Dietzman, D. (2021). Do data security measures, privacy regulations, and communication standards impact the interoperability of patient health information? A cross-country investigation. *International Journal of Medical Informatics, 148,* 104401. https://doi.org/10.1016/j.ijmedinf.2021.104401

Solove, D. J., & Schwartz, P. M. (2023). *EU Data Protection and the GDPR: [Connected EBook].* Aspen Publishing.

Spanakis, E. G., Sfakianakis, S., Bonomi, S., Ciccotelli, C., Magalini, S., & Sakkalis, V. (2021). Emerging and established trends to support secure Health Information Exchange. *Frontiers in Digital Health, 3,* 636082. https://doi.org/10.3389/fdgth.2021.636082

Stahl, B. C., & Coeckelbergh, M. (2016). Ethics of healthcare robotics: Towards responsible research and innovation. *Robotics and Autonomous Systems*, *86*, 152–161. https://doi.org/10.1016/j.robot.2016.08.018

Taha, A. R., Shehadeh, M., Alshehhi, A., Altamimi, T., Housser, E., Simsekler, M. C. E., Alfalasi, B., et al. (2022). The integration of mHealth technologies in telemedicine during the COVID-19 era: a cross-sectional study. *PLoS One*, *17*(2), e0264436. https://doi.org/10.1371/journal.pone.0264436

Tariq, M. U. (2024). Enhancing cybersecurity protocols in modern healthcare systems: strategies and best practices. In *Transformative Approaches to Patient Literacy and Healthcare Innovation* (pp. 223–241). IGI Global. https://doi.org/10.4018/979-8-3693-3661-8.ch011

Tsohou, A., Karyda, M., & Kokolakis, S. (2015). Analyzing the role of cognitive and cultural biases in the internalization of information security policies: recommendations for information security awareness programs. *Computers & Security*, *52*, 128–141. https://doi.org/10.1016/j.cose.2015.04.006

Unver, M. B., & Asan, O. (2022). Role of trust in AI-driven healthcare systems: Discussion from the perspective of patient safety. In *Proceedings of the International Symposium on Human Factors and Ergonomics in Health Care*, *11*(1), 129–134. Sage CA: Los Angeles, CA: SAGE Publications. https://doi.org/10.1177/2327857922111026

Vanaparthi, R., & Rao, S. V. A. (2023). Revolutionizing health care: ai-enabled disease diagnosis, outcome prediction& operational efficiency. *Turkish Journal of Computer and Mathematics Education (TURCOMAT)*, *14*(03), 993–1001. https://doi.org/10.17762/turcomat.v14i03.14198

Voigt, P., & Von dem Bussche, A. (2017). The eu general data protection regulation (gdpr). *A Practical Guide, 1st Ed., Cham: Springer International Publishing*, *10*(3152676), 10–5555.

WHO. (2021). *Global Strategy on Digital Health 2020–2025*. Geneva: World Health Organization. Retrieved from https://www.who.int/docs/default-source/documents/gs4dhdaa2a9f352b0445bafbc79ca799dce4d.pdf

Wiwatkunupakarn, N., Aramrat, C., Pliannuom, S., Buawangpong, N., Pinyopornpanish, K., Nantsupawat, N., . . . Angkurawaranon, C. (2023). The integration of clinical decision support systems into telemedicine for patients with multimorbidity in primary care settings: scoping review. *Journal of Medical Internet Research*, *25*, e45944. https://doi.org/10.2196/45944

Zou, J., & Schiebinger, L. (2021). Ensuring that biomedical AI benefits diverse populations. *EBioMedicine, 67*, 103358. https://doi.org/10.1016/j.ebiom.2021.103358

14 Cybersecurity Challenges in Healthcare Informatics

Smitha Shivshankar, Neeraj Makhija,
and Premkumar Mathusudhanan

14.1 INTRODUCTION

14.1.1 OVERVIEW OF DIGITALIZATION IN HEALTHCARE

Digital technologies have facilitated seamless communication with patients and access to treatments through the integration of smart devices and the development of modern information systems, thereby transforming the healthcare industry. The modern information system components play a significant role in increasing the quality and availability of health services, with electronic health records (EHRs) replacing the paper records and the telecommunication networks supporting seamless communication across the patients and health workers.

The information system components that significantly contribute to increasing the quality and availability of health services are as follows:

1. **EHRs** replaced paper records and increased the efficiency of health services. These are digital systems that collect, store, and share comprehensive health information of patients. The purposes include documentation, retrieval, and processing of health data supporting efficient healthcare (Dimitrios et al., 2006).
2. **Telecommunication networks and services** to support communication and cooperation between patients and health workers.
3. **mHealth, telehealth, and telemedicine** have improved the process of patient management as well as improving the quality of services (Sendelj & Ognjanovic, 2022).
   mHealth, referred as mobile health, refers to the use of mobile devices to support medical and health practices. It encompasses applications such as health monitoring, data collection, patient education, and remote consultation. It provides increased access to healthcare services, improving patient engagement and adherence to treatment plans and enhanced data collection (El-Sherif & Abouzid, 2022).
   Telehealth/telemedicine is the use of telecommunications technologies and electronic information to extend care for a patient remotely. The technologies include videoconferencing, streaming, and store and forward imaging. Some of the benefits of telemedicine include continued care and extended access, although less appropriate for health concerns that require a procedure (Eswaran, 2024; AlOsail et al., 2021; Razali et al., 2020).

14.1.2 CURRENT CYBERSECURITY POSTURE IN HEALTH

Nevertheless, the application of modern technologies has supported the collection of patient data with simultaneous contribution to an increase in the quality of services in healthcare. Furthermore, all actions performed on the personal data represent a potential vulnerability of the system that can arise from software vulnerabilities, human error, or security flaws (He et al., 2021).

DOI: 10.1201/9781003485629-14

Despite the increased potential of mHealth and telemedicine, they experience security and privacy challenges, and the need for regulatory framework and ensuring equitable access to technology (Dimitrios et al., 2006). Although the integration of telemedicine has revolutionized patient access, the field experiences significant vulnerabilities that can be exploited by malicious actors (Eswaran, 2024; AlOsail et al., 2021; Razali et al., 2020).

Cybersecurity is an obligation and crucial for all stakeholders contributing to health including health service providers, insurance institutions, pharmaceuticals, and biotechnology institutions, as well as companies for medical devices and the production of software and other hardware components (Jalali & Kaiser, 2018). In this context, the basic tasks of cyber protection of health organizations can be defined as (i) ensuring service availability, (ii) ensuring operational conditions of the systems and devices, (iii) preserving confidentiality and integrity on patients' information and services, and (iv) ensuring timely response and prevention from sources of cyberattacks (Nifakos et al., 2021).

The taxonomy of cybersecurity challenges in healthcare encompasses various critical aspects. The reliance on electronic health information exposes healthcare organizations to significant cybercrime risks and makes them attractive targets for cyberattackers (Shingari et al., 2023; Sendelj & Ognjanovic, 2022). The increasing digitization and use of advanced technologies makes them a prime target for cybercriminals exploiting weak security controls and accessing confidential patient data (Besenyő & Kovács, 2023). It is imperative for healthcare organizations to prioritize alertness, awareness, preparedness, and rapid response to mitigate security risks effectively. It is crucial to understand and implement protection mechanisms aligned with best practices in enhancing cybersecurity posture within the healthcare industry.

14.2 CYBERSECURITY STATISTICS AND TRENDS

Cybersecurity incidents have the potential to cause devastating impacts on organizations and individuals. The compromise of business emails and ransomware presents high-impact threats to the health sector. The threat actors significantly interfere and threaten the delivery of health services and the lives of patients, causing reputational and financial damage. The malicious actors have significantly taken advantage of pandemic times to tailor their criminal activities.

14.2.1 HEALTH SECTOR THREAT OVERVIEW

Malicious actors target organizations for a variety of reasons. They may seek information and intellectual property relating to vaccine developments, treatments, and research. The sensitive nature of the medical and personal data and their extent of being crucial to maintain business operations and patient care become the reasons for the healthcare sector being viewed as a lucrative target for ransomware attacks. They seek access to sensitive personal information held by health organizations (such as names, dates of birth, addresses, medical histories, Medicare details, and healthcare fund information) to commit identity theft or sell the data in cybercrime marketplaces. Malicious actors may seek to target a wide range of entities in the health sector, including hospitals, general practice services, pathologists, research facilities, aged care providers and other medical service providers, the respective clients, and the vendors in the medical transport and supply chains.

There are several control systems in the health sector that are vital to their operations; however, they provide opportunities for malicious cyber activity. Medical devices have been reported for identified vulnerabilities. Common sources of compromise include hardcoded passwords, improper authentication, or passwords held in a recoverable area. Often regular patches are avoided in specialized devices for fear of rendering critical systems or devices becoming unavailable. However, these devices can possibly impose potential risk on individuals in the case of compromise. It is imperative to take steps to update vulnerabilities, or isolate vulnerable devices if they cannot be patched. The changes to the business model of the health sector are also a significant reason for the

TABLE 14.1

Cyber Incident Breakdown Source

Type	Percentage (%)
Phishing (compromised credentials)	28
Compromised or stolen credentials	27
Ransomware	27
Hacking	10
Malware	5
Brute-force attack	3

Source: (OAIC, 2024)

evolving cyber threats. The increased reliance on remote work also adds as an additional attribute to the "attack surface" for these organizations.

Remote access solutions connect new network segments to the Internet, exposing critical devices. The operational imperative has not given enough time for organizations to consider cybersecurity. Remote access solutions need to be reviewed and segmented from the remaining network. Solutions such as enabling multi-factor authentication (MFA), ensuring appropriate logging, and regularly patching remote access clients ensure effective management of remote access solutions. Additionally, logs should be routinely reviewed and monitored regularly, and attention should be given to the locations and access times to ensure remote access is being utilized by legitimate staff only (Australian Cybersecurity Centre, 2020).

14.2.2 CURRENT STATISTICS

The average cost of a healthcare data breach was $10.93 million, with a 239% increase in large data breaches reported to the US Department of Health and Human Services (HSS) over the last 4 years. According to the HHS, there was a rise of 60% in people affected by the data breaches in 2023. Almost four in five breaches are caused by cyberattacks, and the most reported cause was malicious attacks. However, only 20% of incidents account from human failure, the lowest of any root cause (USAToday). According to the Office of the Australian Information Commissioner, the highest data breaches reported was by healthcare sector service providers, with 67% from malicious or criminal attack, 30% from human error, and 3% from system fault. In 2023, the healthcare reported data breaches costing an average of $10.93 million per breach. While technologies such as EHRs, telemedicine, and Internet of Things (IoT) bring numerous benefits for the sector, they also expand the attack surface, opening up more entry points for cybercriminals. The confidentiality, integrity, and availability of patient information can be maintained only by protecting the digital assets. Table 14.1 presents the breakdown of the cyber incidents, which is demonstrated using Figure 14.1.

14.3 HEALTHCARE ORGANIZATIONS: TARGET FOR CYBERSECURITY ATTACKS

According to the federal and local cybersecurity experts, healthcare has become a top target in the last few decades. The massive amount of patient data—including medical records, financial information, social security numbers, names, and addresses—project the sector as the top target of malicious actors. They are also among the few businesses that stay open 24/7, meaning they might be more likely to prioritize avoiding disruptions and, therefore, more likely to pay a hacker's ransom (The Seattle Times, 2024). "They're basically a one-stop shop for an adversary," said

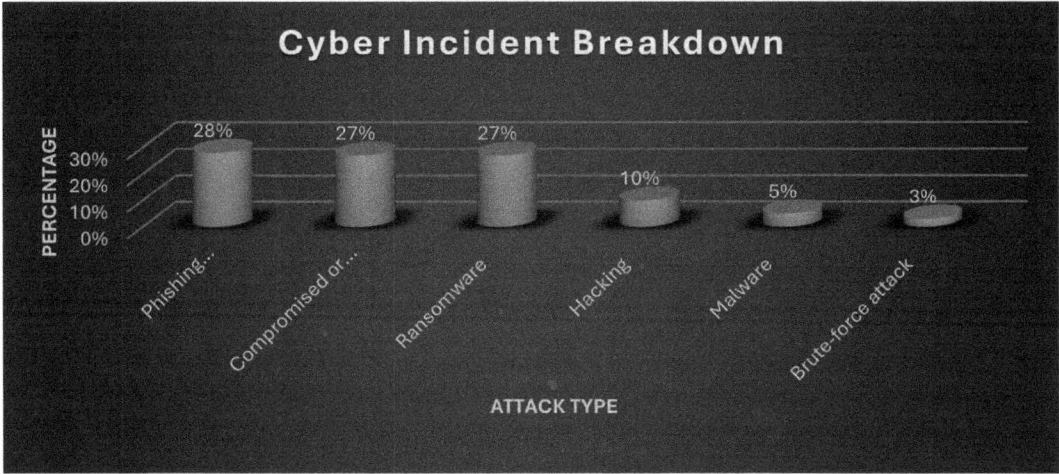

FIGURE 14.1   Cyber incident breakdown.

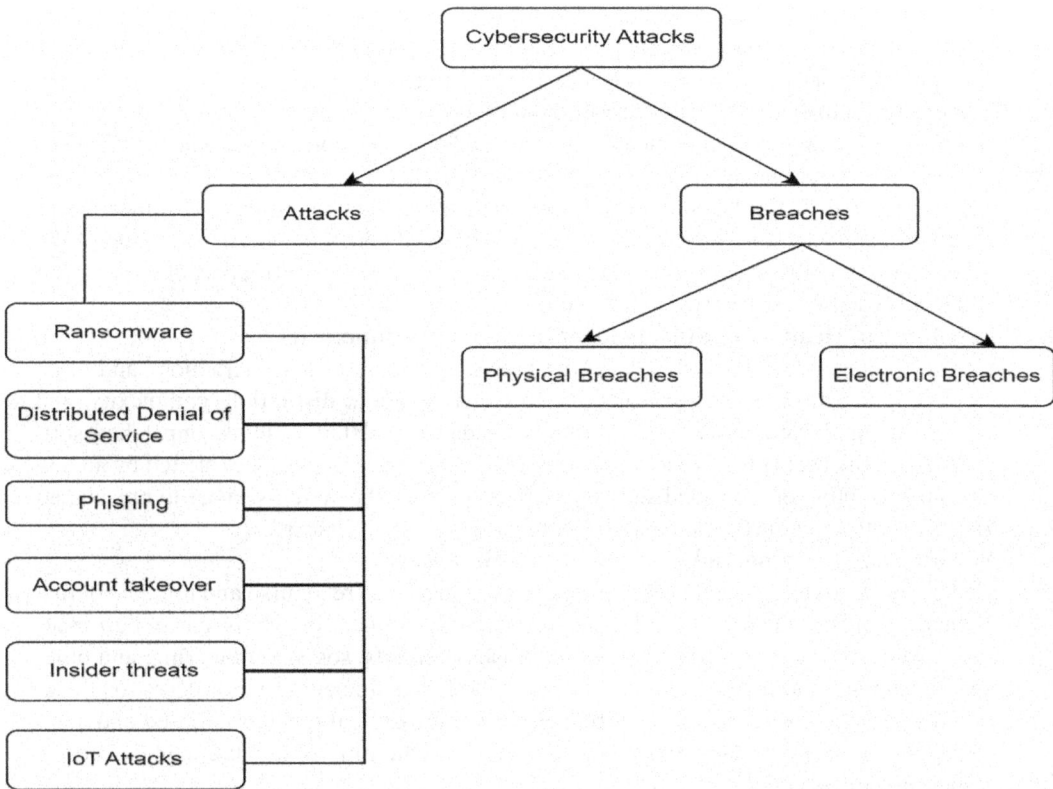

FIGURE 14.2   Cybersecurity attacks.

Chris Callahan, chief of cybersecurity for the Northwest region of the federal Cybersecurity and Infrastructure Security Agency (CISA). Healthcare is now the biggest target for online attacks for the reasons listed below:

1. **Patient Information—a Source of Financial Gain for Attackers**
   The increasing trend of breaches in the healthcare sector is enabled by the health information and the health practices allowing the hackers to sell the incredible amount of patient data that are worth a lot of money making the industry a growing target. Financial penalties for not cooperating with the General Data Protection Regulation (GDPR) or paying to retrieve their data from ransomware are alarming for a healthcare industry that is already struggling with financing daily work demands.
   IT professionals realize that the cost of securing their data with solutions like MFA, requiring more than one authentication information to identify a user, is far less than the payout from ransomware or similar attacks.

2. **Medical Devices Acting as Vulnerable Entry Points**
   The increasing number of medical devices and patient wearables forms a part of IoT and storing patient data directly. Although hackers know that medical devices such as x-rays, insulin pumps, and defibrillators do not contain any patient data, they are considered easy targets and open more entry points. Security is not a primary concern in the design of medical points. Although they do not hold patient data, these devices can be leveraged to launch an attack on a server that holds valuable information. In a worst-case scenario, medical devices can be completely compromised, preventing healthcare organizations from providing services and giving hackers access to other devices.

3. **More Opportunities for Attack through Remote Data Access**
   With the increasing use of telehealth and telemedicine, telecommunication technologies are used to provide healthcare services and health education. Collaborative and remote working is vital in the healthcare industry, with units working together. Connecting to a network remotely from new devices is risky, due to the lack of security in some of the devices. It is imperative to ensure that the compromised devices are not part of the network as it can leave the entire network compromised.

4. **Resistance of Healthcare Stakeholders to Modern Technologies**
   Medical professionals need slick working practices with minimal distractions and often resist adopting modern technologies due to concerns about disruption, complexity, and the cost of implementation. This reluctance leads to outdated systems, unpatched software, and weak security protocols, creating vulnerabilities that can be exploited by attackers. Slow adoption of advanced security measures leaves the systems easier to breach and harder to defend against evolving cyber threats.

5. **No Sufficient Training and Awareness of Online Risks**
   Medical professionals do not have the necessary expertise to recognize and mitigate online threats, and it is impossible for all healthcare staff to be fluent in cybersecurity best practices. Many stakeholders do not recognize phishing emails, social engineering, and other types of threats leading to accidental exposure of data and unauthorized access to attackers. The gap in knowledge and preparedness leaves the critical systems exposed and more susceptible to breaches. Nevertheless, cybersecurity solutions, although complex, need to have a simple interface.

6. **Proliferation Makes Hospitals Hard to Stay on Top of Security**
   Modern healthcare organizations are responsible for an extensive network of connected devices and massive amounts of patient data. Technological advancements in the healthcare sector including wearable medical devices, telehealth services, and EHRs result in a large amount of health information being stored and transmitted electronically (https://www.allens.com.au/insights-news/insights/2018/10/

pulse-data-breaches-in-the-healthcare-sector-the-reality-the/). Each of the device act as a potential threat from attackers. If one device is compromised, it leaves the entire network open to data breaches and medica device hacks.

7. **Healthcare Information Needs to Be Open and Shareable**
   EHRs have been adopted internally within specific practices and in hospitals through the My Health Records (MHR) system. The staff on-site and remote need to be able to access confidential patient data on multiple devices. The emergency service delivery requirements of the medical industry need seamless information sharing. There is no time to pause and consider the security implications of their devices. However, the devices are not always protected.

8. **Smaller Healthcare Entities Are Also at Risk**
   All healthcare organizations are at risk from online threats. Both large and small enterprises across the healthcare sector have their security budgets. The large firms holding the large amount of data become the common targets for attackers. But smaller enterprises have smaller security budgets. Less complex and up-to-date cybersecurity solutions mean smaller enterprises are often seen as an easy target and a backdoor-access opportunity to target larger companies.

9. **Outdated Technology—Unprepared for Attacks**
   Not every aspect of healthcare has kept the pace with the incredible advances in medical technology. The medical technology becomes outdated with limited budgets and users being hesitant to learn new systems. All the hospital systems should keep all software equipped with the most recent version to be secure and free from bugs. When an upgrade is not feasible, there is a need for a more secure software or additional layers of security (Swivelsecure).

14.3.1 THE ALLURE OF HEALTHCARE DATA

The healthcare industry is one of the most targeted industries for cyber threat actors due to the vast amount of sensitive information managed by the sector, including personally identifiable information (PII), medical records, insurance details, and payment data. The healthcare data holds high value in the black market. This section will explore the key reasons why healthcare data are so alluring to cyber criminals and the business challenges experienced in the healthcare mission that contributes to the industry being the target for the cyber attackers. Table 14.2 presents the list of challenges and how it contributes to the data being targeted.

1. **Identity Theft:** The wealth of personal information present in the patient records makes them an ideal source of identity theft. The information can be used by criminals to open fraudulent accounts, access financial information, or commit other criminal activities.
2. **Insurance Fraud:** Cybercriminals can make false insurance claim by exploiting the data and make substantial financial gains.
3. **Fraudulent Billing:** Criminals can bill insurance companies for fictitious treatments or services using the stolen patient data.
4. **Black Market:** Attracts cybercriminals motivated by financial gain, enabling them to sell stolen records for a premium.
5. **Critical Infrastructure:** The healthcare sector is more likely to meet attackers' demands due to the need for the critical infrastructure to restore operations as quickly as possible to provide critical care.
6. **Internet of Medical Things (IoMT):** Healthcare organizations are increasingly reliant on networked devices to provide care. The poor security of the networked devices provides attackers with easier access to sensitive data and the organization's networks.

TABLE 14.2

Cybersecurity Challenges to Healthcare Mission

Challenge	Description
Risk in cloud transition	With a motive to improve the efficiency and scalability, the healthcare industry is transitioning to cloud for their operations from billing to remote patient care options, online patient portals, and more. While the efficiency and scalability are achieved, they also increase the risks with data on the cloud.
IoT security is an emerging issue	The proliferation of highly interconnected medical devices enlarges the attack surface, enabling attackers to gain access to sensitive data and/or disrupt patient care. This proliferation of IoT devices, along with the increase in the sophisticated tools and techniques that threat actors use to hack them, means that healthcare providers have to secure more equipment than ever before—and the stakes have never been higher.
Serious risk to patients due to the staggering cost of disruption and downtime	Healthcare organizations highly rely on electronic data exchange for business operations and patient care delivery. Given that, the healthcare sector can least afford to experience disruptions in essential systems and networks. As they rely increasingly on electronic data exchange, system downtime not only results in huge costs but can also bring delays in accessing critical patient health information.
Monitoring regulators	The Health Insurance Portability and Accountability Act (HIPAA) places additional responsibility on healthcare organizations to protect individuals' electronic personal health information. The security configurations safeguard the confidentiality, integrity, and security of health information using appropriate administrative, physical, and technical rules. They are required to provide notification to affected individuals if they lost control of their data.
Remote work security assurance	Malware and distributed denial of service (DDoS) attacks are targeting innumerable wireless connected devices in healthcare through the security vulnerabilities with remote desktop protocols and virtual private networks.
Endpoint device management	An endpoint device acts as an entry point to larger healthcare networks. An outdated, legacy, or unsupported operating system compromises interoperability, thereby increasing vulnerability.
Human factors in cybersecurity	Majority of information security breaches are related to human errors, leading to a significant correlation between workload and the probability of healthcare staff opening a phishing email.
Inadequate risk assessment communication at the board level	There is lack of understanding of security risks and their impact on organization-wide risk management. There is a need for a matrix that translates strategic requirements of healthcare into prioritized cyber improvement needs.
Inadequate business continuity plans	Risks will continue if security is not designed into the product from the beginning of the development life cycle. Vendor dependence, inappropriate encryption configurations, and inability of seamless information sharing are the key risks challenging information sharing and exchange with third-party partners. There is a lack of sophisticated data security tools.
Uncoordinated incident response	Current defense is reactive, and there is a lack of coordinated incident response to counteract constantly emerging threats. Healthcare experiences time lag between an attack and detection of breach.
Trade-off with a limited budget and the need to deliver an undisrupted service	Value-based systems need to be in place to weigh and balance benefits and risks from the perspective of security, privacy, and adoption of technology.

TABLE 14.2 (*Continued*)
Cybersecurity Challenges to Healthcare Mission

Challenge	Description
Limited budget	Healthcare providers have limited budget to manage cybersecurity risks due to competing financial priorities. Fragmented IT services and ownership of security control can be expensive to acquire and maintain. Fragmentation leads to high operational costs, decreased productivity, and a lack of required provision of security controls.
Lack of awareness	Limited training and awareness activities for staff, a focus on patient care over security, and a misconception that healthcare data are not a primary target result in inadequate investment and preparedness for cyber threats.

Source: (InfoTrust, 2023; Argaw et al., 2019, 2020)

14.4　TAXONOMY OF CYBERSECURITY CHALLENGES FOR HEALTHCARE

While the healthcare sector continues to offer life-critical services with improved treatment and patient care by embracing net technologies, criminals and cyber threat actors look to exploit the vulnerabilities that are coupled with these changes. The healthcare industry is plagued by a myriad of cybersecurity-related issues ranging from malware that compromises the integrity of systems and privacy of patients, to DDoS attacks that disrupt facilities' ability to provide patient care. Ransomware, for example, is a particularly egregious form of malware for hospitals, as loss of patient data can put lives at risk (Centre for Internet Security, 2024; Ministry of Health 2023).

14.4.1　Challenges to the Healthcare's Mission

The industry experiences ramifications beyond monetary loss and breach of privacy. The healthcare sector, increasingly reliant on digital technologies, faces a myriad of cybersecurity challenges that jeopardize patient safety, data integrity, and operational continuity. With EHRs, telemedicine, and connected medical devices nevertheless becoming integral to modern healthcare delivery, they also become prime targets for cyberattacks. These challenges are exacerbated by the sensitivity of medical data, the high financial value of healthcare information on the black market, and the potential life-or-death consequences of disrupted services. While other critical infrastructure sectors are also victims of these types of attacks, the nature of the healthcare's mission has unique cybersecurity challenges.

14.4.2　Cyberattacks in the Healthcare Sector

In the complex landscape of healthcare cybersecurity, various attributes of healthcare systems are vulnerable to a spectrum of cyberattacks. Cybercriminals exploit the vulnerabilities in the digital infrastructure, targeting sensitive patient data, medical devices, and operational systems. Ransomware attacks, for instance, encrypt critical data and demand high ransoms for their release, significantly disrupting healthcare operations and potentially putting lives at risk. Phishing attacks persuade healthcare employees into divulging confidential information or downloading malicious software, often leading to broader system breaches. These attacks can have devastating effects, compromising patient privacy, disrupting care delivery, and causing significant financial losses.

Additionally, insider threats pose a unique challenge as they are individuals within the organization misusing their access privileges, intentionally or unintentionally. DDoS attacks flood healthcare networks with traffic, overwhelming systems and resulting in essential services being inaccessible.

TABLE 14.3

Cyberattacks Targeting Healthcare Organizations

Type of Attack	Description
Ransomware	Ransomware attacks hold hostage the data and infrastructure on which the healthcare organizations are heavily reliant to provide services. The attackers hold hostage these systems until the organization meets the attacker's demands. The attack tricks an unsuspecting user to open an infected email attachment or click a malicious link leading to a compromised website. Once the organization is compromised, malware is installed on the system, rendering it useless and inaccessible until a ransom payment is made.
	Impact: These attacks usually have serious monetary losses as the organizations cannot easily recover from the loss of data and damage. Although organizations agree to make payments to attackers, there is no guarantee that the data will be returned. These types of attacks are becoming more and more sophisticated, and the attackers significantly increase the requested amounts as they are aware of the value of the health information and how imperative it is to protect the interests of patients.
	Example of an Impact: The first known human fatality occurred when the computer systems of a German university affiliated with a hospital was disrupted, experiencing the DoppelPaymer ransomware attack. It penetrated through the unpatched vulnerability in the VPN system. An individual being transported to the hospital by ambulance was re-routed to another hospital 30 kilometers away, passing away en route (CyberWardens; CyberCX, 2020).
	Some vendors sold legitimate medical products to project a legitimate reputation, whereas other vendors exploited the COVID-19 pandemic and public demand for medical products by importing fake and unapproved COVID-19 test kits. Additionally, the increased demand for personal protective equipment, sanitizers, and masks also resulted in a spike in scams from companies and individuals purporting to sell these products.
	The Universal Health Services, one of the largest US healthcare networks, suffered a ransomware attach in 2020, leaving over 400 healthcare providers not being able to access their EHRs for about 3 weeks. The US Department of Homeland Security's CISA released a public alert to provide warning to healthcare providers against an increased and imminent cybercrime threat to US hospitals and healthcare providers. The attack and subsequent alert highlight the significant impact ransomware can have on organizations and customers. To avoid these incidents, effective logging and monitoring are crucial to enable early remediation after the detection of a potential compromise (Cyber Incident Response Plan).
DDoS	DDoS uses a network of compromised systems to overwhelm a target by sending excessive requests to an online platform to exhaust its bandwidth and cause a slowdown or a total shutdown. The attacker demands a ransom to restore the organization's operations. DDoS attacks are executed by sending excessive requests to an online platform to exhaust its bandwidth and cause a slowdown or total shutdown.
	Impact: Prevent access to critical IT tools and systems. The attack takes away the hospital's ability to access its records, hampering research capabilities and disrupting communications with healthcare facilities (CurrentWare, 2024).
Phishing	This is a type of social engineering attack that tricks the recipient into handing highly sensitive information or infecting their systems with malware. The attack involves an inbound phishing email comprising an active link or file, which appears to have originated from a legitimate sender, accessing which will either direct to a website that solicits sensitive information or lead to malicious software download.
	Impact: Phishing attacks assist attackers to obtain sensitive patient data, which can then be misused in terms of impersonation, selling on the black market, and harming healthcare institutions.
Account takeover	Takes advantage of weak passwords or compromised ones through phishing or other types of attacks. Once access is obtained to a legitimate user account, the attacker can steal sensitive data or implement other malicious actions.

TABLE 14.3 (*Continued*)
Cyberattacks Targeting Healthcare Organizations

Type of Attack	Description
Loss of device data and insider threats	Sensitive information stored in mobile devices and laptops can be more critical to healthcare sector if the devices are lost and end up being held by attackers. The consequences are even more significant if such devices do not have adequate encryption.
	Causes of Data Leaks: Cybercriminals gain unauthorized access to IT systems. Insiders transfer protected health information (PHI) to a portable storage device, lost laptops, or portable storage hardware with unencrypted records, which can be accessed via accidental disclosure to unauthorized people via misaddressed emails or phishing.
	Impact: Loss of sensitive patient data can lead to a large-scale loss that directly tarnishes the reputation of the organization and the doctor and can lead to the identity theft of all patients.
Insider leak/threat	A trusted individual of authority being able to steal confidential data and download patient records with their access privileges and disclose to unauthorized parties.
	There are two types: intentional and unintentional.
	Intentional: Attacks from disgruntled employees aiming to purposefully expose or misuse sensitive information as a form of retaliation
	• Sell company IP to competitors for monetary gain • Retrieving PHI from databases and selling it to fraudsters • Deleting data, tampering equipment, sabotaging business processes, and causing damage to the employer
	Unintentional: Attacks due to poor employee training and a lack of cybersecurity awareness, leading to accidental data exposure or leak
	• Fall victim to phishing and social engineering attacks • Non-maliciously break company policy to expedite processes • Sharing sensitive data with unauthorized recipients unintentionally • Misplacing printed documents and data storage devices containing sensitive information
	Impact: Whether accidental or malicious, insider attacks can have serious consequences for patients, healthcare services, and organizations. Also, this type of attack can be realized in a short period of time and immediately shows consequences, while it can continue for a long-time interval.
IoT attacks	IoT device attacks are popular because these devices are unsecured, unencrypted, and not updated. Their connections to the WiFi open a potential entry point for hackers to access.
	Impact: Medical devices are often of vital importance for patients, and disruption of their operation can have direct consequences in the form of health impairment, significantly undermining the organization's reputation.

Source: (Sendelj & Ognjanovic, 2022).

Advanced persistent threats (APTs) involve prolonged and targeted cyber intrusions, often orchestrated by sophisticated actors aiming to steal valuable research data or intellectual property. Each type of attack leverages specific vulnerabilities within healthcare systems. Table 14.3 presents the range of attack types, highlighting how they compromise healthcare missions by exploiting specific vulnerabilities within the sector.

14.4.3 Taxonomy of the Data Breaches in Healthcare

A data breach is not an attack or threat on its own. A data breach is a result of a cyberattack allowing criminals to gain access and steal personal data from a system without the knowledge or authorization of the system's owner, or due to a human error or an insider threat. Broadly, there are two types of data breaches (Ministry of Health, 2023). Data breaches or, in other words, unauthorized access

TABLE 14.4

Types of Data Breaches in Healthcare

Type of Breach	Description
Physical breach	Involves physical theft of documents and equipment containing data. Physical assets are at risk of physical breach, while threat actors can also go hunting for documents that are not disposed of properly, a practice termed "dumpster diving".
Electronic breach	Involves unauthorized access or a deliberate attack on a system or network where data are stored. Phishing, malware, and DDoS are common techniques employed in an electronic breach.

Source: (Ministry of Health, 2023).

to data and patient information is achieved using one or more of the above discussed methods. Table 14.4 presents the classification of breaches, explaining the target of the breaches.

14.5 BARRIERS TO HEALTHCARE CYBER RESILIENCE

Health organizations face several challenges when seeking to improve cybersecurity, including cost, skill shortages, aging infrastructure, multiagency healthcare delivery, and new legislation and reporting requirements. Additionally, the ever-increasing threat landscape and lack of cybersecurity expertise enhance the sector's vulnerability. Understanding these barriers is crucial for developing effective strategies to protect sensitive health data and ensure the continuity of patient care. This section delves into the key challenges impeding the improvement of cybersecurity in healthcare, highlighting the urgent need for comprehensive and adaptive security measures. Let's look at each of these in detail:

1. **Cost**
    A robust security setup comes with an equally robust price tag. Nevertheless, the average cost of a ransomware attack including downtime and network cost is infinitely greater. However, it is impossible to guard against all cybersecurity attacks, and hence, a comprehensive understanding of the critical assets and the risk exposure is imperative to be strategic about your cybersecurity spend.

2. **Workforce**
    Cyber literacy is relatively low in healthcare. For instance, 89% of initial hospital compromises still occur through emails, and 57% of cyberattacks begin with trusted insiders. It is important that healthcare organizations must sufficiently educate, equip, and motivate their people to be vigilant to achieve a cyber-conscious workforce. It is important for every employee to understand their contribution to cybersecurity in their specific job. The security frameworks, training, and work environments need to be tailored with a solid understanding of human behavior that undermines cybersecurity. To achieve this, it is vital for leaders to understand the critical behaviors that drive people's decision-making (e.g., low attention, cognitive bandwidth, and self-control).

3. **Aging infrastructure**
    Globally, 83% of medical imaging devices still rely on legacy technologies that are too old to update, which are vulnerabilities that are known to cybercriminals and make the sector an attractive target for opportunistic attacks. It is imperative for healthcare leaders to upgrade and update the systems wherever possible. As applicable, the operating systems and software should be patched regularly. If not patching, re-platforming should be considered.

4. **Multiagency Healthcare Delivery**
    Healthcare incorporates a vast network involving interactions with multiple health institutions and providers, from medical equipment manufacturers to insurance providers to

government agencies. Each organization possibly becomes a potential entry point for a threat actor. The higher the amount of unsecure transmission of health information shared with third parties, the greater is the risk.

To engage reliable third parties and establish transparency over the end-to-end supply chains, it is vital to perform background checks of suppliers, understand their policies around reporting and data privacy, and conduct testing periodically to ensure that all third-party providers are upholding their service-level agreements.

5. **Legislation and Reporting Requirements**

Health leaders are well versed in matters of regulation and compliance as it is part of healthcare institutions. It is evident that the regulation will keep evolving as cybercriminals are constantly evolving their strategies and tactics. So, proactive health leaders are already thinking ahead, to anticipate and pre-empt future compliance requirements (Richa et al., 2022).

As an example, in Australia,

- under the Part IIIC (notification of eligible data breaches) of the Privacy Act, 1988 (Cth), a breach affecting a healthcare organization is likely to result in "serious harm" to the affected individuals than breaches affecting other sorts of data, and the *My Health Records Act 2012* (Cth) imposes a specific data breach regime for participants in the MHR system, to broadly cover situations where
  - there may have been unauthorized collection, use, or disclosure of health information included in an individual's MHR; or
  - an event may have occurred, or circumstances may have arisen that compromise (or could compromise) the security or integrity of the MHR system.
- the *Health Insurance Portability and Accountability Act 1996 (HIPAA)* requires reporting breaches where there is the acquisition, access, use, or disclosure of personal health information that affects more than 500 personal records; and
- guidance issued by the US HHS provides that most ransomware attacks, including any breach where health information is encrypted by the ransomware, will constitute a data breach under HIPAA and therefore must be reported.

6. **Securing the Healthcare Industry**

Cybersecurity has become imperative for the healthcare sector, driven by the increasing integration of technology and the sensitive nature of healthcare data. EHRs, telemedicine platforms, and connected medical devices are now foundational elements of modern healthcare delivery, enabling improved patient care and operational efficiency. Healthcare organizations have extremely valuable data, and the growing complexity of healthcare IT networks provides cyber threat actors with a variety of potential attack vectors. The digital transformation also exposes the healthcare system to a myriad of cyber threats, attacks, and breaches. The highly sensitive personal and medical information makes them lucrative targets for cybercriminals, who can exploit these vulnerabilities for financial gain, to obtain confidential information, or to disrupt services.

A successful cyberattack can lead to the theft of confidential patient data, financial loss, reputational damage, and even the interruption of critical medical services, putting patient lives at risk, and hence is devastating. Moreover, regulatory requirements impose stringent obligations on healthcare providers to protect patient information, with severe penalties for noncompliance. Therefore, robust cybersecurity measures are essential not only for protecting patient data and ensuring the smooth operation of healthcare services but also for maintaining public trust and adhering to legal and regulatory standards. In this context, investing in advanced cybersecurity solutions, continuous monitoring, and comprehensive staff training becomes crucial for the resilience and reliability of healthcare institutions.

Healthcare organizations struggle with many of the same security challenges as companies in other industries. With the need for monitoring and protecting a diverse mix of technology, security teams are overwhelmed by large volumes of security data. The complexity significantly increases with the array of security products that are complex to monitor and manage. Healthcare chief information security officers looking to ensure that their organizations are protected against cyber threats must focus on simplifying the problem that their security teams face. To achieve this goal, it is imperative to have a security platform that integrates security functionality and centralizes security monitoring and management (Checkpoint).

According to the IBM report (IBM, 2023), organizations should ensure that they

- implement a "privacy by design" approach to business operations;
- understand the data flows and the regulatory framework of their operations;
- identify and address any vulnerabilities resulting from outdated systems and perform appropriate due diligence on third-party vendors;
- create staff awareness on cybersecurity risks and data/privacy best practice;
- inculcate dedicated cybersecurity-risk quantification, assessment, and ongoing management and continuous monitoring capability;
- ensure that disclosed information is de-identified and not capable of re-identification;
- ensure regular audit of data storage processes and compliance with data storage policies and procedures; and
- develop a comprehensive data breach response plan through a response team to respond to potential data breaches quickly and efficiently and minimize harm.

14.5.1 Cybersecurity Imperative for Healthcare

Given the high stakes in healthcare, robust cybersecurity measures are not an option: they are an imperative. To protect patient data and ensure the continuity of healthcare services, the following measures are crucial:

- **Regulatory Compliance:** Ensure regulatory compliance and other relevant regulations to maintain the security and privacy of patient data.
- **Encryption:** Protect patient data at rest and in transit using encryption.
- **Access Control:** Implement strict access controls to limit data access to only perform the jobs.
- **Training and Awareness:** Train healthcare employees on recognizing and mitigating cybersecurity threats.
- **Regular Patches:** Update the software and systems with regular security patches to address vulnerabilities.
- **Network Security:** Address network security and protect the network through firewall configuration, intrusion detection systems, and segmentation.
- **Incident Response Plan:** For a swift containment and recovery, develop a clear incident response plan to guide through a security breach.
- **Device Security:** Secure devices with strong authentication and encryption.
- **Vendor Risk Management:** Assess and manage the cybersecurity risks posed by third-party vendors that have access to healthcare systems and data.

The healthcare data, combined with vulnerabilities in the infrastructure, make healthcare a top target for cybersecurity threats. Protecting patient data and ensuring the continuity of healthcare services are of paramount importance. By implementing strong cybersecurity measures and staying vigilant about emerging threats, the healthcare sector can continue to provide the best care for patients while keeping their data and operations secure. The Global Cybersecurity Association recognizes the importance of healthcare cybersecurity and encourages industry stakeholders to collaborate and share knowledge to ensure a safer and more secure healthcare environment (Nehra, 2023).

14.5.2 HEALTHCARE SECTOR-WIDE CYBER RESILIENCE

No single organization or government entity can tackle cybersecurity alone with the scale and inter-connectedness of the healthcare industry. It is imperative to take a collaborative and systematic approach within the ecosystem. Cyber resilience must be viewed beyond the limits of one organization. Collaboration between the public and private sectors is crucial for building cyber resilience in the healthcare industry. It is imperative to recognize that the healthcare ecosystem is an interconnected network of organizations, technologies, and individuals while taking a systematic approach to cybersecurity. Beyond protecting individuals, cyber resilience also ensures the robustness of the entire ecosystem to withstand and recover from cyber incidents.

Some of the important steps to elevate the resiliency of healthcare cybersecurity are as follows (Paloalto, 2024):

1. Assist the security team's efforts to rely on a standard framework
2. Adopt best practices of the selected framework
3. Meet regularly with the chief information security officer, chief information officer, and other technical leadership to do in-depth risk mitigation planning
4. Get the facts on your key metrics and how your organization matches up against those metrics at any point in time
5. Recognize that more and more of your day-to-day healthcare operations are potentially affected by cyberattacks and
6. importantly, acknowledge and accept that security and cyber resiliency are everyone's responsibility.

Action Plan for Cyber Resilience (Marc, 2023):

1. Cyber Roadmap: Align your organization on guiding principles, create a cyber roadmap, and prioritize investments based on critical assets and risk exposure.
2. Security by Design: Embed cybersecurity principles in the design of software, products, and capabilities from the outset, fostering a security-by-design culture throughout the organization.
3. Create an Ecosystem of Expertise: Establish a collaboration with internal and external specialists, forming an ecosystem of expertise to address the global shortage of cybersecurity talent.

14.5.3 CYBERSECURITY APPLICATIONS IN HEALTHCARE

The high values of sensitive data make healthcare organizations a prime target for cyberattacks. The industry's complex networks and numerous connected devices create multiple potential entry points for hackers. There is pressure to maintain rigid cybersecurity standards due to the highly regulated nature of the healthcare sector as breaches can lead to severe financial and reputational damage. To mitigate these risks, healthcare firms must invest in robust cybersecurity measures, educate employees on recognizing threats, and implement advanced strategies like MFA and disaster recovery plans to safeguard critical systems and data. Table 14.5 presents the list of cybersecurity applications that need to be considered for enhancing the security of the healthcare sector.

TABLE 14.5

Cybersecurity Application

Criteria for Application	Need for the Application
Protecting information	Cybersecurity enhances the detection, evaluation, and response to cyberattacks, improving efficiency and data protection. Advanced technologies like robotics and machine learning analyze vast data to detect risks, becoming more accurate over time. High reliance on technology makes cybersecurity crucial for healthcare to protect patient safety and privacy from threats like ransomware, unauthorized access, and data manipulation, which can severely impact patient health.
Protecting devices	Medical devices need protection through encryption, vulnerability assessments, and software updates to counter evolving cyber threats. As healthcare's reliance on software grows, so does the risk of cyberattacks exploiting system flaws, especially with increased telecommuting.
Protecting patient data	Fundamental security measures such as antivirus, backup, encryption, and firewalls are crucial for protecting highly valuable data, especially with the high reliance on remote healthcare services. The vulnerability of IoT devices further exacerbates risks. With often small IT teams, securing healthcare technology and maintaining effective IT support are essential for swift recovery from system failures.
Securing stakeholder access	Robust authentication and strong security measures are essential for protecting healthcare systems and data. As cyberattacks become more frequent, securing devices with passwords and biometrics, and evaluating new mHealth apps are key to preventing unauthorized access and defending against potential threats as attackers exploit vulnerabilities in the supply chain and interconnected systems.
Check and control treatment process	To limit user access and identify risks, it is essential for implementing controls and checks. Improving software patching and vulnerability discovery is critical. Federal agencies need to closely work with healthcare partners to develop robust contingency plans for serious cyber incidents.
Improving daily tasks	Healthcare IT teams use cybersecurity to enhance or replace routine tasks like monitoring and patching medical devices and configuring network security. Data breaches or ransomware attacks can severely impact patient care and reputation, making it crucial for healthcare organizations to work closely with cybersecurity experts to protect data and maintain operational integrity.
Preventing medical fraud	The healthcare industry must prevent legal issues, medical fraud, and damage to its reputation from breaches. Organizations should enforce strong authentication and carefully manage access based on employees' roles. Restricting access to data and systems will enhance overall security.

Source: (Javaid et al., 2023)

14.6   CONCLUSION

In the rapidly evolving landscape of cybersecurity, the healthcare sector stands as a particularly vulnerable and high-stake target for cyberattacks. This chapter has delved into the multifaceted reasons behind the targeting of healthcare systems, the intrinsic value of healthcare data, and the sector-specific challenges that complicate cybersecurity efforts. Through examining the various types of attacks and breaches, and highlighting the critical importance of cyber resilience, a clearer understanding emerges of the urgent need for robust cybersecurity measures in healthcare.

The allure of healthcare data cannot be overstated. The comprehensive nature and the significant financial value of PHI and EHRs in the black market make them highly sought by cybercriminals. PHI includes immutable personal identifiers, such as social security numbers and medical histories that cannot be changed, making it a lucrative target for identity theft and fraud unlike other types of data. Healthcare's unique operational environment presents distinct cybersecurity challenges. The integration of legacy systems, the necessity of uninterrupted access to patient data for clinical care, and the proliferation of connected medical devices (IoT) contribute to an expanded attack surface. Additionally, the sector's stringent regulatory requirements mandate rigorous data protection standards that impose difficulty in maintenance amid resource constraints and IT infrastructure complexity.

Healthcare organizations experience diverse and increasingly sophisticated types of cyberattacks and breaches. Ransomware attacks, data breaches, phishing schemes, and insider threats cause significant disruption to healthcare services by exploiting different vulnerabilities, and thereby jeopardizing patient safety. Given these challenges, the imperative for cyber resilience in healthcare cannot be overstated. Cyber resilience encompasses not only robust preventive measures but also the ability to swiftly respond to, recover from, and adapt to cyber incidents. Strategies such as regular security assessments, employee training, incident response planning, and investment in advanced cybersecurity technologies are essential components of a resilient healthcare system.

In conclusion, the intersection of healthcare and cybersecurity is fraught with challenges but also ripe with opportunities for innovation and improvement. As cyber threats continue to evolve, healthcare organizations must adopt a proactive and comprehensive approach to cybersecurity. This includes not only technical defenses but also fostering a culture of security awareness and resilience. By prioritizing cybersecurity, the healthcare sector can better protect sensitive patient data, ensure continuity of care, and maintain the trust and confidence of the patients it serves.

REFERENCES

AlOsail, Deemah, Noora Amino, and Nazeeruddin Mohammad. "Security issues and solutions in e-health and telemedicine." *Computer Networks, Big Data and IoT: Proceedings of ICCBI 2020*. Springer Singapore, 2021.

Argaw ST, Bempong N, Eshaya-Chauvin B, Flahault A. The state of research on cyberattacks against hospitals and available best practice recommendations: a scoping review. *BMC Med Inform Decis Mak.* 2019 Jan 11;19(1):10. doi: 10.1186/s12911-018-0724-5.

Argaw ST, Troncoso-Pastoriza JR, Lacey D, Florin M, Calcavecchia F, Anderson D, Burleson W, Vogel J, O'Leary Chana, Eshaya-Chauvin B, Flahault A. Cybersecurity of Hospitals: Discussing the challenges and working towards mitigating the risks. *BMC Med Inform Decis Mak.* 2020 Jul 03;20(1):146. doi: 10.1186/s12911-020-01161-7.

Australian Cybersecurity Centre. "Sector Snapshot: Health". 2020. Available at https://www.cyber.gov.au/sites/default/files/2023–03/2020%20Health%20Sector%20Snapshot%20-%2020210210.pdf (Accessed May 20, 2024)

Besenyő, János, Attila Máté Kovács. Healthcare cybersecurity threat context and mitigation opportunities. *Security Science Journal.* 2023;4(1): 83–101. doi: 10.37458/ssj.4.1.6

Centre for Internet Security. 2024. "Cyber Attacks: In Healthcare Sector", Available at Cyber Attacks: In the Healthcare Sector. (Accessed 20th May 2024).

CurrentWare. Cyberattacks on the Healthcare Sector (Cyberattacks on the Healthcare Sector—Check Point Software). Available at https://www.checkpoint.com/cyber-hub/cyber-security/what-is-healthcare-cyber-security/cyberattacks-on-the-healthcare-sector/

CurrentWare. "The Impact of Cyberattacks on Healthcare." 2024. Available at The Impact of Cyberattacks on Healthcare | CurrentWare (Accessed on May 22nd 2024)

CyberIncident Response Plan https://www.cyber.gov.au/sites/default/files/2023–03/2020%20Health%20Sector%20Snapshot%20-%2020210210.pdf

CyberCX, Cyber Intel Report, 2020 https://cybercx.com.au/resource/australian-healthcare-and-aged-care-threat-report/

CyberWardens, https://cyberwardens.com.au/4-most-common-cyber-attacks-in-healthcare/#:~:text=One%20extreme%20example%20involves%20a,and%20passed%20away%20en%20route.

Dimitrios G, Katehakis, Manolis Tsiknakis. "Electronic Health Record." 2006. doi: 10.1002/9780471740360.EBS1440.

El-Sherif DM, Abouzid M. Analysis of mHealth research: Mapping the relationship between mobile apps technology and healthcare during COVID-19 outbreak. *Global Health.* 2022;18(67). https://doi.org/10.1186/s12992-022-00856-y

Eswaran, Ushaa. "Fortifying Cybersecurity in an Interconnected Telemedicine Ecosystem." *Improving Security, Privacy, and Connectivity among Telemedicine Platforms,* edited by Nuno Geada, IGI Global, 2024, pp. 30–60. https://doi.org/10.4018/979-8-3693-2141-6.ch002

He Y, Aliyu A, Evans M, Luo C. Health care cybersecurity challenges and solutions under the climate of COVID-19: Scoping review. *Journal of Medical Internet Research*. 2021 Apr 20;23(4):e21747.

IBM. "Cost of a Data Breach Report." 2023. Available at https://www.ibm.com/reports/data-breach (Accessed 18th May 2024).

InfoTrust. "Cybersecurity in the Australian Healthcare Sector." 2023. Available at Cyber Security in the Australian Healthcare Sector | InfoTrust (Accessed 25th May 2024).

Jalali MS, Kaiser JP. Cybersecurity in hospitals: A systematic, organizational perspective. *Journal of Medical Internet Research*. 2018 May 28;20(5):e10059

Javaid, Mohd, et al. Towards insighting cybersecurity for healthcare domains: A comprehensive review of recent practices and trends. *Cyber Security and Applications*. 2023;1: 100016.

Marc, D. "Enhancing Cyber Resilience in Healthcare Sector: A Strategic Imperative." November 2023. Available at Enhancing Cyber Resilience in the Healthcare Sector: A Strategic Imperative | LinkedIn, (Accessed 27th May 2024).

Ministry of Health. 2023. "Common Cyberthreats and Data Breaches in the Healthcare Sector." Available at MOH | Common Cyber Threats and Data Breaches in the Healthcare Sector (Accessed 25th May 2024).

Nifakos S, Chandramouli K, Nikolaou CK, Papachristou P, Koch S, Panaousis E, Bonacina S. Influence of human factors on cyber security within healthcare organisations: A systematic review. *Sensors*. 2021 Jul 28;21(15):5119.

OAIC. Notifiable Data Breaches Report: July to December 2023, Available at Notifiable Data Breaches Report: July to December 2023 (Accessed May 24, 2024)

Paloalto. "Making Cyber Resiliency a Priority in healthcare: My Advice for Leaders—Palo Alto Networks." 2023. Available at Making Cyber Resiliency a Priority in Healthcare: My Advice for Leaders—Palo Alto Networks (Accessed on 28th May 2024)

Raj Singh Nehra. "Healthcare Sector Is the Biggest Target for Cyber Attacks." 2023. Available at (1) Healthcare Sector Is the Biggest Target for Cyber Attacks | LinkedIn, (Accessed on 25th May 2024)

Razali, Rina Azlin, and Norziana Jamil. "A quick review of security issues in telemedicine." *2020 8th International Conference on Information Technology and Multimedia (ICIMU)*. IEEE, 2020.

Richa Arora, Jason Smart and Jamie Wiggins. "Proven Precautions to Help Protect Health Organisations and Patients from Cyberattacks." 2022. Available at Cyber Security—The Healthcare Sector (pwc.com.au) (Accessed 20th May 2024).

The Seattle Times. "Why health care has become a top target for cybercriminals." February 2024, Available at Why health care has become a top target for cybercriminals | The Seattle Times (Accessed May 15, 2024)

Sendelj, Ramo, and Ivana Ognjanovic. "Cybersecurity challenges in healthcare." In *Achievements, Milestones and Challenges in Biomedical and Health Informatics*, pp. 190–202. IOS Press, 2022.

Shingari, Nitinkumar, Seema Verma, Beenu Mago, and Muhammad Sheraz Javeid. "A review of cybersecurity challenges and recommendations in the healthcare sector." In *2023 International Conference on Business Analytics for Technology and Security (ICBATS)*, pp. 1–8. IEEE, 2023. doi: 10.1109/icbats57792.2023.10111096

Swivelsecure. "9 Reasons Healthcare Is the Biggest Target for Cyberattacks." Available at 9 Reasons Healthcare Is the Biggest Target for Cyberattacks (swivelsecure.com) (Accessed May 18th, 2024)

15 Impact of Cybersecurity and Artificial Intelligence on Healthcare Operations

Lola A. Osawe and Benjamin A. Osawe

15.1 INTRODUCTION

This chapter will discuss opportunities to use technology more effectively to deliver and protect healthcare services empowered by cybersecurity and artificial intelligence (AI). Rapidly emerging technologies such as AI and the more critical discipline of cybersecurity are fields required as force enablers of all other technologies used in our daily lives, especially as consumers of health services.

In the AI section, we will also explore opportunities to amplify virtual medicine through AI and minimize the risk of human error in care environments that usually include risks to providers and patients, such as rendering care in a pandemic in both clinical and nonclinical functions. We will address challenges such as machine bias and opacity that come with AI because of bias in society on human developers, which complicates matters due to the significant damages machine bias and opacity can cause to institutions and patients without proper guardrails. We will also discuss use cases and future opportunities in AI for clinical and nonclinical functions to improve healthcare operations. We will also review the ethical impact of AI in healthcare, considering the design and implementation of AI technologies that are vulnerable to bias in design and function.

In the cybersecurity sections, we will review the impact of cybercrime on healthcare institutions, and discuss cybersecurity frameworks (CSFs) and the impact of cyber vulnerabilities in real-world examples. Threats like cyber terrorists who already can infiltrate AI, disrupt it, and even redesign it for mass impact against their targets are real threats that will exploit our lack of urgency to have practices such as "zero trust" in the development and use of advanced technology with any form of AI capabilities. Without sound cybersecurity rules, laws, and industry standards, machine bias and other manipulation of AI will happen, in addition to its being used as a weapon that negatively affects our society socially and economically, and even our national security. This is also a developing field that needs integration with AI systems, and more is to come as we seek to protect all these systems.

Ultimately, both cybersecurity and AI are on a rapid growth path and power the fastest-growing platforms like ChatGPT, OpenAI, and generative AI. They will continue to define what happens in health information technology applications as they affect healthcare delivery through governance, policy development, operations, and fiscal management practices.

15.2 AI IN HEALTHCARE: OPPORTUNITIES AND CHALLENGES

15.2.1 MACHINE BIAS

Over the past decade, there has been evidence of discrimination based on race and gender by various technological companies, which resulted in litigation or formal government investigations. These top IT firms, Amazon, Google, and Apple, have found themselves in hot water related to their products and bias built into their algorithms (Véliz, 2023). Like other technologies, AI through algorithms is

DOI: 10.1201/9781003485629-15

a product of human design and reflects their human creators' decision-making. Opacity contributes to the problem of machine bias when autonomous systems lack full transparency on how they make decisions; machine learning (ML) can and does inherit bias through the data used to train them.

AI without data ethics creates machine bias that reflects the human biases of the people who produced it. It is not ethical to delegate accountability and responsibility for machine bias to the technology. Responsibility and moral obligation to address biases generated by biased algorithms lie squarely on the owners, creators, coders, and anyone associated with creating the algorithms. It is also important to note that all manufactured technologies reflect the culture of the creators and their preferences and biases.

Examples of machine bias in AI in the United States showing algorithms that favor White, male, and Western European demographics have resulted in bias in digital products and services, especially from the use of ML platforms (Binns, 2018). ML cannot offer normative justifications for their outputs or make decisions from ethical considerations, resulting in a "responsibility gap" where human stakeholders try to absolve themselves of responsibility, claiming the algorithm is at fault when things go wrong.

This is technically correct. AI responds to how it was designed by an engineer or coded by a developer. Underlying factors in socioeconomic realities are fraught with discrimination, so it is no surprise that learning systems are also subject to bias in their design and results (Binns, 2018). Digital discrimination, just like physical discrimination, creates excellent harm to people in society and preventable disparities we have spent years combating in civil society.

15.2.2 SOCIAL MEDICAL INJUSTICE AND ML

In high-stake sectors like medicine and healthcare, machine bias can be devastating, which may explain caregivers' reluctance to broaden the acceptance of AI in healthcare. One of the controversial areas where there is social injustice in using medical ML is the prediction drug monitoring programs (PDMP) used for drug addiction monitoring and forecasting and also used in medical testimonials where it was discovered that these algorithms do harm patients by silencing their voices and provide pessimistic predictions based on social biases (based on age, race, and gender) on whom the algorithm predicts as drug abusers (Pozzi, 2023).

Opioid abuse is a silent epidemic and a significant contributor to bad health (addictions and mental health challenges) and social problems (homelessness and unemployment) in America today and has overwhelmed communities across the country in rural, suburban, and urban communities with over 560,000 deaths in the United States since 1999 (Connect2Health, 2024). Social injustice does occur with algorithms as predictive tools based on ML on social issues like drug abuse; other areas of injustice can be wrong predictions of genetic predisposition for cancer, heart disease, and other health problems based on the use of algorithms for healthcare forecasting. Healthcare already challenged with healthcare disparities in both care outcomes and care delivery based on race, gender, and even level of income is vulnerable to machine bias. Without the guardrails required in physical medicine, healthcare disparities will only worsen without any governance or application of healthcare ethics.

So, how do we protect ourselves and society against machine bias? One of the ways is to engage people on the positive and negative aspects of using AI. It is vital that we also start educating our younger generation, who are growing up in this digital age with the intersection of social media and every facet of life; they must be digitally literate so they can be better custodians of this technology for the preservation of both individual liberties and communities. Personal rights to privacy will continue to erode due to the increased use of big data required for ML.

Protection of personal privacy is critical to maintaining a "free" society and constitutes a democratic society. The more advanced we become with the use of AI, the more we should focus on rapidly investing in training our communities, investing in training ethicists, and making it mandatory for all careers involved in technology to avoid ethical pitfalls. In medicine, we teach "do no harm," and it is the framework for patient safety and patient engagement, and it is part of the framework of medical law to include a whole career of medical litigation to protect people from unethical physicians, nurses, and support staff trusted with the care of people in their most vulnerable state due to disease, emergency, and other health issues that degrade our bodies.

In the "moral determinant of health" discussion, it is essential that medical ethics is the foundation of providing quality and ethically sound healthcare services (Berwick, 2020). When medical workers violate ethics by harming patients, ignoring their moral determinants of health, including their socioeconomic determinants of health, they are subject to scrutiny and potentially lose their license, depending on the gravity of such violations. The same paradigm applies to the field of AI, its experts, and anyone in the business of ML, development, and marketing of AI-enabled systems and environments for both private and public sectors.

Licensed humans are accountable for malpractice and criminality in their profession; however, unlike healthcare workers, we cannot prosecute machines, and we cannot prosecute AI, even the most advanced, due to opacity. We can prosecute the engineers, data experts, investors, company owners, and governments who design, fund, and promote them, and we should when they are irresponsible and cause harm to others. ML is structurally opaque, and I do not see any changes in the future no matter how advanced it gets; without "explainability" of every output and action it produces, we will have bias, unintended consequences that will always create chaos, and we should always have consequences of such results and put safeguards around ML and all forms of AI now and in the future.

A moral demand for accountability, explainability, and transparency calls for justice and constant human oversight; without it, we are creating a destructive system of technology adaptation that will harm us and our future society. We do not trust professionals without training, constant monitoring through board certifications, and continued education; why would we trust the professions behind AI without the same level of scrutiny and accountability we expect from licensed professionals?

15.3 PRACTICAL APPLICATIONS OF AUTONOMOUS AI IN HEALTHCARE CLINICAL OPERATIONS

Autonomous AI holds an auspicious future in its capacity to help humanity solve problems backed up by cybersecurity protocols that make it dependable and safe. Autonomous AI can be a force multiplier of human abilities and a safe alternative for high-risk endeavors humans have traditionally performed, such as rendering clinical services, including pharmaceutical, surgical, imaging, and other areas that support clinical operations, such as nutrition services, housekeeping, and facilities management. Autonomous AI in hospitals transforms healthcare delivery by enhancing diagnosis, treatment, and patient care. Here are some notable examples.

15.3.1 Robotic Surgery

Da Vinci Surgical System: This well-known system is widely used for minimally invasive surgeries. It provides surgeons with a 3D high-definition view of the surgical area and allows for precise movements of miniaturized instruments. While the surgeon controls the system, the AI assists in improving the precision and consistency of the procedures.

15.3.2 Medical Imaging and Diagnostics

- Zebra Medical Vision: This AI-powered tool analyzes medical imaging data such as x-rays, CT scans, and MRIs to detect various conditions, including cancers, cardiovascular diseases, and liver diseases. It can flag abnormalities and provide diagnostic insights to radiologists.

Aidoc: Another AI tool used in radiology, Aidoc helps identify acute abnormalities across the body, such as strokes or blood clots, in real time, improving the speed and accuracy of diagnosis.

15.3.3 CLINICAL DECISION SUPPORT

- IBM Watson Health: Watson for Oncology leverages AI to analyze patient data against a vast array of medical literature and clinical trial data to provide evidence-based treatment recommendations for cancer patients.
- DeepMind's Streams: Initially developed for kidney injury detection, Streams provides clinicians with real-time alerts and decision support, ensuring timely and effective intervention.

15.3.4 AUTONOMOUS MONITORING AND CARE

- Moxi by Diligent Robotics: Moxi is a robot designed to assist hospital staff by performing non-patient-facing tasks such as fetching and delivering supplies, allowing nurses to spend more time on direct patient care.
- TUG by Aethon: TUG robots autonomously transport medications, lab specimens, and other materials throughout the hospital, reducing the workload on staff and improving operational efficiency.

15.3.5 MEDICATION MANAGEMENT

Pharmacy Automation Systems: These are systems like Omnicell and BD. Pyxis uses AI to manage medication dispensing, ensuring accurate dosages and reducing the risk of medication errors. These systems can automate inventory management and restocking as well.

15.3.6 PATIENT MANAGEMENT AND FLOW

Qventus: This AI platform optimizes hospital operations by predicting patient admission and discharge patterns, managing bed allocation, and reducing emergency department overcrowding. It helps streamline hospital workflows and improve patient throughput.

15.3.7 VIRTUAL NURSING ASSISTANTS

Catalia Health's Mabu: Mabu is a conversational robot that engages with patients to monitor their health, provide medication reminders, and offer emotional support. It helps manage chronic conditions and ensure adherence to treatment plans.

15.3.8 TELEMEDICINE AND REMOTE MONITORING

TytoCare: This system includes an AI-powered device that enables remote physical exams by capturing vital signs and images of the patient. The AI assists in the initial assessment, which a healthcare professional then reviews.

15.4 AI IN BUSINESS OPERATIONS

In nonclinical environments, there are so many opportunities for AI to streamline administration of healthcare services to benefit patients and healthcare institutions, areas like fraud detection, simplified billing with the use of AI to find errors in provider coding, and potential mismatches with medical record documentation and services billed to patients (Kilanko, 2023). Historically patients complain about high medical charges that are inconsistent with the care they received; many more believe price gouging exists when healthcare companies have differing charges for the same services, also called surprise billing.

Billing problems have led legislation across states to continue to find ways to mitigate surprise billing for patients (Rosso, Isserman, & Shen, 2021). AI can help mitigate this by standardizing pricing list and conducting smart searches of existing billing platforms to normalize pricing adjustments based on transparency and equity in hospital and practice billing across states and regions to enable fair billing practices. Other opportunities include training AI platforms to detect fraudulent billing and eliminate healthcare fraud that continues to plague the healthcare industry.

Functions like workflow management of medical practices based on number of full time employments, patients, and appointment templates are areas that will enhance patient experience and reduce unnecessary reschedules, cancellations, and long wait times for patients. There is an extensive list of nonclinical functions in medical operations that can benefit from adopting ML to resolve inefficiencies in their institutions; integrating data science in healthcare operations provides a platform for new innovations in healthcare administration.

These examples demonstrate how autonomous AI is enhancing the efficiency, accuracy, and quality of healthcare in hospitals, leading to better patient outcomes and optimized hospital operations. With the above examples, it is inevitable that "strong" AI will happen sooner rather than later. We now have sophisticated ML and reinforcement learning (RL) platforms to develop a strong AI based on massive data representing human experiences. Intentionality in AI requires the subject to intentionally connect the representation and the object and have previous experience and knowledge. One can make the argument that an extensive library of medical files through computer vision of disease tissue (cancer, e.g.) or healthy tissue in the case of surgery constitutes an "experience" no different than the knowledge and experience of a seasoned radiologist or surgeon (although void of instincts and unconscious ability to make decisions).

It is conceivable that we can train AI to recognize cancer tissue in its many forms through both ML and RL coupled with computer vision and imagery. It is predicted that by 2030, AI systems will be designed to address social issues, and AI-driven solutions can impact how we educate (tailored versus "one-size-fits-all" model) and how we provide medicine to all populations. This has the most significant potential to improve access to care, cut costs, and free up time for both health systems and patients (AI Uncovered, 2024). None of the innovations will have positive and lasting results if implemented without responsible AI. These autonomous AI systems perform according to ethics and human values and are required for autonomous AI to function in making life-and-death decisions that affect humans since the entity dying or living is us humans affected by machines (Dubber et al., 2020).

So how do we protect all these innovations through AI? Healthcare, if plagued with IT vulnerabilities, and the next section will discuss how we can address them through cybersecurity concepts, available cybersecurity constructs, and frameworks IT professionals can review to mitigate cyber vulnerabilities.

15.5 CYBERSECURITY IN HEALTHCARE: IMPLICATIONS AND OPPORTUNITIES

According to Dasgupta et al. (2022), cybersecurity is the set of activities associated with securing data, computer devices, and users' privacy in cyberspace. All organizations, including healthcare organizations, must take cybersecurity very seriously as they deal with sensitive personal identifiable data and systems that handle such data daily 24/7. Healthcare organizations handle personal identifiable information (PII) and personal health information (PHI), which, if they fall into wrong hands, could be used to carry out destructive activities against the targeted individuals. Mahmoud and Al Najjar (2024) stated that cybersecurity at this moment in time is very important to healthcare organizations because they are vulnerable to data breach, data theft, and ransomware attacks. Banu et al. (2024) stated that cyberattacks in the healthcare industry are the highest, with 28% of the total cyberattacks as of the year 2020 when this information was gathered.

Data show that the healthcare sector requires strong cybersecurity governance to keep malicious actors at bay now and in the future. The future of quantum computing and the dangers to computer systems must also be taken into consideration to enable better security protocols. According to SaberiKamrposhti et al. (2024), the current objective of healthcare researchers and practitioners is to ensure that post-quantum cybersecurity technologies are incorporated into pre-existing infrastructure to ensure interoperability and adherence to regulatory requirements. This essentially is talking about cybersecurity in the age of quantum computing. It is projected that when quantum computing becomes ubiquitous, current cybersecurity mechanisms will be inadequate to protect computer systems and enterprise networks. The primary objective of healthcare cybersecurity is to secure healthcare data either at rest or in transit, the network, and the reputation of the healthcare organization.

There are different types of healthcare data, and the type determines how they are protected. Nong et al. (2024) stated that there are 15 types of data that are grouped into 3 broad categories for ease of use; these categories are listed as personal characteristics data, health related data, and sensitive data. The name of a category determines how each category of data is protected by the cybersecurity team of a healthcare organization.

The regulatory requirement for each category differs. Some of the main regulatory requirements that affect healthcare include the Health Insurance Portability and Accountability Act (HIPAA) and General Data Protection Regulation (GDPR). Healthcare regulations such the American HIPAA and the European Union (EU) GDPR emphasize transparency, consent, and data breach notification, but differ in enforcement and penalties. GDPR, in the EU, imposes strict fines for noncompliance, up to 4% of global annual revenue. In contrast, US enforcement under HIPAA varies by state, with penalties typically arising reactively following data breaches.

15.5.1 THREAT LANDSCAPE IN HEALTHCARE CYBERSECURITY ENVIRONMENT

According to Tariq (2024), the "cybersecurity landscape has indeed changed" when compared to just 5 years ago without going too far back. According to Clarke and Martin (2024), Internet of things (IoT) and its uses in healthcare delivery have completely changed the way cybersecurity will be practiced in healthcare going forward. The IoT is the connection of physical health devices, which could be fixed operational devices or mobile devices, to digital networks, enabling pair to pair communication between them. In healthcare, this encompasses patient monitoring, diagnostics, and robotic surgery devices. As connectivity grows, the need for agile and robust cybersecurity measures becomes increasingly critical. The threat with IoT devices has to do with the size of the equipment drive, as there is not enough space for high-capacity security software, which leads to security vulnerability for these IoT devices.

The advent of COVID-19 was another serious challenge for the healthcare sector, as remote work became prevalent, the norm rather than the exception, which became a vulnerability. Endpoint devices became a cybersecurity challenge to the enterprise and a point for malicious actors to compromise a network not prepared for such attacks. Shen and Shen (2024) stated that enterprise endpoint security has emerged as a major challenge. The prevalent threat to cybersecurity in all sectors since 2019 has been phishing/social engineering. However, by the year 2023, ransomware was the most prevalent in healthcare. According to Li and Madisetti (2024), in the year 2023 the incidence of ransomware attack among healthcare organizations across America was well over 60%. This far exceeds all other cyberattack incidences across various sectors.

The key targets of malicious actors in the healthcare sector are mainly PII and PHI. PII in the hands of malicious actors can be used to access and steal the identity of victims, while PHI could be used for the same, but more so for blackmail if the potential victim is exposed politically or economically. Specifically, if such an exposed individual just so happens to be the CEO of an organization, it could affect share prices negatively in a for-profit healthcare organization (HCO). Below are the most recent examples of cybersecurity breaches in HCOs.

15.5.2 RECENT SIGNIFICANT HEALTHCARE CYBERSECURITY BREACHES

According to Abuasal et al. (2024), malicious actors often target PHI because it can be used to obtain prescription drugs legally. The Metropolitan Health Systems (MHS), a hospital system based in Ohio, has continuously experienced cyberattacks on five different occasions within the last 8 years from calendar years 2015 to 2023 (Klatt, 2024). The hospital and its third-party vendors have experienced data theft, leaving the hospital system vulnerable to future cyberattacks. Alder (2024) reported that Change Healthcare was hit by a ransomware attack on February 21, 2024. The ALPHV/BlackCat group is claiming responsibility for stealing 4TB of data. Despite paying a $22 million ransom for data deletion, the group conducted an exit scam, and the stolen data were passed to another group, RansomHub, which demanded another ransom. This is an ongoing saga as of the time of writing this book. Other examples include Kaiser Foundation Health Plans with breach affecting 13 million individuals, and Concentra Health Services Inc, with 3.9 million individuals affected; these two incidents in 2024 cost the HCOs productivity and financial resources and affected their reputation to protect patient information (Alder, 2024).

15.5.3 LESSONS LEARNED FROM PAST BREACHES

The ransomware attack on Change Healthcare, for example, offers several important lessons:

1. **Ransom Payments Don't Guarantee Data Safety**: Despite paying a $22 million ransom, Change Healthcare's data were not deleted as promised, highlighting that paying a ransom does not ensure data security or resolution.
2. **Trust Issues with Ransomware Groups**: The exit scam by ALPHV/BlackCat underscores the inherent unreliability of criminal groups. Organizations should be wary of trusting that attackers will honor their word.
3. **Risks of Double Extortion**: The stolen data being passed to another group, RansomHub, for further extortion shows the risk of double or multiple extortions, where attackers continue to exploit the same data.
4. **Importance of Robust Cybersecurity**: Preventing such attacks in the first place is critical. This incident highlights the need for stronger cybersecurity measures, regular updates, and employee training to avoid breaches.
5. **Need for Comprehensive Incident Response Plans**: Organizations should have a well-prepared incident response plan that includes steps to handle ransomware attacks, communications, and potential legal consequences.
6. **Consideration of Alternative Strategies**: Rather than paying ransoms, organizations might consider alternative strategies such as data backups, collaboration with law enforcement, and investment in cybersecurity insurance.
7. **Legal and Regulatory Compliance**: This incident serves as a reminder of the legal and regulatory implications of data breaches, emphasizing the need for compliance with data protection laws and regulations.

Equally, the continuous breach of the network infrastructure over a period of 8 years of MHS in Ohio, along with its third-party vendors, offer several critical lessons:

1. **Continuous Vulnerability Awareness**: Repeated attacks indicate that MHS and its vendors may not have fully addressed the underlying vulnerabilities in their systems. Regular security assessments and updates are essential to close these gaps.

2. **Importance of Vendor Management**: The involvement of third-party vendors in these breaches highlights the need for rigorous vendor management. MHS should ensure that all vendors meet strict cybersecurity standards to prevent indirect vulnerabilities.

3. **Strengthening Cybersecurity Infrastructure**: The frequency of attacks suggests that MHS's cybersecurity infrastructure may be insufficient. Investing in advanced security technologies, such as threat detection and response systems, could help prevent future breaches in healthcare institutions.

4. **Incident Response and Recovery Planning**: MHS should have a robust incident response plan that includes immediate actions to mitigate damage, communication strategies, and long-term recovery efforts. Regular drills and updates to these plans are crucial.

5. **Employee Training and Awareness**: Cyberattacks often exploit human error. Continuous training for employees and vendors in identifying and responding to phishing attempts, malware, and other threats is vital.

6. **Data Encryption and Protection**: Ensuring that all sensitive data are encrypted both in transit and at rest can reduce the impact of data theft. Implementing strict access controls can also limit exposure.

7. **Learning from Past Incidents**: Analyzing previous breaches and understanding how they occurred is crucial. MHS should use these lessons to improve their security measures and prevent similar incidents in the future.

8. **Legal and Regulatory Compliance**: Repeated breaches can lead to legal consequences and damage to the hospital's reputation. MHS should ensure compliance with healthcare regulations like HIPAA to protect patient data and avoid penalties.

9. **Collaboration with Cybersecurity Experts**: Engaging with cybersecurity experts and adopting best practices from the industry can help MHS stay ahead of emerging threats.

10. **Building Resilience against Ransomware**: Given the rise in ransomware attacks in the healthcare sector, MHS should focus on building resilience, including having reliable data backups, incident response strategies, and possibly cybersecurity insurance.

15.6 CSFS, STANDARDS, AND LAWS

15.6.1 CSFs

According to Syafrizal et al. (2020), cybersecurity framework is a set of guidelines for companies to follow so they are better equipped to identify, detect, and respond to cyberattacks. Taherdoost (2022) stated that a CSF is a general guideline that covers many components or domains that can be adopted by businesses, companies, and institutions, which does not specify the steps that are required to be taken (how to implement a standard):

1. COBIT: This is a high-level IT standard that focuses on broad IT management decision-making rather than specific details. It covers 34 key IT processes and includes best practices for managing processes, infrastructure, resources, responsibilities, and controls. Each IT process is linked to detailed control objectives (DCOs) and control objectives (COs), which are grouped into planning, implementing, supporting, and monitoring and evaluating categories. However, although well-suited as an integrated solution due to its comprehensive nature, it may not be the best choice when the main priority is the effective implementation of security controls, mainly because it does not provide specific guidelines for achieving predefined control objectives.

2. NIST CSF: The NIST CSF, established after a 2014 executive order and expanded by the Cybersecurity Enhancement Act of 2014, provides a structured approach for organizations to improve their cybersecurity measures. It integrates best practices, standards, and recommendations to address cybersecurity concerns and can be used to develop new

programs or enhance existing ones, helping organizations identify and fill gaps in their cybersecurity practices.

15.6.2 Cybersecurity Standards

According to Standards Australia, "Standards are voluntary documents that set out specifications, procedures and guidelines that aim to ensure products, services, and systems are safe, consistent, and reliable." Taherdoost (2022) stated that "Cybersecurity standards determine the requirements that an organization should follow to achieve cybersecurity objectives and prevent cybercrimes." Cybersecurity standards explain and provide methods one by one, specify what is expected to be done to complete the process, and clarify methods to coincide with the standard for compliance. The different types of standards are described below:

1. ISO/IEC 27000: Focuses on information security management (ISM) and is published by the International Organization for Standardization (ISO) in collaboration with the International Electrotechnical Commission (IEC). The first in this series, ISO 27001, was initially published in 2005. Four key standards—ISO 27001, ISO 27002, ISO 27005, and ISO 27006—are widely implemented across various industries and countries worldwide.
2. The Standard of Good Practice (SoGP): This was created by the Information Security Forum (ISF) in 1996 and is a widely recognized framework for information security best practices. Updated every 2 years, it guides companies across various industries in six key areas, including computer installation, business processes, security management, system development, and end-user security.
3. BSI: The Bundesamt für Sicherheit in der Informationstechnik (BSI), a German government agency, publishes the BSI IT, which focuses on computer and communication security for the German government. BSI offers guidelines on cybersecurity approaches, covering key areas like cryptography, Internet security, and security products, to help companies and public authorities develop effective security strategies. The series includes the following: BSI Standard 100-1, BSI Standard 100-2, and BSI Standard 100-3.
4. Industry-Related Standard: In addition to the general classification of cybersecurity standards, this study also addresses a category of standards specifically focused on their application in business and technology, including IEC 62443, ISO/SAE 21434, and ETSI EN 303 645.

15.6.3 Cybersecurity Healthcare Laws

According to MERIPLEX, there is the mandatory healthcare cybersecurity compliance laws and the un-mandatory healthcare cybersecurity compliance laws. The mandatory healthcare cybersecurity compliance laws include HIPAA and the quality system regulation (QSR). HIPAA has three rules: the privacy rule, the security rule, and the breach notification rule. The privacy rule addresses the limitation on the release of an individual's health data, while the security rule mandates a risk assessment by hospital systems. This is usually conducted by a compliance officer, with the objective of finding risks if any exist. The security rule mandates that HIPAA-covered entities complete a risk assessment. A risk assessment is conducted by a compliance officer and is intended to find security risks within a health organization. The breach rule makes it mandatory to report any breach of private health information.

The QSR is a food and drug agency (FDA)-led initiative, to drastically improve the cybersecurity of medical devices. This compliance law was created because of ransomware attacks that shutdown hospital systems. Medical devices such as pacemakers, drug infusion pumps, or insulin pumps could stop functioning, possibly leading to patient harm. QSR standards require medical device manufacturers to incorporate data encryption or authentication on their devices. While these standards mostly apply to medical device manufacturers, the FDA states that healthcare establishments share the responsibility. Penalties for QSR noncompliance include fines of up to $500,000 and criminal prosecution.

15.6.4 INCIDENT RESPONSE AND RECOVERY

- Developing an Incident Response Plan: According to Johansen (2020), not all incidents are the same in severity and threat to an organization. A high-level incident is an incident that is expected to cause significant damage, corruption, or loss of critical and strategic data. Assume data have been exfiltrated to a source outside the organization. This is a high-level incident. According to the Scottish government data loss playbook published in the year 2019, "a data breach is defined as an incident, breach of security or wider privacy violation that leads to the accidental or unlawful destruction, unauthorized retention, misuse, loss, alteration, unauthorized disclosure of, or access to, data transmitted, stored or otherwise processed by the organization, its employees, contractors or service providers." The Cybersecurity and Infrastructure Security Agency (CISA) cybersecurity incident and vulnerability response playbook published in the year 2021 mentioned exfiltration of data as one of the incidences that should trigger this playbook.

These two playbooks, gleaned from both the Scottish and American incidence response playbooks, list the following steps as necessary in response to a data breach such as exfiltration of data, which often is the target of malicious actors targeting hospital systems and medical practices.

1. Detection and analysis
2. Communications
3. Containment
4. Eradication and recovery
5. Post-incident activities
6. Preparation.

The above figure starts with the first stage in any incident response scenario, which is the detection stage either by a staff member who should promptly inform the security operations staff or a security operation center (SOC) operative. Logs are scrutinized to ascertain if indeed the alert received is a breach. The communications center of the organization is promptly informed of a suspected breach. The second stage is where the decision to qualify the intrusion as a breach is made by relevant responsible parties depending on the structure of the firm under attack. This decision is equally communicated to the communications team in a timely manner, depending on whether a breach is confirmed or not. If a breach is confirmed, an incident response team further analyzes the breach data and the equipment affected is enumerated so that containment activities like isolating affected equipment in a segment or Vlan can be carried out. Next is the eradication and recovery stage where a system administrator reformats the equipment affected; if it is still fit for use, it can then be reconfigured using the backup data of the organization. The next stage is the post-incident activities of the incident response team of the organization, like what were the reasons that would likely have left the organization vulnerable and how to stop it from happening again. Another issue at this stage is finding out what worked as it should during any response and what did not work. All this and more can be incorporated into the next stage. That stage is the preparation for future incidents stage that gets ready for any future breach incidence, incorporating results from the post-incident activities stage. A more detailed breakdown of the steps from Figure 15.1 can be found below.

1. Detection and analysis:
   a. Detection: Usually, folks who make first contact with an incidence such as users, help desk analyst, and SOC analyst. Other times it could be federal agencies informing

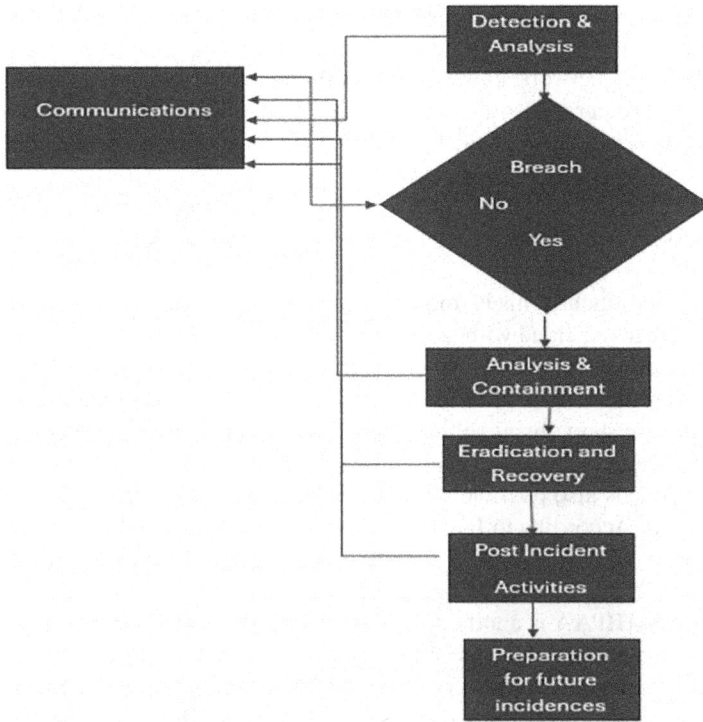

FIGURE 15.1 Conceptual Framework for Cybersecurity Breach Response.

organizations of the discovery of malware in the wild or of zero-day malware (Johansen, 2020). It has been established that data have been exfiltrated. Confidentiality, integrity, and availability have been compromised.

b. Analysis:
I. Identify the Scope: This basically involves analyzing data from the firewall and web proxy server, to identify the internal database system or systems that had been communicating with the fingered source of the data breach under investigation.
II. Identify the Impact: This is about finding out if the breach has had an impact on any of the elements of the security triad referred to as the confidentiality, integrity, and availability (CIA) triad. In this instance, availability and confidentiality have been impacted by exfiltration; if data are encrypted, then it will take a while, if at all, before the thieves can access the data stolen.
III. Identify the Root Causes: These steps need to happen to ensure that any lapses are discovered, and it can be mitigated, or the risk transferred to insurance firms.
IV. Incident Attribution: This is where the computer security incidence response team (CSIRT) team attempts to determine the adversary that was responsible for the breach be it an individual, organization, hacktivist group, or nation state. This is time consuming, so the best-case scenario is to pass it off to a third-party organization with historical data on attacks to compare artifacts supplied with patterns of groups to give a most likely group or state responsibility.

2. Containment: Containment strategies refer to strategies and actions taken during an incident to contain, limit, or stop damage to database systems and networks within an organization. These strategies are of four forms:
a. Physical Containment: Simply unplugging the system or network from the Internet to contain or stop the attack. In this instance, damage has been done and the CIA triad breached.

    b. Network Containment: This is where the network engineers and architects use their knowledge of the network to curtail packets from the identified source of breach to the areas of the network under attack at the network packet forwarding level on the switches and routers. Also due to the exfiltration, the CIA triad has been breached for sure, and steps must now be taken to block the known IP address or address discovered to have been responsible for the breach.

    c. Perimeter Containment: This involves using the perimeter firewall to filter the source (IP addresses) of the breach at the perimeter of the network using the firewall filtering capabilities.

    d. Virtual Containment: This is important as most organizations have moved or are planning to move to the cloud with the flexibility available to remove network connection to multiple systems at once. Virtual switching can also be used in the cloud the same way as physical switches can be used to segregate VLANS. Virtualization software allows for pausing a system during an incident. This capability to pause a system enables that system to preserve evidence that can be examined later. Blocking the offending IP addresses here is also possible after full restoration from backup sources.

3. Communications: According to Johansen (2020), the GDPR Article 33 has a 72-hour break notification requirement; essentially it is law that within 72 hours, cyber breach incidents must be made public, with steps being taken clearly listed without jeopardizing operational exigencies. HIPAA is another government regulation that stipulates notifications be made in the event a breach occurs in an organization holding the health data of residents of America. The main responsibility of the CSIRT team is to provide techniques to mitigate breaches and bring recovery of systems. Also, the CSIRT team provides information about any breach to individuals responsible for disseminating breach information to the public Villegas-Ch et al. (2021). Johansen (2020) state that during crises, there are three types of communication: internal communication, external communication, and public communication.

    a. Internal Communication: Must be from a single source to avoid miscommunication and confusion, and that communication link must be the CSIRT lead. Individuals to be informed should include the CEO, legal department, marketing and communications, and HR if internal staff is suspected of being part of the breach. Also, a cadence for information dissemination about the incident in a timely manner must be established, every 4 hours is the norm.

    b. External Communication: When incidents occur, often there might be external organizations with connections to the IT systems of the breached organization to be able to carry out their duties. These need to be informed about the breach in a timely manner as well. Depending on their relationship, they could be involved in the communication list along with internal stakeholders.

    c. Public Communication: This is required by laws such as GDPR Article 33 and HIPAA, with a timeline attached of no later than 72 hours after discovery. However, this public communication must be handled by a specific group of professionals within an organization to prevent legal and image issues. The CSIRT team is to explain and advise on the incident but not coordinate the external communication. Rather, the legal, communications, and marketing teams working together are better placed to handle the external communication (Johansen, 2020).

4. Eradication and Recovery:

    • Eradication: This involves the first step of eradicating malware from systems by simply reimaging the systems that have been compromised. These systems are then brought back online via a quarantine system where three VLANs are provided: first, for all the infected systems; second, for the systems being reimaged; and lastly, the VLAN that contains the production systems that were never infected or breached.

- Recovery Strategies:
  - All systems (both infected and not infected) must be patched with up-to-date patches.
  - Additional detection and prevention alerts must be put in place based on the finding during the incidence handling.
  - Changes to infrastructure made during the handling of the incidence must be reviewed whether they are fit for current and continuous production environment. If fit, then the changes must go through the already established change control process, ensuring that the CIA triad is taken into consideration.
  - A full vulnerability scan must be conducted to ensure that a proper eradication and recovery of systems and data have taken place.

5. Post-incident Activities: According to CISA (2021), this step must be the documentation of the incidence and the responses, highlighting what worked and what did not work during the incidence response process. This information will be used for adjusting network sensors to better detect early future breaches. All documentation goes into preparing for any future anticipated breach, with the aim of either responding better or being able to stop the next breach in its track. A review of the response as whole must be done to check if all steps in the incident response plan were followed, and if not, why. All the outcomes will then be used to revamp the incident response plan for future responses (Johansen, 2020).

6. Preparation for Future Incidents: This is where all the lessons learnt from previous breaches and the incidence response plan executed during that incidence are revamped and made better for future use. Also, adjustments to detection instruments are made so they have better sensitivity based on patterns and techniques of threat actors during the current breach. Tactics, techniques, and procedure (TTP) of threat actors must influence future response to data breaches (CISA, 2021).

15.7 CYBERSECURITY TRAINING FOR HEALTHCARE STAFF

It is anticipated that as technical protections mature within an enterprise environment, the vulnerability shifts to human factors (Waddell, 2024). Humans become the weak link that malicious actors can exploit to infiltrate an enterprise using social engineering tactics. Tariq (2024) defined social engineering as the psychological manipulation of people into performing actions or divulging confidential information. In healthcare cybersecurity, social engineering is a threat that has bad ramifications for the hospital system, if attackers succeed. Social engineering can be successful at making healthcare workers reveal sensitive patient information or granting access to secure systems where PII or PHI about patients reside.

Training is required so healthcare workers can be aware and be able to take appropriate defensive steps when confronted with social engineering tactics. Fratti et al. (2024) made clear that applicable cybersecurity training tailored to organizational needs is required in the healthcare sector as PII and PHI are very valuable to criminals. Each organization is different, so no one-size-fits-all training will do. According to Jerry-Egemba (2024), 95% of healthcare sector breaches are due to human errors. Therefore, it is suggested that cybersecurity training be tailored to specific job roles, putting into consideration how each job group in healthcare interacts with the enterprise network in doing their job daily.

15.8 FUTURE OF HEALTHCARE CYBERSECURITY

Tripathy et al. (2024) stated that quantum computing is the future of computing, and these pose a grave danger to two areas of healthcare cybersecurity. One of the areas happens to be the security of IoT devices, devices that are now so prevalent and will continue to increase in their use and popularity going into the future. Nevertheless, ML is being used to increase the resilience of IoT devices to quantum computing. The other area where quantum computing will create challenges for healthcare cybersecurity is in security algorithms used for encryption and decryption as quantum computing will be able to break most keys easily via brute force tactic deployable because of quantum computing power. Therefore, security key lengths would have to be increased drastically to 128-bit key length to be able to keep keys that secure computer systems safe. Quantum computing poses significant dangers to healthcare cybersecurity due to its potential to break existing cryptographic systems. The key concerns include the following:

1. **Breaking Encryption:**
   - **Vulnerability of Current Cryptography:** Quantum computers could easily break widely used encryption algorithms like Rivest, Shamir, Adleman, which protect patient data and communications. This could lead to unauthorized access to sensitive medical information, financial details, and other confidential data.
   - **Healthcare Data Breaches:** Quantum computing capabilities could allow attackers to decrypt vast amounts of healthcare data, resulting in privacy breaches, identity theft, and financial fraud.

2. **Threats to Data Integrity:**
   - **Tampering with Medical Records:** Quantum attackers could alter medical records, leading to misdiagnoses, incorrect treatments, and loss of trust in EHR systems.
   - **Impact on Research:** Quantum attacks could target and corrupt large datasets used in medical research, potentially derailing studies and hindering medical advancements.

3. **Vulnerability of IoT Devices:**
   - **Medical IoT Devices:** Many healthcare devices rely on encryption for secure data transmission. Quantum computing could break this encryption, leading to unauthorized control over critical medical equipment like pacemakers or insulin pumps.
   - **Smart Hospital Systems:** Quantum threats could compromise the integrated systems of smart hospitals, disrupting patient monitoring, automated treatment protocols, and more.

4. **Risk to the Pharmaceutical Industry:**
   - **Intellectual Property Theft:** Quantum computing could be used to steal proprietary research and drug formulations by decrypting communications and data storage systems.
   - **Supply Chain Disruption:** Attackers could manipulate or sabotage the pharmaceutical supply chain by breaking the encryption used to secure logistics and inventory data.

5. **Challenges in Implementing Quantum-Resistant Solutions:**
   - **Cost and Complexity:** Transitioning to quantum-resistant cryptography is expensive and complex. Many healthcare institutions may struggle to implement these solutions quickly, leaving them vulnerable during the transition period.
   - **Interoperability Issues:** Adopting new quantum-safe encryption methods may present challenges in interoperability with existing healthcare infrastructure, potentially leading to security gaps.

6. **Increased Sophistication of Cyberattacks:**
   - **Advanced Attack Strategies:** Quantum computing could enable more sophisticated cyberattacks that are difficult to detect and mitigate, such as quantum-enhanced phishing schemes or advanced persistent threats (APTs).
   - **Enhanced AI in Attacks:** Quantum computing could enhance AI capabilities in cyberattacks, making them more effective and harder to defend against.

To mitigate these risks, the healthcare industry must begin adopting quantum-resistant encryption and develop strategies to protect critical infrastructure from potential quantum-based threats.

15.8.1 EMERGING CYBERSECURITY TREND

According to Edo et al. (2024), with the prevalence of insider attacks and recurring data breaches in the healthcare sector, addressing system vulnerabilities requires a more nuanced approach to mitigate insider threats effectively. The idea of adopting the zero-trust model, which is a new trend in cybersecurity, is fast gaining popularity among cybersecurity practitioners. Stephen and Abbas (2024) defined zero trust architecture (ZTA) as a model based on the principle of "never trust, always verify," which results in every user and device accessing the network being continuously authenticated and authorized.

Zero trust architecture (ZTA) is a cybersecurity model based on the principle of "never trust, always verify." It requires continuous authentication and authorization of every user, device, or application attempting to access the network. Key principles include continuous verification, least privilege access, micro-segmentation, multi-factor authentication, and context-aware access. Also, training of both users and technical staff is important for the successful implementation of this model in any healthcare setting (Stephen & Abbas, 2024).

ZTA enhances security by reducing the attack surface and improving resilience against modern threats. However, implementing ZTA can be complex and may require significant changes to existing infrastructure and processes. Despite these challenges, ZTA offers robust protection against unauthorized access and insider threats.

15.9 CONCLUSION

Without cybersecurity, our society at large is vulnerable to attacks by internal and external actors, and the healthcare industry continues to experience vulnerabilities that will need robust cybersecurity protocols and practices to prevent and recover from cyberattacks when they happen. Like all other technologies, AI needs cybersecurity to protect our society, and healthcare industry will benefit greatly if both technologies are integrated into every healthcare organization to ensure the continuity of healthcare services and protection of patients and organizations alike. The future of healthcare operations will need to explore how much AI we need and how we will control it. The question of why humans are creating robotic systems that can mimic humans needs to be filtered through the lens of how robotic systems can enhance human life but not replace it. Fundamentally, like any other technology, AI needs both ethical considerations and design considerations. What about companionship using robotics in elder care? Is this ethical, given that the robot lacks emotions and cannot be held responsible legally for any actions interacting with humans? What about medical liability using AI-enabled technology in care settings? These questions are both cultural and technological; we have yet to determine our appetite for AI and the human experience in healthcare delivery that will transform related services.

REFERENCES

Abuasal, S., Alsarayra, K., & Alyabroodie, Z. (2024). Designing a standard-based approach for the Security of healthcare systems. *Journal of Statistics Applications & Probability Letters*, *13*(1), 419–434.

AIUncovered (2024). How Powerful Will AI Be In 2030? *YouTube video* https://youtu.be/XKMvk5hWDfo ?si=7BR5NgWLayDz4opW

Alder, S., (2024). Healthcare Data Breach Statistics. The HIPAA Journal. https://www.hipaajournal.com/healthcare-data-breach-statistics/

Banu, S. A., Al-Alawi, A. I., Padmaa, M., Priya, P. S., Thanikaiselvan, V., & Amirtharajan, R. (2024). Healthcare with datacare—a triangular DNA security. *Multimedia Tools and Applications*, *83*(7), 21153–21170.

Berwick, D. M. (2020). The moral determinants of health. *JAMA*, *324*(3), 225–226.

Binns, R. (2018, January). Fairness in machine learning: Lessons from political philosophy. In *Conference on Fairness, Accountability, and Transparency* (pp. 149–159). PMLR.

Clarke M, Martin K. Managing cybersecurity risk in healthcare settings. (2024) *Healthcare Management Forum*, 37(1), 17–20. https://doi.org/10.1177/08404704231195804

Connect2Health. (2024). Federal Communications Commission: Focus on Broadbands and Opioids. Retrieved from https://www.fcc.gov/reports-research/maps/connect2health/focus-on-opioids.html#:~:text=More%20than%20560%2C000%20people%20in,82%25%20involved%20synthetic%20opioids%3B%20and

Cybersecurity & Infrastructure Security Agency. (2021). *Federal Government Cybersecurity Incident & Vulnerability Response Playbooks*. Retrieved from https://www.cisa.gov/sites/default/files/publications/Federal_Government_Cybersecurity_Incident_and_Vulnerability_Response_Playbooks_508C.pdf

Dasgupta, D., Akhtar, Z., & Sen, S. (2022). Machine learning in Cybersecurity: a comprehensive survey. *The Journal of Defense Modeling and Simulation*, 19(1), 57–106.

Dubber, Markus D., Frank Pasquale, and Sunit Das (eds), The Oxford Handbook of Ethics of AI (2020; online edn, Oxford Academic, 9 July 2020), https://doi.org/10.1093/oxfordhb/9780190067397.001.0001, accessed 16 Apr. 2024.

Edo, O. C., Ang, D., Billakota, P., & Ho, J. C. (2024). A zero-trust architecture for health information systems. *Health and Technology*, 14(1), 189–199.

Frati, F., et al. (2024). Cybersecurity training and healthcare: the AERAS approach. *International Journal of Information Security*, 1–13.

Jerry-Egemba, N. (2024, January). Safe and sound: Strengthening Cybersecurity in healthcare through robust staff educational programs. In *Healthcare Management Forum* (Vol. 37, No. 1, pp. 21–25). Sage CA: Los Angeles, CA: SAGE Publications.

Johansen, J. (2020). *Digital Forensics and Incident Response*. Packt, UK, India.

Kilanko, V. (2023). The Transformative Potential of Artificial Intelligence in Medical Billing: A Global Perspective.

Klatt, M. K. (2024). Case Study Analysis: Cybersecurity Breach at Metropolitan Health Systems. In *Multisector Insights in Healthcare, Social Sciences, Society, and Technology* (pp. 115–135). IGI Global.

Li, X., & Madisetti, V. K. (2024). ERAD: Enhanced ransomware attack defense system for healthcare organizations. *Journal of Software Engineering and Applications*, 17(5), 270–296.

Mahmoud, R., & Al Najjar, Y. (2024). Cybersecurity in healthcare industry. *GSJ*, 12(2).

Nong, P., Adler-Milstein, J., Kardia, S., & Platt, J. (2024). Public perspectives on the use of different data types for prediction in healthcare. *Journal of the American Medical Informatics Association*, ocae009.

Pozzi, G. (2023). Testimonial injustice in medical machine learning. *Journal of Medical Ethics*, 49(8), 536–540.

Rosso, R. J., Isserman, N. D., & Shen, W. W. (2021). Surprise Billing in Private Health Insurance: Overview of Federal Consumer Protections and Payment for Out-of-Network Services. *Congressional Research Service (CRS) Reports and Issue Briefs*, NA-NA.

SaberiKamrposhti, M., Ng, K. W., Chua, F. F., Abdullah, J., Yadollahi, M., Moradi, M., & Ahmadpour, S. (2024). *Post-Quantum Healthcare: A Roadmap for Cybersecurity Resilience in Medical Data*. Heliyon.

Shen, Q., & Shen, Y. (2024). Endpoint security reinforcement via integrated zero-trust systems: a collaborative approach. *Computers & Security*, 136, 103537.

Standard Australia. https://www.standards.org.au/standards-development/what-is-standard

Stephen, T., & Abbas, A. (2024). Zero Trust Architecture for Securing Digital Health Technologies: Insights from Healthcare Workers in Pandemic Times.

Syafrizal, M., Selamat, S. R., & Zakaria, N. A. (2020). Analysis of cybersecurity standard and framework components. *International Journal of Communication Networks and Information Security*, 12(3), 417–432.

Taherdoost, H. (2022). Understanding cybersecurity frameworks and information security standards—a review and comprehensive overview. *Electronics*, 11(14), 2181.

Tariq, M. U. (2024). Enhancing cybersecurity protocols in modern healthcare systems: strategies and best practices. In *Transformative Approaches to Patient Literacy and Healthcare Innovation* (pp. 223–241). IGI Global.

Tripathy, B. K., Goel, S., & Guha, A. (2024). Quantum Computing for IoT Security. In *Fostering Cross-Industry Sustainability with Intelligent Technologies* (pp. 1–20). IGI Global.

Véliz, C. (2023). Oxford Handbook of Digital Ethics. Oxford University Press.

Villegas-Ch., W., Ortiz-Garces, I., & Sánchez-Viteri, S. (2021). Proposal for an Implementation Guide for a Computer Security Incident Response Team on a University Campus. *Computers*, 10(8), 102. http://dx.doi.org/10.3390/computers10080102

Waddell, M. (2024, January). Human factors in Cybersecurity: Designing an effective cybersecurity education program for healthcare staff. In *Healthcare Management Forum*, 37(1), 13–16. Sage CA: Los Angeles, CA: SAGE Publications.

16 Healthcare Cyberattacks over the 2014–2023 Period
Trends, Lessons Learned, and Potential Paths Forward

David J. Ranney

16.1 INTRODUCTION

We have been witnessing a decreasing number of cyberattacks (CAs) with increased costs to patients (and their data) and the facilities (both direct and indirect) involved. What this tells us is the attackers may be fewer in number, but their knowledge of health systems (and their weaknesses) is growing. In short, attackers have become subject matter experts (SMEs) on the cybersecurity software and IT/IS operations of healthcare organizations. The odd thing, however, is if we experience fewer attacks (although more costly), shouldn't the companies and IT departments "protecting" the hospitals be better at fighting the attackers? If not, why not? The driving research questions of this chapter is: Does analysis of available information of CAs on healthcare organizations during the 2014–2023 timeframe show a trend? If so, what conclusions can be drawn? Second, the chapter provides decision-makers with a "here's what's happening in the world of hackers" perspective, allowing them to build effective cyber programs.

16.2 BACKGROUND

The push to make patient information available to everyone requiring a need (the rationale behind making electronic medical/health records available on-demand in any location) created an opportunity for illegal activity, especially identity theft and the market for buying and selling this once private information. Cybersecurity providers have been playing catch up with tech-savvy hackers (both individuals and groups), hoping to stem the outflow of private data to the black market.

In their efforts to stem illegal data flow, governments and professional bodies have tried (with mixed results) to create easy reporting requirements and structures. The belief being if facilities report on breaches and attacks, the oversight structures will be able to find patches (or fixes) and quickly implement changes to catch or stop hackers. Governments use a carrot and stick approach, without the carrot. In essence, if your organization failed to properly prepare (e.g., lacked or lacks a fully functioning cybersecurity operation) for a preventable (e.g., the hacker used a known tactic) breach, then on top of the public damage of being attacked, you "get" to pay the government a fine.

16.3 ISSUES WITH COMPLIANCE

Regulatory and Reporting Agencies: Ask ChatGPT 4 "who are the reporting and regulatory agencies for cybersecurity attacks" and you'll get the following:

- Cybersecurity and Infrastructure Security Agency (CISA)
- Federal Bureau of Investigation (FBI)

- Department of Health and Human Services (HHS), Office for Civil Rights (OCR)
- Federal Trade Commission (FTC)
- U.S. Securities and Exchange Commission (SEC)
- National Institute of Standards and Technology (NIST)

Not listed are the numerous sub-reporting agencies and programs. For example, the FBI has an Internet crime complaint center (IC3), a recovery asset team (RAT) for financial institutions, and an asset-freezing program (Financial Fraud Kill Chain or FFKC).

The above points to a central concern when looking for trends in cyberattacks: "Is there a single source or repository of truth?" Choosing the "wrong" repository may lead well-intentioned researchers to problematic conclusions.

16.4   TRANSPARENCY

The stigma of being attacked has both social (people may have second thoughts about coming to your facility if you've been in the news for losing patient data) and economic (fewer patients equate to lower revenue) impacts. If regulations require the facility to disclose only incidents above a certain threshold, is there a duty to tell all patients? This dilemma may lead some facilities to release only what is mandatory. In turn, if only mandatory disclosures are made, it becomes impossible to know the true number of cyberattacks.

Healthcare providers and systems are highly susceptible to "word of mouth" damage. One bad action (or actor) can impact an organization for years to come. Just one example is Group Health (a healthcare provider/health plan), which for years (in the 1980s) was known as Group Death by many practitioners. Whether this was fair or reasonable is irrelevant: the "stain" of a bad perception tends to stay with healthcare systems.

16.5   COMMON TERMS AND CLARIFICATIONS

16.5.1   Cyberattack or Cyber-Attack

A cyberattack is "an attempt by cybercriminals, hackers, or other digital adversaries to access a computer network or system, usually for the purpose of altering, stealing, destroying, or exposing information" (Crowdstrike, 2022). Others (Fortinet, 2024) go a step further and include language indicating the attack is the first step in the overall plan to gain access to the target organization, suggesting larger questions: (1) is a cyberattack solely the gaining of access to the system, or (2) is cyberattack the full process (i.e., from gaining entry to the system, to finding the target data, to changing or manipulating the data, to taking or theft of that data, to the exiting of the target network, and finally, to any demands/ransoms requested or paid by the targeted organization? For our purposes, we will look at a more robust definition and will discuss aspects thereof. To ensure clarity of terms, "cyberattack" versus "cyber-attack" is used.

16.6   WHAT A CYBERATTACK IS NOT

For clarification, it is necessary to understand that a cyberattack isn't necessarily a breach. When a hacker attempts to break into a system, you have a cyberattack. If a hacker successfully breaks into the system, you have a cyber breach. Unless otherwise indicated, this section focuses on cyber breaches.

16.7 AI

ChatGPT-4 (and updated versions) and Consensus 2.0 (and updated versions) are used and cited in accord with the APA 7th edition. Harvard library's interpretation of APA guidance suggests the back and forth nature of "talking or chatting" with AI isn't personal communication, but rather algorithmic output (Harvard Library, 2024), and will be cited as such.

16.7.1 BASIC DEFINITIONS

Problematic to any discussion on health facility attacks are the basic definitions. Although commonalities exist across borders, there are many differences. When is a clinic not a clinic? In Ethiopia, for example, many rural communities have facilities run solely by personnel with limited medical training and education. Is this a clinic? In Ethiopia, yes. In the United States, the answer would be no.

Who or what defines a cyberattack? Must patient data be at risk? Must the data be stolen? Must access to the system be denied until a ransom is paid? Does the government tell hospitals to pay the ransom? Are data-destroying viruses (without demand for money) cyberattacks? Does the government mandate a certain level of cybersecurity by individuals or facilities? If the facility or individual is not up-to-date with their cybersecurity, is there a government-imposed penalty? Who pays for cybersecurity software?

16.8 OVERVIEW OF THE PREVALENCE OF GLOBAL CYBERATTACKS

Few, if any, would argue cyberattacks aren't affecting health facilities. Unfortunately, most argue over the details, from what defines a health facility to reporting requirements. The author uses data from international organizations (e.g., the World Health Organization or WHO), domestic organizations (e.g., Health and Human Services or HHS in the United States), to professional organizations (e.g., the American Hospital Association or AHA in the United States) and, where differences are present, makes conservative assumptions.

Globally, the average cost of a data breach has risen from USD $3.86 million in 2020 to USD $4.45 million in 2023 (IBM, 2023). IBM points to a shorter "time to discovery and containment of breach" as well as a "USD $1.76 M lower data breach cost" as justification for a robust cybersecurity program. There is no mention of the cost to develop and maintain a cybersecurity program (e.g., cost of ensuring staff is appropriately trained, cost of hardware and software for security monitoring, and cost of cybersecurity insurance) or the cost of training employees on cybersecurity best practices—a notable exclusion as many (e.g., Protenus, 2024) point to internal missteps as the primary factor in data breaches.

16.9 PURPOSE AND SCOPE OF THE STUDY

At best, understanding the past and present cyber landscape will prevent future attacks. At worst, building a cybersecurity strategy around what we currently know is a solid baseline and will prevent many attacks by new, lazy, or "old school" hackers and their tools (Witts, 2024). In essence, something is far superior to nothing. A key purpose of this section is to provide decision makers with information on what hackers have been doing over the covered decade to help ensure they are minimally prepared for ongoing and future cyberattacks.

Furthermore, this section will present the facts regarding past cyberattacks (numbers per/year, types, and possible trends) as provided by recognized bodies. Speculation on the rationale behind the attacks is beyond the scope of this section.

16.10   TRENDS IN GLOBAL CYBERATTACKS

16.10.1   Historical Context of Cyberattacks over the Past Decade

ChatGPT-4o was asked to provide the top five types of cyberattacks over the 2014–2023 timeframe. Although the answer supplied did not result in a list of top five attacks, the information provided highlighted the most predominant attack type:

> 2014: Data breaches; 2015: Advanced persistent threats (APTs); 2016: Ransomware; 2017: Ransomware; 2018: Supply chain attacks; 2019: Phishing; 2020: Ransomware; 2021: Supply chain attacks; 2022: Phishing and ransomware; and 2023: Ransomware and Cloud attacks (OpenAI, 2024).

> Interestingly, the information provided by AI limits the attack types used by hackers to six: data breaches, APTs, ransomware, supply chain attacks, phishing, and cloud attacks. Based on this question alone, one could incorrectly assume cyberattacks could be thwarted solely by countermeasures designed to identify and stop the above attack types. The thinking behind this statement is a single cyberattack makes use of numerous tools, for example, a hacker's use of email containing a link. The email in this instance is a phishing tool (or technique); the link, when clicked on by the user, opens harmful software (i.e., malware). This action then releases the malware onto the users' system. This use of mixed methods is why cybersecurity efforts must be both robust (i.e., cover a wide range of potential attacks) and adaptive (i.e., able to "see" and adjust for attack changes). It is this line of thought that demands AI have a "seat at the table" for any cybersecurity or cyberattack discussion.

To expand upon the trends provided by AI, here are the year-by-year trends and/or highlights:

2014: ChatGPT-4o provides the following for 2014: "Major data breaches, such as the Yahoo breach that exposed 500 million accounts, dominated the year. This type of attack involved unauthorized access to large volumes of personal data stored by organizations" (OpenAI, 2024).

2015: In a 2015 blog post highlighting the top trends of 2015, healthcare makes an appearance as a hacker target: (a) attackers continue to increase in reach and creativity, (b) the healthcare industry emerges as the top target for cybercriminals, (c) a major increase in state-sponsored cyberattacks, and (d) cybersecurity goes mainstream (Lord, 2015).

2016: "93 major cyberattacks hit healthcare organizations this year (2016), up from 57 in 2015" (Sheridan, 2016). Furthermore, "researchers pinpointed two major trends . . . continued discovery and evolution of medical device hijacking . . . and increase of ransomware across a variety of targets" (Sheridan, 2016).

2017: The US government developed a program to identify high-value targets (known as the HVA program and developed by the Office of Management and Budget and Department of Homeland Security in 2015). In 2017, the program stated the following risk and vulnerabilities assessment (RVA): spear phishing weaknesses; patch management; sensitive data exfiltration; cleartext password disclosure, and easily guessable credentials (Office of Management and Budget [OMB], 2018).

2018: In the fiscal year 2018 FISMA report, the following findings (risks) were presented:
- Lack of data protection
- Lack of network segmentation
- Inconsistent patch management
- Lack of strong authentication
- Lack of continuous monitoring, including audit and logging capabilities (OMB, 2019).

2019: The American Medical Collection Agency (AMCA) data breach, 8 months (August 1, 2018, to March 30, 2019) in the making and over 25 million individuals were affected. One of the highlights of this particular breach was that external (or third) parties were also affected (Davis, 2019).

2020: "239.4 million cyberattack attempts; 816 attempted attacks per healthcare endpoint (nearly 10,000% increase over 2019); Approximately 1 million healthcare records breached each month, and 80 ransomware incidents" (HHS Cybersecurity Program, Office of Information Security, 2021).

2021: Of the top 10 data breaches in 2021, Jercich (2021) highlights the Florida Health Kids Corporation (over 3.5 million individuals were affected by "significant vulnerabilities") and the 20/20 Eye Care Network (over 3.2 million individuals were affected by "suspicious activity").

2022: Cyber Incident Reporting for Critical Infrastructure Act of 2022 introduced two major points: (1) covered entities must report cyberattacks to the Cybersecurity and Infrastructure Security Agency (CISA) within 72 hours and (2) covered entities must report ransomware payments made to attackers within 24 hours.

2023: According to one compliance corporation, 171 million patient records were breached in 2023. Of these breached records, "unauthorized access, including insiders, represents 93% of the cause of reported incidents" (Protenus, 2024). It should be noted the report by Protenus blurs the line between reportable (incidents involving 500 or greater individuals) and unreportable. Further complicating the figures are the outlier events (such as the Anthem data breach affecting approximately 80 million individuals). Drawing conclusions based solely on this data is therefore problematic.

16.11   KEY TYPES OF CYBERATTACKS AND THEIR PURPOSE

Fortinet (www.fortinet.com) lists the following types of cyberattacks: malware, phishing, ransomware, denial-of-service, man-in-the-middle, cryptojacking, SQL injection, and exploits.

Aside from the above-mentioned attacks, there are many others (and subtypes). For example, phishing attacks consist of many subtypes such as spear phishing (hackers posing as relatives or close friends), clone phishing (a copy of a trusted email, but containing harmful links or attachments), whaling (targeting executives of companies or high-profile people), and pop-up phishing (when an online pop-up contains a link to harmful malware).

The focus here is not on listing all attack types but understanding (at least at a 30,000-foot level) the volume of attacks.

16.12   ANALYSIS OF CYBERATTACK FREQUENCY, SEVERITY, AND EVOLUTION

In a recent article on ransomware trends, Neprash et al. (2022) asked the topical question, "How frequently do health care delivery organizations experience ransomware attacks, and how have the characteristics of ransomware changed over time?" The study covered the 2016–2021 timeframe. The study concluded ransomware attacks have increased in frequency and sophistication, but more work is needed.

16.13   WHAT THE DATA ARE TELLING US

Any effort to place a dollar figure or attack number in the future will be met with more push back than the effort itself. That said, understanding whether/not a trend is in place could help cybersecurity teams better prepare for 2024.

Using data from the HHS, OCR, and HA–OCR (hhs.gov), we have the following breach information.

Of note, the above data include only resolved providers (health plan, business associate, healthcare provider, and others) and breach types (hacking/IT incident, unauthorized access/disclosure, improper disposal, loss, theft, and other). The data were downloaded (and accurate) as of May 29, 2024.

TABLE 16.1
OCR Breach Data, January 1, 2014 through December 31, 2023

Year	# of Breaches	Affected Individuals	Median
2023	293	24,976,513	3,833
2022	570	37,100,990	7,820
2021	716	59,563,327	5,048
2020	663	34,999,777	4,501
2019	512	44,970,906	3,992
2018	369	15,236,139	2,393
2017	358	5,314,987	2,075
2016	328	16,711,004	2,380
2015	270	112,466,720	2,030
2014	314	19,073,551	2,674

TABLE 16.2
Year over Year % Change in Number of Resolved/Targeted Cyberattacks.

Year	# of Breaches	Year over Year % Change
2023	293	−48.60
2022	570	−20.39
2021	716	+7.99
2020	663	+29.49
2019	512	+38.75
2018	369	+3.07
2017	358	+9.15
2016	328	+21.48
2015	270	−14.01
2014	314	

Using the information from the OCR, we are tempted to divide individuals by breaches. Performing this operation just once shows the error we would be making: If we look at 2016 numbers, we would suggest the mean of affected individuals per breach is just shy of 51,000. Calculating the median for these same data gives us a much different number: 2,380. The use of the median appears to be a much better gauge of central tendency in this case.

With 2023 showing decreases across the board (i.e., number of breaches, affected individuals, and median), it is difficult to say with any certainty whether/not there is an upward or downward trend. The years 2019–2022 coincide with the COVID-19 pandemic and associated/contributory events. The year 2015 includes the Anthem cyberattack in which 78.8 million people were affected. Should 2024 data stay above the 2018 median of 2,393, one could argue the cyberattack trend is in place, and we are likely to see higher numbers in the future.

The initial review of online materials suggested we would see the greatest number of attacks occurring during the "COVID years" of 2020–2022. However, the data show 2019 (versus 2018) as the single-highest jump in attacks (38.75%), and 2020 and 2021 show the highest number of successful (and resolved) cyberattacks on healthcare systems—suggesting hackers were busy while the economy was struggling with pandemic-related issues.

16.13.1 HORIZONTAL AND VERTICAL ANALYSIS

Although more common to the financial arena (specifically, financial statement analysis), horizontal and vertical analyses are less sophisticated (versus in-depth statistics) methods for understanding data that change over time and interpreting/viewing what those changes may mean.

16.13.2 HORIZONTAL ANALYSIS

The year-over-year column allows us to understand the overall changes taking place year over year. For example, from 2014 to 2015, the number of breaches decreased from 314 to 270, representing a decrease of 14.01%. By itself, these data tell us the OCR resolved approximately 14% fewer breaches in 2015 (versus 2014). What this doesn't tell us is where or why those breaches occurred.

- Is the decrease due to fewer cases being reported?
- Were the number of agents working on these cases the same?
- Were regulations introduced that loosened reporting rules (e.g., if a regulation mandates reporting of breaches greater than 500 was changed to 1,000, one expects a drop in reported breaches).
- Did all areas and attack types drop? Did some attack types increase?
- What do we know about the organizations that were attacked? Large health systems? Small, independent clinics?

16.13.3 VERTICAL ANALYSIS

Unlike HA, which looks at changes from one period to the next, vertical analysis (VA) looks at changes within the same reporting period. It answers the following questions:

- Was there a drop in all areas and attack types?
- Did some attack types increase?

If we look at the data over our covered period (2014–2023), HA allows us to quickly see the year-over-year changes. To see which attack types increased (or reduced), we need to dig in and use VA. Here's a quick look at 2023:

- The attacks in which $> 1,000,000$ individuals were affected were seven. These seven attacks represent 2.4% of all cases for the year.

16.13.4 TREND ANALYSIS USING HA AND VA

For trend analysis, actionable VA requires one to look at various time frames. Looking at 2022, we see there were seven incidents, affecting $> 1,000,000$ individuals. These seven attacks represent 1.2% of all cases.

Question: Although we saw a 100% increase in % change for the $> 1,000,000$ affected individual category for 2022 (1.2%) to 2023 (2.4%), we saw a total decrease in attacks of 48.9%. Can we say hackers are spending more effort on targeting large organizations (or those with large patient populations) than smaller, sub-million patient populations?

The answer to the above question has too many variables to readily answer. It takes the OCR time to address all cyberattacks, and it is highly likely the numbers will increase over time.

TABLE 16.3

VA of Affected Individuals by Year

	2014	2015	2016	2017	2018	2019	2020	2021	2022	2023
500–1000	80	76	88	99	92	96	114	118	83	55
	(25.4%)	(28.1%)	(26.8%)	(27.7%)	(24.9%)	(18.8%)	(17.2%)	(16.5%)	(14.6%)	(18.77%)
1001–5000	123	113	129	132	145	185	232	238	159	108
	(39.2%)	(41.9%)	(39.3%)	(36.9%)	(39.3%)	(36.1%)	(35.0%)	(33.2%)	(27.9%)	(36.9%)
5001–10000	35	31	29	44	31	68	66	79	67	31
	(11.1%)	(11.5%)	(8.8%)	(12.3%)	(8.4%)	(13.3%)	(10.0%)	(11.0%)	(11.8%)	(10.6%)
10001–20000	28	20	32	43	37	58	57	65	73	16
	(8.9%)	(7.4%)	(9.8%)	(12.0%)	(10.0%)	(11.3%)	(8.6%)	(9.1%)	(12.8%)	(5.5%)
20001–50000	24	10	26	19	32	44	61	96	74	28
	(7.6%)	(3.7%)	(7.9%)	(5.3%)	(8.7%)	(8.6%)	(9.2%)	(13.4%)	(13.0%)	(9.6%)
50001–100000	13	8	10	12	9	19	59	39	51	15
	(4.1%)	(3.0%)	(3.0%)	(3.4%)	(2.4%)	(3.7%)	(8.9%)	(5.4%)	(8.9%)	(5.1%)
>100001	11	12	14	9	23	42	74	81	63	39
	(3.5%)	(4.4%)	(4.3%)	(2.5%)	(6.2%)	(8.2%)	(11.2%)	(11.3%)	(11.1%)	(13.3%)
TOTAL	**314**	**270**	**328**	**358**	**369**	**512**	**663**	**716**	**570**	**293**

Sums > or < 100% due to rounding error(s).

By combining VA and HA, we can make a few quick comments:

- Incidents involving 5,001–10000, 10,0001–20,000, and > 100,000a are increasing; each of the groups has increased at least five of ten previous years, with the > 100,000 group increasing six of the last ten years.
- The combined incidents for groups 500–1,000 and 1,001–5,000 were greater than 50% of the total breaches except during the high COVID-19 years of 2021 and 2022.
- Except for 2022, the group > 100,000 increased from a low of 2.5% in 2017 to a peak of 13.3% in 2023. This is suggestive of hackers targeting larger health organizations and helps explain the decreased incidents of attacks on smaller facilities.

16.13.5   COST OF CYBERATTACKS

In a 2023 report, IBM states, "the global average cost of a data breach in 2023 was USD 4.45 million, a 15% increase over 3 years" (IBM, 2023). The same IBM report lists the United States as the nation/region with the highest cost per data breach at USD $9.48 million in 2023 and USD $9.44 million in 2022. In terms of healthcare, the IBM report states the United States held the title for highest cost per breach at USD$ 10.93 million in 2023 and USD$ 10.10 million in 2022.

Of note is the cost (impact) on patient outcomes or safety. There is little information on this subject, but examples exist. One such instance occurred in Germany (2020) when a patient died while being routed from one facility to another. The initial destination facility was under a ransomware attack (HHS Cybersecurity Program, Office of Information Security, 2021).

16.14   IMPACT ON HEALTHCARE

16.14.1   NOTABLE HEALTHCARE BREACHES

During the covered period, there have been numerous significant healthcare breaches.

TABLE 16.4

Date	Company	No. of Patients Impacted	Attack Type	Source
April–June 2014	Community Health Systems	4.5 Million	Software vulnerability, malware	https://www.databreachtoday.com/community-health-systems-faces-lawsuit-a-7238
March 2015	Anthem	79 Million	Unknown, patient info compromised	https://www.hhs.gov/guidance/document/anthem-pays-ocr-16-million-record-hipaa-settlement-following-largest-us-health-data-breach
July 2015	UCLA Health	4.5 Million	Unknown, patient info compromised	
July 2015	Medical Informatics Engineering	4 Million	Compromised usernames and passwords	
July 2016	Newkirk Products	3.8 Million	Server access, patient info compromised	
August 2016	Banner Health	3.6 Million	Server access, patient info compromised	
May 2020	Trinity Health	3.3 Million	Third-party vendor ransomware, patient info compromised	
March 2022	Shields Healthcare Group	2 Million	Network server accessed, not certain of patient data loss	

16.15 CRITICAL AREAS OF CONCERN IN HEALTHCARE CYBERSECURITY

16.15.1 ELECTRONIC MEDICAL RECORDS

Electronic medical and health records (EMRs/EHRs) are here to stay, and so too are the security issues they have raised: Making patient data available to providers (across the system or globe) creates opportunities for bad actors. Worse yet, the more encompassing a health record (i.e., bringing in third parties such as laboratories, pharmacies, and radiology firms), the more opportunities there are for the bad actors. Legacy systems (i.e., older systems without the latest and greatest hardware and software) cannot be fully trusted as they may be targeted as "easy prey." However, upgrading hardware and software is extremely expensive (aside from the cost of the physical hardware, any new system must work with existing systems) and requires skilled personnel (many times these are consultants who demand high pay) to implement. Until such a time when computers are made that last forever, have continuous upgrades, and come with assurances such as always on, this "legacy versus upgrade to new" battle will continue to grow.

16.15.2 MEDICAL DEVICE SECURITY

Medical device management in hospitals (e.g.) is off limits for all but biomedical staff. The devices are expensive, highly calibrated, and require in-depth bioengineering knowledge. On the positive side, these devices provide a vast array of provider-needed information for patient care. On the negative side, the communication of data from devices to health records is a potential opportunity for bad actors.

16.15.3 Successful Attacks versus Attempts

It is impossible to know the effectiveness of your cybersecurity efforts if you don't know the number of attempts. Although, arguably, the numbers don't really matter, it only takes one successful attack to bring an organization to a standstill. However, this is a practical study and for those looking to fully understand the issue, it is important to understand cybersecurity effectiveness.

Although we are able to find data showing successful data breaches, it is more difficult to find information on cyberattacks. In a blog post by cybersecurity firm Check Point, we have the following 2022 information on global cyberattacks: Global cyberattacks averaged 1168 weekly attacks per organization, with education/research, government, and healthcare being top targets. Africa experienced the highest number of weekly attacks, at 1,875 per organization (Check Point Research Team, 2023).

If we consider the data provided earlier by OCR, and the number of successful breaches, versus the 1,463 cyberattacks per week (in 2022, according to Check Point) against healthcare organizations, it appears our cybersecurity teams and software are doing an amazing job at preventing data breaches. Taking this information "as gospel," however, is difficult as the authors of the blog make no mention of their sources.

16.16 RESEARCH GAPS AND PREDICTIONS FOR FUTURE CYBERSECURITY CHALLENGES IN HEALTHCARE

Protecting organizations from future cyberattacks is unlikely to get easier on those charged with keeping the organization safe. Immediate issues include the use of ever-improving artificial intelligence, economic pressure on the majority of the population will ensure continued interest in risky ventures (e.g., hacking activities), lack of national or global regulations preventing true attack figures from coming to light, lack of cooperation between like-minded organizations, and an ever-changing technological environment will create both positive and negative opportunities for hackers and cybersecurity professionals.

16.16.1 Ever-Improving AI

The use and proliferation of artificial intelligence (AI), the improved large-language models, and the increased specialization and niches of AI will serve both "good and bad" actors in the cybersecurity arena. As governments continue to struggle with finding cooperative stances, it is likely we will see more AI-related confusion before any practical solutions come to fruition.

16.16.2 Economic Pressure

The cost of data breaches is more than zero, but likely far less than what many have suggested. For corporations, and for the current moment, the cost of cybersecurity is being passed to the consumer. This may or not last. One thing for certain, a data breach negatively impacts any targeted organization. Whether they like it or not, corporations will need to maintain a serious cybersecurity footprint if they wish to stay out of the public's attention.

16.16.3 Lack of Governance

There are many regulatory and governing bodies across the globe (e.g., CISA in the United States and ECSO in the European Union), but the Internet (and therefore cybersecurity) is worldwide. Short of implementing Chinese-like firewalls, these governing bodies are fighting an uphill battle to prevent external cyberattacks. The problem of solutions as bold as the Chinese firewall is the fact that many attacks are domestic in nature. Will locking out external nations and players help?

16.16.4 Lack of Cooperation

Whether governmental, regional, or local, there is little cooperation among institutions. This may be related to a fear of sharing data (thereby opening oneself to a third-party attack) or simply economic (i.e., "we paid millions for this cybersecurity solution, and we're not sharing" mentality), or something else. It is unlikely any government will demand corporate cooperation.

16.16.5 Technological Changes

Physically, computers of today bear minimal resemblance to their ancestors of 30 years ago. Their size has shrunk, internal memory and storage have grown astronomically, and the speed at which calculations are completed is nearly incomprehensible. These differences (size aside) do have an impact—as a hacker, the processing power of today's mobile phones makes breaking encrypted information (once thought impossible) as easy as tapping the phone screen. Adding to the processing power and compact size is the cost. Although a high-performance computer will cost thousands of dollars, a capable system only dreamed of a few years ago will cost less than USD $1,000. Considering the number of businesses across the globe, the lack of comprehensive cybersecurity for most organizations, the expense of new computers, availability of hacking tutorials and software, and the "help" of AI, it is not much of a leap to see why hacking is such a big business.

16.17 PRACTICAL STEPS FOR HEALTHCARE ORGANIZATIONS

16.17.1 Cooperation

Perhaps scared by the thought of opening their IT departments (and the data of their patients) to competing entities, organizations need to take the step of working together. Well-drafted agreements, continuous monitoring, and trust-over-time will allow organizations to share resources and reduce costs—ultimately making for a safer data environment.

16.17.2 AI and Associated Technology

AI is a useful add-on tool. That is, it is not a tool you can "give the keys" to and walk away. AI integration with complex cybersecurity solutions will help provide a holistic approach to threat discovery/assessment. Other technologies (e.g., blockchain) have been/are being developed to help ensure secure transmission and storage of highly sensitive information.

16.17.3 Training, Training, Training

It is no surprise that our greatest resource is also the weakest link in the cybersecurity chain. People can be too quick to click on "bad" links in email, too easily tricked into giving away credentials, and often fail to do even the simplest of cybersecurity chores (e.g., change passwords every 3 months). Through ongoing cybersecurity training and awareness, people can become better cyber detectives.

16.18 PROPOSED AREAS FOR FUTURE RESEARCH AND DEVELOPMENT

16.18.1 True Costs

The true cost of cyberattacks remains highly subjective. Although IBM claims healthcare attacks (in the United States) cost nearly USD $11 million, this is certainly an average which takes into consideration the largest outliers. Any guess at a true cost is no more than a guess.

16.18.2 GOVERNANCE AND REGULATION

Until such time reporting becomes less disciplinary in nature (i.e., the reporting parties are not given fines on top of the actual dollars lost), it is highly unlikely that researchers will have solid numbers for data breaches. This author, for one, is not pushing for a "no fines" system as this would create a system of unaccountable behavior and "oh well" responses from executives. Policymakers must be willing to put the effort into piloting various efforts and coming together to push for the best solution(s).

16.19 CONCLUSION

16.19.1 FINAL THOUGHTS ON THE EVOLUTION OF CYBERSECURITY MEASURES IN HEALTHCARE

Currently, it is impossible to know the extent of cyberattacks. There are too many loopholes, too many reporting bodies, and too many regulations. This is not to say any single body is superior to another body. Rather, there needs to be a reporting chain of command that allows for clear data. If, for example, the HHS is overall responsible for ensuring cyberattack reporting, there must be a very clear reporting mechanism. As it stands today, this mechanism does not exist.

REFERENCES

Check Point Research Team. (2023, January 5). *Check Point Research Reports a 38% Increase in 2022 Global Cyberattacks*. Check Point. Retrieved July 1, 2024, from https://blog.checkpoint.com/2023/01/05/38-increase-in-2022-global-cyberattacks/

Crowdstrike. (2022). *What Is a Cyberattack?* Crowdstrike.com. https://www.crowdstrike.com/cybersecurity-101/cyberattacks/

Davis, J. (2019, July 23). *The 10 Biggest Healthcare Data Breaches of 019, so Far*. Health IT security. https://healthitsecurity.com/news/the-10-biggest-healthcare-data-breaches-of-2019-so-far

Fortinet. (2024). *What Is a Cyber Attack?* fortinet.com. https://www.fortinet.com/uk/resources/cyberglossary/what-is-cyber-attack

Harvard Library. (2024). *Artificial Intelligence for Research and Scholarship: Citing Generative AI*. library.harvard. https://guides.library.harvard.edu/c.php?g=1330621&p=10046069

HHS Cybersecurity Program, Office of Information Security. (2021). *2020: A Retrospective Look at Healthcare Cybersecurity (No. 202102181030)*. https://www.hhs.gov/sites/default/files/2020-hph-cybersecurty-retrospective-tlpwhite.pdf

IBM. (2023). *Cost of a Data Breach Report 2023*. https://www.ibm.com/reports/data-breach

Jercich, K. (2021, November 16). *The Biggest Healthcare Data Breaches of 2021*. Healthcare IT news. https://www.healthcareitnews.com/news/biggest-healthcare-data-breaches-2021

Lord, N. (2015). *The Top 4 Cybersecurity Trends of 2015*. Data Insider. https://www.digitalguardian.com/blog/top-4-cybersecurity-trends-2015

Neprash, H. T., McGlave, C. C., Cross, D. A., Virnig, B. A., Puskarich, M. A., Huling, J. D., Rozenshtein, A. Z., & Nikpay, S. S. (2022). Trends in ransomware attacks on US hospitals, clinics, and other health care delivery organizations. *JAMA Health Forum*, 3(12). https://doi.org/10.1001/jamahealthforum.2022.4873

Office of Management and Budget. (2018). *Federal Information Security Modernization Act of 2014: Annual Report to Congress: Fiscal Year 2017* [Report]. https://www.whitehouse.gov/wp-content/uploads/2017/11/FY2017FISMAReportCongress.pdf

Office of Management and Budget. (2019). *Federal Information Security Modernization Act of 2014: Annual Report to Congress: Fiscal Year 2018* [Report]. https://www.whitehouse.gov/wp-content/uploads/2019/08/FISMA-2018-Report-FINAL-to-post.pdf

OpenAI. (2024). *ChatGPT* (Version 4o) [Computer software]. https://chatgpt.com

Protenus. (2024). *2024 Breach Barometer: A Look Back at 2023 and Insight on What 2024 Could Hold for Healthcare Data Breaches* [Report]. https://www.protenus.com/breach-barometer-report

Sheridan, K. (2016, December 22). *Major Cyberattacks on Healthcare Grew 63% in 2016*. Dark Reading. https://www.darkreading.com/cyberattacks-data-breaches/major-cyberattacks-on-healthcare-grew-63-in-2016

Witts, J. (2024, February 9). *Healthcare Cyber Attack Statistics 2022: 25 Alarming Data Breaches You Should Know*. Expert Insights. https://expertinsights.com/insights/healthcare-cyber-attack-statistics/

17 Intelligent Transportation System for Healthcare Improvement

Angayarkanni S.A., Rajaram V, Pandimurugan V,
Balakiruthiga B, Umamageswaran C., and Rajesh Babu

17.1 INTRODUCTION

The rapid advancement of technology should not compromise human health, which is a very important part of life. Transportation is one of the areas where technology can greatly affect human health: millions' mobility, safety, and general well-being depend on it daily [1]. Therefore, transportation systems are becoming increasingly intelligent and connected because of the information and data exchange between different vehicles, infrastructure, and other things. This can lead to enhanced efficiency, more excellent dependability, and more secure transportation services as well as better user experience and satisfaction. However, using intelligent transportation systems (ITS) for addressing medical emergency service delivery and life support, among others, poses both opportunities and challenges [2].

In the world of ITS, vehicular ad hoc networks (VANETs) are a rare breed of wireless networks that facilitate exchange among vehicles and between cars and roadside units (RSUs) [3]. Services that VANETs may open up to drivers, passengers, pedestrians, and authorities are diverse: traffic management, navigation, entertainment, and safety, to name a few. Not only can VANETs serve these groups, but they may also provide timely health-related information and services for various stakeholders, such as blood banks, RSUs, emergency vehicles, and hospitals [3]. For example, by leveraging VANETs, hospitals and ambulances near an accident or emergency can receive an alert and help faster. Additionally, VANETs can make possible remote health monitoring of patients as they move in their vehicles and ensure smoother transport of emergency medical services (EMS) and life support vehicles [4].

In a world where many cities are adopting smart technology, the possibility of linking hospitals, blood banks, and RSUs presents a promising opportunity for faster and more efficient emergency response [5]. This innovative approach could potentially save lives and reduce health risks. However, this integration brings up various challenges and inquiries regarding data privacy and security, the ability to expand and rely on networks, the development of protocols and algorithms for routing, the quality and effectiveness of service, and the reception and confidence of users [6].

17.1.1 IMPACT OF ROAD TRAFFIC MANAGEMENT ON HEALTH

Road transportation is one of the key means of transportation in India. Traffic congestion in Indian roads may be due to dynamic traffic signal failure, less disciplined driving ethics, heterogeneous traffic load, and bilateral movements of two-wheeler vehicles in mixed lanes. Despite well-planned traffic measures, there are more fatal road accidents [7].

It has been studied that road accidents are mainly caused by careless driving, sleepiness of the driver, and less disciplined driving behavior. In densely populated cities of India, a large number of accidents occur on curved undivided roads, in which the length and degree of the curvature have a high impact [8]. Employment of road traffic management for the healthcare industry is a doubtful advantage. When not properly deployed, poor road traffic management will cause many road accidents and lead to death. Meanwhile, when properly planned, proper road traffic management can enhance the betterment of healthcare.

When the road lanes are cleared from traffic congestion and have well-planned connectivity between on-road vehicles and RSUs, it will be helpful for treating patients with trauma injury, road accidents, cardiac issues, and burn cases. It will be more instrumental in providing on-time treatment for pregnancy cases and neonatal cases.

Road traffic management can significantly impact public health in both constructive and destructive ways. Let us examine both in detail:

1. **For Betterment of Healthcare:**
   - **Reduced Air Pollution**: Efficient traffic management, such as traffic flow optimization and congestion reduction, can lead to decreased vehicle emissions, thus improving the quality of air. Increase in air quality results in decrease in respiratory diseases.
   - **Accident Prevention:** Effective road traffic management strategies like speed limits, traffic signals, and signage can decrease the likelihood of accidents, thereby reducing injuries and fatalities.
   - **Promotion of Active Transportation:** Implementing pedestrian-friendly infrastructure, bike lanes, and safe crossings encourages walking and cycling. This contributes to increased physical activity levels, leading to improved cardiovascular health and reduced obesity rates.
   - **Noise Reduction:** Traffic management measures can also mitigate noise pollution, which has been linked to stress, sleep disturbances, and cardiovascular problems.
2. **For Deterioration of Healthcare:**
   - **Exposure to Air Pollution:** Despite efforts to reduce emissions, traffic congestion in urban areas can still lead to high exposure to pollutants for pedestrians, cyclists, and those living near busy roads.
   - **Stress and Mental Health:** Congested roads, long commute times, and traffic-related stress can negatively impact mental health by causing frustration, anxiety, and fatigue.
   - **Physical Inactivity:** Areas where road designs prioritize cars over pedestrians or cyclists may discourage physical activity and contribute to a sedentary lifestyle.
   - **Road Traffic Accidents:** Inadequate road infrastructure, poor signage, or inefficient traffic management can increase the risk of accidents, leading to injuries and fatalities.

17.1.2 OVERALL IMPACT

Proper road traffic management is crucial for public health. Efforts aimed at reducing congestion, improving air quality, promoting active transportation, and ensuring road safety through efficient traffic management policies and infrastructure play a vital role in creating healthier communities.

However, the effectiveness of these measures depends on various factors such as urban planning, policy implementation, public awareness, and technological advancements in transportation systems. Collaboration between urban planners, policymakers, healthcare professionals, and the community is essential to mitigate the negative health impacts of road traffic and maximize the positive outcomes for public health.

Section 17.2 explains the role of VANETs in healthcare with a clear listing of challenges and benefits of using VANETs. Few successful case studies are discussed. Driver health monitoring for safe driving and mobility of emergency medical service vehicles are discussed in Sections 17.3 and 17.4, respectively. Section 17.5 presents the protocols and architectures for ITSs assisting healthcare services. Technologies for ITSs assisting healthcare service are given in Section 17.6. Section 17.7 addresses the challenges and solutions in integrating intelligent systems for healthcare. Section 17.8 addresses the challenges and scope of research.

17.2   ROLE OF VANETS IN HEALTHCARE

Providing healthcare facilities to everyone is the primary goal in human society to avoid any mishap. Due to the rapid development of the Internet of Things (IoT), medical Internet of Things (IoMT) can detect signs of fatigue or health issues early and give the best medication to people. Healthcare vehicle ambulance plays a significant role in protecting people's lives from all aspects, like accidents and emergency situations. Traffic management is important in the healthcare vehicular network to avoid mishaps and save the lives of patients. Sensors play a major role in all applications of modern world technology, especially in the healthcare field; wearables are used for tracking and measuring health parameters in humans.

According to the survey, Industry 4.0 applications rely on the IoT, cloud, and mHealth. Intelligent transportation system such as cloud-based ambulance tracking system that aims to bridge the communication gap between ambulance drivers and hospital management, particularly during emergency cases. It utilizes real-time ambulance location tracking to notify hospitals when an ambulance is within a 3-kilometer range, enabling timely patient treatment and potentially saving lives. Ambulance Tracking System is motivated by the urgent need to bridge the gap between emergency medical service demands and the existing capabilities. The tracking system provides a profound commitment to saving lives and creating safer communities through the potential of real-time tracking and optimized resource management. For storing information about ambulances and data about patients in a secure and timely transfer manner, a better storage environment and cloud can be used. Ambulance services available versus required in India are shown in Figure 17.1.

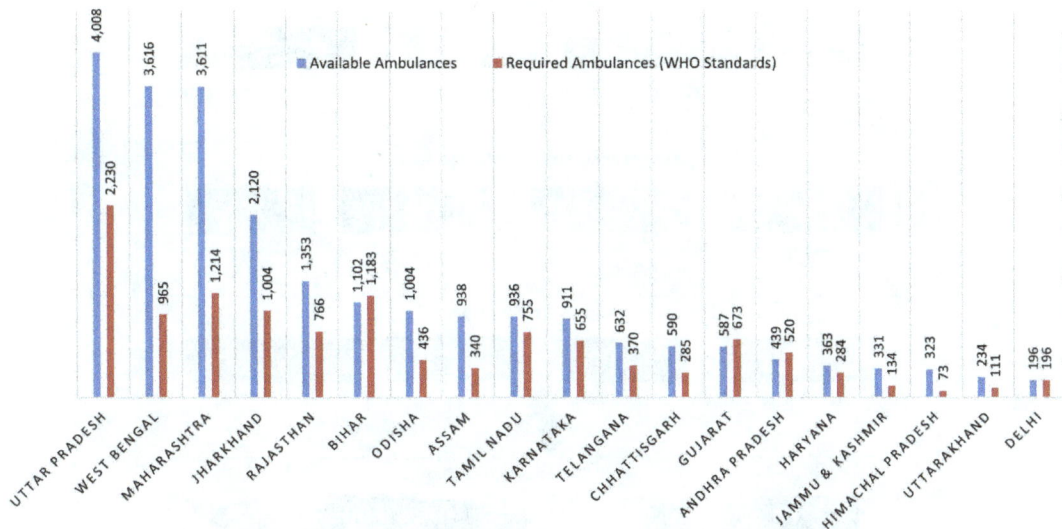

FIGURE 17.1   Ambulance Services Available vs Required in India.

17.2.1 COMMUNICATION BETWEEN HOSPITAL AND AMBULANCE

Due to many vehicles, the number of accidents is increasing daily, and the need for assistance for people in accidents are also growing, so to provide better facilities to them, we need a regularized traffic system or clearing or alternate routes displayed for the ambulance drivers to save people's life, as shown in Figure 17.2. Communication between vehicles can be classified into two types: vehicle-to-vehicle (V2V) communication and vehicle-to-hospital communication. Exchange of vehicle information like speed and position of the surrounding vehicles can be used in V2V communication to avoid crashes, ease traffic congestion, and improve the environment if the entire vehicle communicates efficiently with help of standard protocols. Comparison of different tracking methods and their pros and cons are shown in Table 17.1.

V2V communication has some constraints, which are listed below.

- Receive and transmit a required message.
- A protocol-based communication platform is required.
- Security-based communication is required.
- Provide alternative technologies when it is necessary.

Vehicle to Infrastructure (**V2I) Communication**

- Advanced road marking
- Smart signs
- Wireless communication

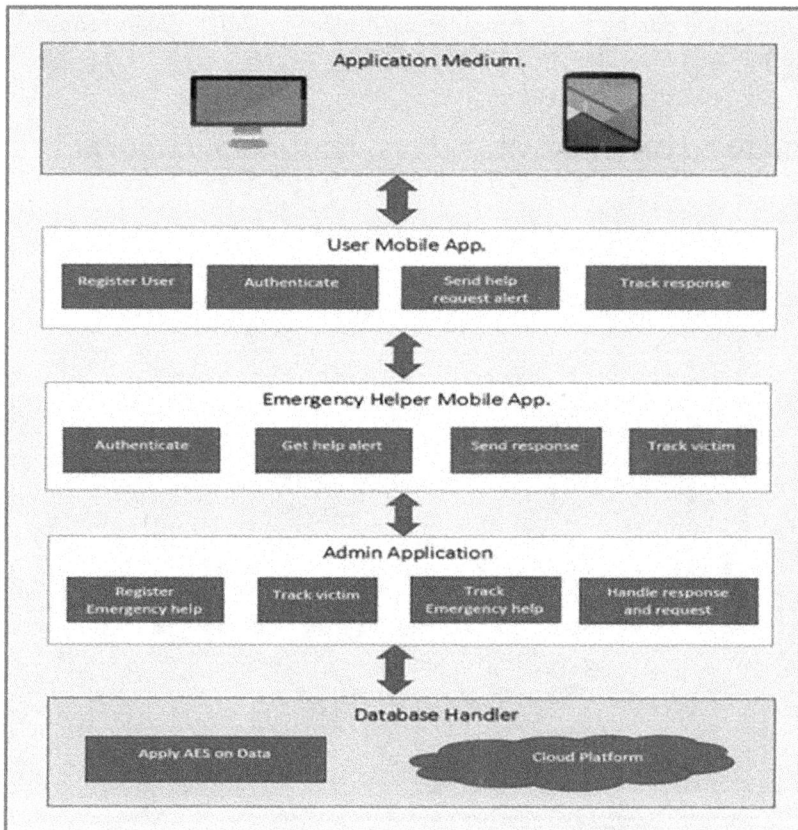

FIGURE 17.2 Ambulance Tracking System with Cloud Environment.

TABLE 17.1

Comparison of Different Tracking Methods and Their Pros and Cons

Existing Techniques	Algorithm Used	Parameters, If Any	Drawbacks
"GPS-Based Ambulance Tracking System in Cloud"	Global Positioning System (GPS) tracking, cloud server	Data transmission rate, data encryption	Limited scalability due to cloud costs, limited network coverage in remote areas
"Machine Learning Approach for Ambulance Routing"	Machine learning, cloud-based data storage	Training data size, cloud-based data storage	Requires substantial training data, potential privacy concerns
"Real-time Mobile Ambulance Tracking System"	Mobile app, cloud-based data storage	Mobile device, battery life, data, synchronization	Limited to mobile device capabilities, reliance on network connectivity
"RFID-Based Cloud Ambulance Tracking System"	Radio-frequency identification (RFID), cloud computing	RFID tag range, data, processing speed	Limited range of RFID, potential security vulnerabilities
"IoT-Enabled Cloud-Based Ambulance Tracking"	IoT devices, GPS, cloud-based platform	IoT device communication, GPS accuracy	Complexity in managing multiple IoT devices, high initial setup costs
"Machine Learning for Cloud-Based Ambulance Dispatch"	Machine learning, cloud-based data storage	Learning algorithm, accuracy, data volume	Requires continuous retraining, potential data transfer delays
"GIS-Based Cloud Ambulance Tracking System"	Geographic information system (GIS), cloud computing	GIS data integration, real-time data updating	Dependency on accurate and up-to-date GIS data, potential latency in updates
"Real-time Mobile Ambulance Tracking App"	Mobile app, GPS, cloud	Mobile app user, interface, data	Limited to mobile device capabilities, reliance on network connectivity
"Deep Learning for Cloud-Based Ambulance Tracking"	Deep learning, cloud-based data storage	Deep learning model, architecture, data	High computational requirements, training data size

Vehicle to Network Communication

- Transfer the data from the network and receive, vice versa.
- Helping find the patient's location.

Vehicle to Pedestrian Communication

- Broadcasting a warning message to the pedestrian near a moving vehicle.
- Environmental conditions like roadblocks, rainfall, etc.

17.2.2 CHALLENGES AND BENEFITS OF VANETs IN HEALTHCARE

- Inexperienced medical professional in hospitals and healthcare organizations
- High access cost and delivering healthcare
- Population health trends, increasing chronic medical conditions, evolving new diseases, etc.
- High rate of hospital patient admission and avoidable medical emergencies
- Stress and strain associated with healthcare hospitalization
- Increase in the average length of stay (ALOS) in the hospital

17.2.3 Case Studies of VANETs to Enhance Healthcare Services

VANETs can be included in EMS in smart cities to enhance the efficiency of response time in severe medical situations [9]. VANETs are utilized in New York City to facilitate communication and coordination among ambulances, hospitals, and traffic management systems. Upon receiving an emergency call, the EMS system utilizes the VANET technology to ascertain the closest ambulance, utilizing real-time traffic data to find the quickest path to the patient's whereabouts.

A study conducted in rural South Africa explored the use of mobile clinics equipped with VANETs to provide remote healthcare services. The research focused on how VANETs facilitated real-time data transmission between mobile clinics and centralized healthcare providers, improving the quality of care in remote areas.

There is an implementation of VANETs to enhance healthcare delivery in the rural regions of India, particularly in the state of Karnataka. The project aimed to improve the accessibility of healthcare services by deploying mobile health clinics that were connected through VANETs. These clinics provided primary healthcare services and facilitated remote consultation with specialists in urban hospitals.

17.3 DRIVER HEALTH MONITORING FOR SAFE DRIVING

17.3.1 Platform Overview

Ensuring road safety is a paramount concern in the evolving landscape of ITS. One crucial aspect contributing to safer roads is the implementation of Driver Health Monitoring Systems. These systems leverage advanced technologies to assess and monitor the health of drivers in real time, thereby enhancing road safety and response to emergency situations (illustrated in Figure 17.3).

17.3.2 Integration of Health Monitoring in Vehicles

ITS incorporate sophisticated technologies, including sensors, biometric devices, and real-time data analytics, to monitor the health status of drivers. These systems are designed to detect various health indicators such as heart rate, fatigue, and stress levels. The integration of wearable devices and in-vehicle sensors allows for continuous monitoring, providing insights into the driver's well-being during their journey.

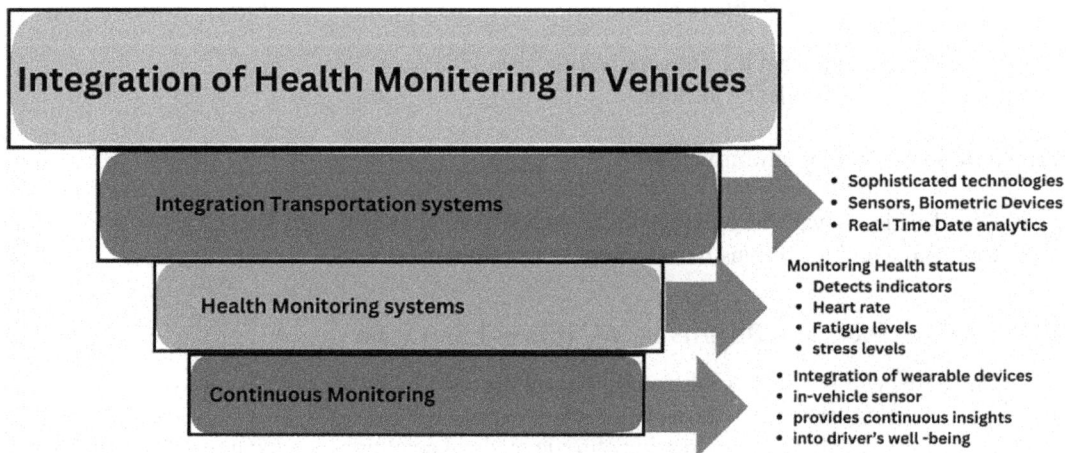

FIGURE 17.3 Driver Health Monitoring Systems.

17.3.3 REAL-TIME HEALTH ASSESSMENT

Driver Health Monitoring Systems enable real-time health assessments, offering a proactive approach to road safety. By continuously analyzing vital signs and driver behavior, these systems can detect signs of fatigue or health issues that may compromise driving capabilities. Immediate alerts can be generated for drivers, prompting them to take necessary breaks or seek medical attention, thus preventing potential accidents caused by health-related issues.

17.3.4 EMERGENCY RESPONSE AND COMMUNICATION

In the event of a health emergency or an accident, Driver Health Monitoring Systems play a critical role in initiating rapid emergency responses. Integrated communication systems can relay vital health information to emergency services and nearby healthcare facilities, ensuring that responders are well-prepared to provide appropriate medical assistance. This real-time communication facilitates a swift and targeted response, potentially saving lives and minimizing the impact of accidents.

17.3.5 CHALLENGES AND FUTURE DIRECTIONS

While Driver Health Monitoring Systems offer significant advantages, challenges such as ensuring data privacy, addressing false positives/negatives, and integrating seamlessly with existing ITS infrastructure need attention. Future directions in research and development should focus on refining algorithms for health assessment, enhancing the interoperability of monitoring systems, and developing standardized protocols for communication between vehicles and emergency services.

17.4 MOBILITY OF EMS VEHICLES

Emergency vehicle signal coordination (EVSC) methodology was proposed to provide the green path to emergency vehicles [10], with improved results obtained by traffic simulations on eight intersections in Qingdao, China. Emergency Vehicle Management System (EVMS) is proposed to identify a prompt and effective vehicle-passing sequence that enables emergency vehicles to pass through the intersections.

VANETs hold significant promise in enhancing emergency vehicle management due to their real-time communication capabilities and the potential to improve response times and overall efficiency in emergency situations. The usage of VANETs for emergency vehicles is beneficial in the following perspectives:

- **Traffic Management:** VANETs can provide real-time traffic information to emergency vehicles, enabling them to navigate through congested or blocked routes swiftly.
- **Priority Access:** These networks allow emergency vehicles to communicate with traffic signals, giving them priority access to intersections, helping reduce response times.
- **Inter-Vehicle Communication**: VANETs enable communication between emergency vehicles and nearby vehicles, helping create temporary lanes or clear paths for emergency response.
- **Communication with Infrastructure:** They facilitate communication with roadside infrastructure, enabling better coordination between emergency vehicles and traffic control systems.
- **Collision Avoidance:** VANETs can help prevent collisions by providing warnings to both emergency and regular vehicles about potential hazards or approaching emergency vehicles.
- **Situational Awareness:** They allow emergency services to have a comprehensive view of the situation by accessing real-time data from various sources, aiding in better decision-making.

- **Centralized Dispatch System**: A central system that monitors and coordinates ambulance locations, statuses, and incoming emergency calls for efficient deployment.
- **Precise GPS and Mapping**: High-precision GPSs with updated mapping data for accurate navigation to emergency locations, especially in complex urban environments.
- **Telemedicine Integration**: Enabling communication between paramedics and healthcare professionals to provide real-time medical guidance before reaching the hospital.
- **Dynamic Routing:** VANETs can dynamically reroute emergency vehicles based on real-time traffic and incident information, guiding them to the quickest and safest routes.
- **Navigation Assistance:** Providing precise navigation instructions to emergency responders, especially in unfamiliar areas or complex urban environments.

VANETs offer immense potential for enhancing emergency vehicle management, improving response times, and, ultimately, saving lives. Implementing these networks effectively involves a coordinated effort between government agencies, emergency services, infrastructure providers, and technology experts to overcome challenges and maximize the benefits of this technology in emergency situations. Despite these benefits, challenges such as network reliability, scalability, and interoperability between different communication technologies need to be addressed. Ensuring robust security measures to prevent cyber threats and maintaining data integrity are also critical in emergency scenarios.

17.5   PROTOCOLS AND ARCHITECTURES FOR ITS ASSISTING HEALTHCARE SERVICES

Healthcare services can benefit greatly from the use of ITS, particularly in situations involving patient transportation, emergency medical response, and general healthcare accessibility. The protocols and architectures listed below can be taken into consideration when incorporating ITS using healthcare services.

17.5.1   VEHICLE-TO-EVERYTHING COMMUNICATION

Protocol: Dedicated short-range communication (DSRC) or cellular vehicle-to-everything (C-V2X).

Communication between automobiles, infrastructure, pedestrians, and other devices is made possible by V2X [11]. Real-time data interchange between ambulances, hospitals, and traffic management systems can be facilitated by this in the healthcare industry. DSRC is a wireless technology purpose-built for automotive applications. Operating in the 5.9-GHz frequency band, DSRC enables low-latency communication, making it particularly well-suited for safety-critical functions such as collision avoidance, emergency braking notifications, and coordination with traffic signals. This technology facilitates direct communication between vehicles (V2V) and between vehicles and infrastructure (V2I) without the need for cellular networks, providing dependable performance even in areas with limited network coverage. DSRC has a communication range of 300 meters to 1 kilometer, allowing vehicles to interact efficiently in various traffic scenarios, including intersections and lane changes.

17.5.1.1   C-V2X

C-V2X is a communication technology that utilizes existing cellular networks to enable V2X interactions. Unlike DSRC, C-V2X supports both direct communication between vehicles (V2V) and infrastructure (V2I), as well as long-range communication through cellular networks (V2N). This dual-mode functionality offers increased flexibility and range, allowing vehicles to communicate over greater distances and access cloud-based services. C-V2X leverages the ongoing advancements in 4G LTE and 5G networks, which provide enhanced bandwidth, low latency, and the capacity to manage a large number of connected devices simultaneously. Consequently, C-V2X is viewed as a scalable solution capable of supporting sophisticated applications, including real-time traffic management, automated driving, and smart city integration.

17.5.2 ELECTRONIC HEALTH RECORD INTEGRATION

Protocol: Health Level Seven International (HL7) or Fast Healthcare Interoperability Resources (FHIR) [12].

ITS integration with defined procedures in healthcare information systems guarantees patient data interchange that runs smoothly. This makes vital medical information accessible to emergency responders while they are on the road. HL7 is a global organization that focuses on creating standards for the exchange, integration, sharing, and retrieval of electronic health information. Established in 1987, HL7 aims to enhance the interoperability of healthcare systems, enabling seamless communication among healthcare providers, organizations, and systems worldwide. HL7 is renowned for its standards, particularly those related to electronic health records (EHRs), clinical data exchange, and messaging protocols that ensure the secure and accurate transfer of patient information across different platforms. These standards are widely used in healthcare to support clinical operations, administrative functions, and research, allowing healthcare providers to access and share vital information efficiently, which contributes to better patient care and outcomes. HL7's efforts are pivotal in the global movement toward more interconnected, efficient, and patient-focused healthcare systems.

17.5.3 GPS AND GIS

Protocol: NMEA 0183 for GPS data [13].

For real-time ambulance tracking and route optimization based on traffic patterns and hospital proximity, use GPS and GIS. GIS can help locate adjacent healthcare facilities as well. NMEA 0183 is a communication protocol established by the National Marine Electronics Association (NMEA) for transmitting GPS and other navigational data between marine electronics devices. It standardizes the way GPS receivers and related instruments communicate, ensuring compatibility across different systems. NMEA 0183 transmits data in a simple serial format, where GPS data are formatted into specific sentences, each beginning with a unique identifier (such as $GPGGA for GPS fix data). These sentences contain various fields separated by commas, including latitude, longitude, speed, and time, with a checksum at the end for error detection. The protocol operates on a single-talker, multiple-listener model, meaning one device (typically the GPS receiver) sends data to multiple receiving devices, such as chart plotters or autopilots. The receiving devices parse the sentences to extract relevant information for real-time navigation, display, or storage. NMEA 0183's structured approach to data transmission ensures reliable and accurate communication between GPS devices and other navigational systems, making it a cornerstone in marine and GPS-based applications.

17.5.4 SENSOR NETWORKS

Protocol: Message Queuing Telemetry Transport (MQTT) [14] *for lightweight sensor data communication.*

Install a variety of sensors in ambulances to track patients' vital signs and send real-time data to medical professionals. This can help with patient monitoring from a distance while in transit. MQTT is a streamlined messaging protocol crafted for effective communication in resource-constrained environments, such as IoT systems. Originally developed by IBM and now established as an open standard, MQTT operates on a publish/subscribe model. In this setup, devices (clients) send messages to a central broker on designated topics, and other devices subscribed to those topics receive the messages. This approach supports scalable and flexible communication by separating data producers from consumers. MQTT is tailored for low-bandwidth, high-latency networks, ensuring efficient message delivery with minimal overhead. It features three quality of service (QoS) levels to balance reliability and performance, making it well-suited for time-sensitive applications. MQTT's versatility has led to its widespread use in various industries, including smart home systems, industrial automation, and other IoT applications, facilitating real-time data exchange and remote monitoring.

17.5.5 TELEMEDICINE INTEGRATION

Protocol: Hypertext Transfer Protocol (HTTP), Secure Real-time Transport Protocol (SRTP) for secure communication.

This integration enables implementation of telemedicine features in ambulances, allowing healthcare professionals to provide real-time guidance and support to paramedics. This requires a reliable and secure communication protocol.

HTTP is the foundational protocol used for transmitting web pages and other data over the Internet. It operates at the application layer of the Internet protocol suite and facilitates the communication between web browsers and servers by defining how requests and responses should be formatted and transmitted. HTTP is stateless, meaning each request is independent of others, and it typically uses transmission control protocol (TCP) to ensure reliable data transfer. Although HTTP is widely used for general web traffic, it does not inherently provide security features, which is why HTTP Secure (HTTPS) was developed to add encryption and secure data transmission.

In contrast, SRTP is designed specifically for securing real-time communications such as voice and video over IP networks. SRTP enhances the Real-time Transport Protocol (RTP) by providing encryption, message authentication, and integrity, ensuring that the transmitted data are secure from eavesdropping and tampering. It is commonly used in applications like Voice over IP (VoIP) and videoconferencing to protect sensitive information during transmission. By combining RTP's capabilities for real-time data delivery with SRTP's security measures, this protocol ensures both timely and secure transmission of media streams across the network.

17.5.6 CLOUD COMPUTING FOR DATA STORAGE AND PROCESSING

Protocol: Representational State Transfer (REST) for cloud API interactions.

Cloud-based solutions can store and process large amounts of healthcare and transportation data. This enables data analysis, predictive modeling, and better allocation of resources. REST is an architectural style used to design networked applications and services, primarily utilizing the HTTP. REST is founded on principles that support stateless communication, scalability, and the use of standard HTTP methods—such as GET, POST, PUT, and DELETE—for interacting with resources. In a RESTful system, resources are accessed via URLs, and operations are carried out through standardized HTTP requests. The approach emphasizes the use of straightforward, predictable URLs and stateless interactions to enhance performance and scalability. REST also accommodates various data formats, including JSON and XML, making it adaptable and compatible with different client and server setups. Its simplicity and effectiveness in providing a clear and organized interface for data access and manipulation have led to its widespread adoption in web development.

17.5.7 CYBERSECURITY MEASURES

Protocol: Transport Layer Security (TLS) for secure communication.

Apply robust cybersecurity measures to safeguard sensitive healthcare data transmitted through the ITS. This includes encryption, secure authentication, and intrusion detection systems. TLS is a protocol designed to secure communications over networks by providing encryption, authentication, and data integrity. It ensures that data transmitted between clients and servers, such as web traffic and email, remain confidential and unaltered. TLS establishes a secure, encrypted connection, protecting against eavesdropping, tampering, and impersonation. Operating at the transport layer of the Internet protocol suite, TLS works on top of protocols like TCP to enhance the security of data exchanges. As the successor to Secure Sockets Layer (SSL), TLS is essential for securing HTTPS connections and is widely used to safeguard sensitive online interactions and communications.

17.5.8 INTERAGENCY COLLABORATION FRAMEWORK

Protocol: Simple Object Access Protocol (SOAP) for web services [15].

Architecture: Establish a framework for collaboration between transportation agencies, emergency services, and healthcare providers. This involves standardizing communication protocols to ensure effective cooperation during emergencies. SOAP is a protocol designed for exchanging structured information in web services across different platforms and networks. Utilizing XML (eXtensible Markup Language), SOAP specifies a standardized message format and processing rules to ensure consistent communication between diverse systems. A SOAP message is composed of an envelope that includes a header, which may contain metadata or control information, and a body that carries the core data or request. SOAP supports multiple transport protocols, including HTTP and Simple Mail Transfer Protocol, offering flexibility in communication methods. Although more complex than REST, SOAP is renowned for its comprehensive standards for security (such as WS-Security), transactions, and reliability, making it ideal for enterprise applications that demand structured messaging and reliable service delivery.

By integrating these protocols and architectures, an ITS can enhance the efficiency of healthcare services, particularly in emergency situations, and contribute to better patient outcomes.

17.6 TECHNOLOGIES FOR ITS ASSISTING HEALTHCARE SERVICE

The symbiotic integration of transportation systems and healthcare services represents a transformative frontier in patient care. This chapter explores the dynamic interplay of cutting-edge technologies, specifically telemedicine, the IoT, GIS, fleet management systems, and AI-driven predictive analytics [16]. Together, these intelligent systems are revolutionizing the accessibility, efficiency, and overall quality of patient healthcare [17], as illustrated in Figure 17.4.

17.6.1 TELEHEALTH: REDEFINING CONSULTATIONS DURING TRAVEL

Telemedicine platforms have transcended traditional boundaries to enable seamless medical consultations while driving [18]. By leveraging videoconferencing and real-time data sharing, healthcare providers can assess a patient's condition remotely, reducing reliance on in-person visits and facilitating timely intervention [19].

Example: Imagine that a senior citizen with limited mobility can now have a video consultation with their healthcare provider while being transported to a clinic. This not only alleviates travel challenges but also ensures timely and consistent medical care [20]. Likewise, pregnant women living in remote areas can have a virtual check-up with their obstetrician while commuting to work, eliminating the hassle of traveling to a clinic.

17.6.2 IoT AND WEARABLE TECHNOLOGY

Continuous Monitoring on the Move: The integration of IoT sensors and wearable devices ensures continuous monitoring of patients throughout their journey. This section explores practical applications of wearable technology and shows how patients, especially those with chronic diseases, can communicate real-time health data to healthcare professionals during their daily commute [21].

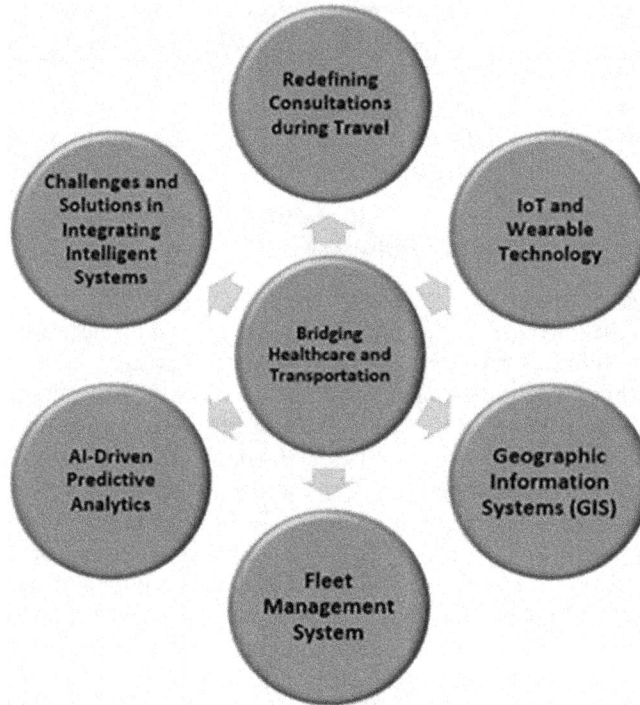

FIGURE 17.4   Bridging Healthcare and Transport.

Example: Imagine a patient with heart disease wearing a smartwatch with an ECG monitor that sends real-time data to a cardiologist during their daily commute. If a cardiologist detects an abnormality, he or she may recommend immediate treatment, potentially preventing a heart attack. Continuous monitoring through IoT and wearable devices ensures a proactive response to medical emergencies.

17.6.3   GIS

Optimizing Emergency Medical Transportation: GIS proves to be an important part of emergency medical transportation as it optimizes the route of an ambulance. This section explains the role of GIS in map analysis that considers hospital location, patient housing, and transportation options [22]. Real-life scenarios illustrate how GIS can dynamically adjust routes based on real-time traffic updates, ensuring fast response times and efficient resource allocation during emergencies.

Example: When an ambulance is dispatched to a busy downtown area, GIS dynamically adjusts the route based on real-time traffic conditions and guides the vehicle to the nearest hospital with available capacity. This strategic deployment expedites critical medical care and ensures rapid response to emergencies.

17.6.4   FLEET MANAGEMENT SYSTEM

Healthcare Logistics Orchestration: Dedicated fleet management systems have proven essential in streamlining the complex logistics of patient transport. Through real-time data analysis, these systems enable healthcare providers to track, plan, and optimize transportation routes [23].

Example: A professional medical transportation service uses fleet management software to coordinate the pickup and drop-off of patients requiring dialysis treatments. The system optimizes routes based on current traffic conditions to ensure patients receive timely treatment. This dynamic fleet management not only improves logistics efficiency, but also adapts in real time to ensure patient health remains a top priority.

17.6.5 AI-DRIVEN PREDICTIVE ANALYTICS

Predicting Patient Needs: Healthcare systems are now able to proactively anticipate and fulfil patient transportation needs, thanks to the combination of AI and predictive analytics. Patient wait times are reduced and resource allocation is optimized by machine learning algorithms that are powered by real-time and historical data [24].

17.7 CHALLENGES AND SOLUTIONS IN INTEGRATING INTELLIGENT SYSTEMS

For instance, a hospital system uses predictive analytics to estimate how much nonemergency medical transport will be needed in various neighborhoods. This makes it possible to allocate resources efficiently, which shortens wait times for patients who require transport to regular doctor's appointments. Empirical instances demonstrate how predictive analytics predict the need for nonemergency medical transport, facilitating the effective use of resources and cutting down on wait times for regular doctor appointments.

The integration of intelligent systems into healthcare presents a set of challenges that necessitate strategic solutions for the establishment of a seamless and effective healthcare ecosystem. One prominent challenge is interoperability, as the integration of diverse technologies may encounter compatibility issues. A key solution to this challenge involves standardizing communication protocols and ensuring smooth interaction between different systems. This can be achieved by adopting widely accepted healthcare data exchange standards, facilitating interoperability across the healthcare landscape. Another critical challenge revolves around safeguarding patient data privacy, considering the significant concerns surrounding the confidentiality of health information. The solution lies in implementing robust encryption protocols, such as end-to-end encryption for transmitted healthcare data, coupled with strict adherence to healthcare data protection regulations to serve as vital safeguards. Moreover, the complexity of regulatory compliance within the healthcare sector poses a formidable obstacle. Navigating through intricate healthcare regulations requires a strategic approach involving collaboration with regulatory bodies, adherence to industry standards, and staying well-informed about evolving compliance requirements. Maintaining open communication channels with regulatory authorities becomes crucial, providing clarity on compliance standards and ensuring a smoother integration process. Addressing these challenges proactively is paramount to unlocking the full potential of intelligent systems in healthcare, safeguarding data security, privacy, and compliance with regulatory standards.

Transit networks integrated with healthcare services have revolutionized patient care. Cutting-edge technologies such as telemedicine, IoT, GIS, fleet management systems, and predictive analytics are improving accessibility, effectiveness, and quality of care.

To realize the full potential of intelligent systems in healthcare, challenges such as regulatory compliance, patient data protection, and interoperability need to be addressed. Collaborative efforts to navigate healthcare legislation, create strong encryption, and standardize communication methods are essential.

By overcoming these obstacles, we can create a smooth, efficient healthcare environment that values patient privacy, data security, and regulatory compliance. Proactive approaches, well-thought-out solutions, and continuous integration of cutting-edge technologies into the healthcare delivery framework are essential to achieve accessible, effective, and high-quality healthcare.

17.8 CHALLENGES AND SCOPE FOR RESEARCH

VANETs offer promising opportunities for healthcare applications, especially in scenarios like EMS, remote monitoring, and disseminating health-related information [25]. However, several challenges persist in utilizing VANETs for healthcare purposes:

Intermittent Connectivity: VANETs rely on vehicular communication, which can be intermittent due to mobility, signal interference, or varying network densities. Maintaining continuous connectivity for healthcare applications is challenging [26].

Network Stability: VANETs face challenges in maintaining stable connections, especially in dynamic traffic environments or areas with limited infrastructure support.

Quality of Communication: VANETs may encounter issues related to latency, packet loss, and bandwidth limitations, affecting the transmission of critical healthcare data in real time [27].

Prioritization of Traffic: Ensuring prioritized communication for healthcare-related data over other types of traffic is crucial. However, achieving this balance without impacting the overall network performance can be challenging.

Data Security: Healthcare data transmitted over VANETs need robust security measures to prevent unauthorized access, tampering, or interception, ensuring patient privacy and data integrity [28].

Authentication and Trust: Establishing trust among vehicles and infrastructure units is essential to avoid malicious attacks or unauthorized access to sensitive health information.

Infrastructure Requirements: VANETs often require a robust and extensive infrastructure, including RSUs and dedicated healthcare-related network components, which might not be universally available.

Standardization Issues: Lack of standardized protocols and interoperability between different VANET systems and healthcare devices can hinder seamless integration and data exchange.

17.8.1 REGULATORY AND ETHICAL CHALLENGES

Handling of healthcare data over VANETs poses challenges as they need to obtain compliance with healthcare regulatory bodies. Health Insurance Portability and Accountability Act (HIPAA) is one of the standard regulatory bodies that regulates the storage and transmission [29].

Ethical Concerns: Ensuring ethical use of healthcare data, consent management, and respecting patient privacy in a highly dynamic and shared network environment is critical.

Deployment Costs: Implementing VANET-based healthcare systems requires substantial investment in infrastructure, equipment, and maintenance, potentially limiting widespread adoption [30].

Scalability: As the number of connected vehicles and healthcare devices increases, ensuring scalability without compromising performance becomes challenging.

Need for Awareness: There is a need to impart confidence about these technologies to the public in advance, before implementation. While applying any means for their health, humans need to be convinced psychologically.

Addressing these challenges requires collaborative efforts among researchers, policymakers, healthcare providers, and technology experts to develop robust solutions that prioritize patient safety, data security, and efficient communication within VANETs for healthcare applications.

17.9 CONCLUSION

An ITS tailored for ambulances has the potential to significantly improve emergency response times, patient outcomes, and overall efficiency in EMS. By harnessing real-time data and advanced communication technologies, such a system can optimize route planning and enhance coordination between responders and medical facilities. Successful implementation of this system will require collaboration among healthcare providers, technology experts, government agencies, and infrastructure developers.

Future research should focus on refining predictive algorithms, ensuring system scalability, and integrating emerging technologies like AI, IoT, and 5G. As we advance, potential developments such as AI-driven decision support and drone-assisted medical deliveries could further enhance the capabilities of ambulance services. While challenges remain, the future of ITS in healthcare is promising, with the potential to revolutionize EMS and improve public health outcomes.

REFERENCES

1. D. Oladimeji, K. Gupta, N. A. Kose, K. Gundogan, L. Ge, and F. Liang, "Smart Transportation: An Overview of Technologies and Applications," *Sensors*, vol. 23, no. 8, Art. no. 8, Jan. 2023, doi: 10.3390/s23083880.
2. D. A. Christian, A. Bachtiar, and C. Candi, "Analysis of Health-Based Transportation System for Health Transformation in DKI Jakarta," *JOSR*, vol. 2, no. 11, pp. 4103–4112, Oct. 2023, doi: 10.55324/josr.v2i11.1568.
3. M. Saad Talib, A. Hassan, B. Hussin, A. Abdul-Jabbar Mohammed, A. Abdulhussian Hassan, and A. Awad Mutlag, "Vehicular Ad hoc Network for Intelligent Transport System: A Review," *IJET*, vol. 7, no. 4.36, p. 350, Dec. 2018, doi: 10.14419/ijet.v7i4.36.23803.
4. N. H. Hussein, C. T. Yaw, S. P. Koh, S. K. Tiong, and K. H. Chong, "A Comprehensive Survey on Vehicular Networking: Communications, Applications, Challenges, and Upcoming Research Directions," *IEEE Access*, vol. 10, pp. 86127–86180, 2022, doi: 10.1109/ACCESS.2022.3198656.
5. K. A. Khaliq, O. Chughtai, A. Qayyum, and J. Pannek, "An Emergency Alert System for Elderly/Special People Using VANET and WBAN," in *2017 13th International Conference on Emerging Technologies (ICET)*, Islamabad: IEEE, Dec. 2017, pp. 1–6. doi: 10.1109/ICET.2017.8281757.
6. J. El Ouadi, N. Malhene, S. Benhadou, and H. Medromi, "Shared Public Transport within a Physical Internet Framework: Reviews, Conceptualization and Expected Challenges Under COVID-19 Pandemic," *IATSS Research*, vol. 45, no. 4, pp. 417–439, Dec. 2021, doi: 10.1016/j.iatssr.2021.03.001.
7. Y. M. Bhavsar, M. S. Zaveri, M. S. Raval, and S. B. Zaveri, "Vision-Based Investigation of Road Traffic and Violations at Urban Roundabout in India Using UAV Video: A Case Study," *Transportation Engineering*, vol. 14, p. 100207, Dec. 2023, doi: 10.1016/j.treng.2023.100207.
8. S. Basu and P. Saha, "Evaluation of Risk Factors for Road Accidents Under Mixed Traffic: Case Study on Indian Highways," *IATSS Research*, vol. 46, no. 4, pp. 559–573, Dec. 2022, doi: 10.1016/j.iatssr.2022.09.004.
9. Juan Carlos Cano, Carlos T. Calafate, and Pietro Manzoni, "VANETs for Smart Cities: Efficient Emergency Services through Traffic Management," IEEE Transactions on Intelligent Transportation Systems, 2019.
10. P. Oza and T. Chantem, "Timely and Non-Disruptive Response of Emergency Vehicles: A Real-Time Approach," in *29th International Conference on Real-Time Networks and Systems*, NANTES France: ACM, Apr. 2021, pp. 192–203. doi: 10.1145/3453417.3453434.
11. A. Rayamajhi, A. Yoseph, A. Balse, Z. Huang, E. M. Leslie, and V. Fessmann, "Preliminary Performance Baseline Testing for Dedicated Short-Range Communication (DSRC) and Cellular Vehicle-to-Everything (C-V2X)," in *2020 IEEE 92nd Vehicular Technology Conference (VTC2020-Fall)*, Victoria, BC, Canada: IEEE, Nov. 2020, pp. 1–5. doi: 10.1109/VTC2020-Fall49728.2020.9348708.
12. C. N. Vorisek *et al.*, "Fast Healthcare Interoperability Resources (FHIR) for Interoperability in Health Research: Systematic Review," *JMIR Med Inform*, vol. 10, no. 7, p. e35724, Jul. 2022, doi: 10.2196/35724.
13. B. Senkus, B. Yaman, H. Aydin, and M. Soyturk, "Implementation of High Performance Multi-Agent Position Feeding Framework," in *2022 24th International Microwave and Radar Conference (MIKON)*, Gdansk, Poland: IEEE, Sep. 2022, pp. 1–5. doi: 10.23919/MIKON54314.2022.9924764.

14. D. Kurniawan, R. J. Putra, A. Bella, M. Ashar, and K. Dedes, "Smart Garden with IoT Based Real Time Communication using MQTT Protocol," in *2021 7th International Conference on Electrical, Electronics and Information Engineering (ICEEIE)*, Malang, Indonesia: IEEE, Oct. 2021, pp. 1–5. doi: 10.1109/ICEEIE52663.2021.9616869.

15. G. Ajvazi and F. Halili, "SOAP Messaging to Provide Quality of Protection through Kerberos Authentication," in *2022 29th International Conference on Systems, Signals and Image Processing (IWSSIP)*, Sofia, Bulgaria: IEEE, Jun. 2022, pp. 1–4. doi: 10.1109/IWSSIP55020.2022.9854476.

16. A. N. Navaz, M. A. Serhani, H. T. El Kassabi, N. Al-Qirim, and H. Ismail, "Trends, Technologies, and Key Challenges in Smart and Connected Healthcare," *IEEE Access*, vol. 9, pp. 74044–74067, 2021, doi: 10.1109/ACCESS.2021.3079217.

17. S. A. Alowais *et al.*, "Revolutionizing Healthcare: The Role of Artificial Intelligence in Clinical Practice," *BMC Med Educ*, vol. 23, no. 1, p. 689, Sep. 2023, doi: 10.1186/s12909-023-04698-z.

18. S. N. Gajarawala and J. N. Pelkowski, "Telehealth Benefits and Barriers," *The Journal for Nurse Practitioners*, vol. 17, no. 2, pp. 218–221, Feb. 2021, doi: 10.1016/j.nurpra.2020.09.013.

19. A. Haleem, M. Javaid, R. P. Singh, and R. Suman, "Telemedicine for Healthcare: Capabilities, Features, Barriers, and Applications," *Sensors International*, vol. 2, p. 100117, 2021, doi: 10.1016/j.sintl.2021.100117.

20. S. Abdi, A. Spann, J. Borilovic, L. De Witte, and M. Hawley, "Understanding the Care and Support Needs of Older People: A Scoping Review and Categorisation Using the WHO International Classification of Functioning, Disability and Health Framework (ICF)," *BMC Geriatr*, vol. 19, no. 1, p. 195, Dec. 2019, doi: 10.1186/s12877-019-1189-9.

21. W.-H. Wang and W.-S. Hsu, "Integrating Artificial Intelligence and Wearable IoT System in Long-Term Care Environments," *Sensors*, vol. 23, no. 13, p. 5913, Jun. 2023, doi: 10.3390/s23135913.

22. L. Zhou, S. Wang, and Z. Xu, "A Multi-factor Spatial Optimization Approach for Emergency Medical Facilities in Beijing," *IJGI*, vol. 9, no. 6, p. 361, Jun. 2020, doi: 10.3390/ijgi9060361.

23. M. Pons, E. Valenzuela, B. Rodríguez, J. A. Nolazco-Flores, and C. Del-Valle-Soto, "Utilization of 5G Technologies in IoT Applications: Current Limitations by Interference and Network Optimization Difficulties—A Review," *Sensors*, vol. 23, no. 8, p. 3876, Apr. 2023, doi: 10.3390/s23083876.

24. A. Bohr and K. Memarzadeh, "The Rise of Artificial Intelligence in Healthcare Applications," in *Artificial Intelligence in Healthcare*, Elsevier, 2020, pp. 25–60. doi: 10.1016/B978-0-12-818438-7.00002-2.

25. M. Maad Hamdi, L. Audah, S. Abduljabbar Rashid, A. Hamid Mohammed, S. Alani, and A. Shamil Mustafa, "A Review of Applications, Characteristics and Challenges in Vehicular Ad Hoc Networks (VANETs)," in *2020 International Congress on Human-Computer Interaction, Optimization and Robotic Applications (HORA)*, Ankara, Turkey: IEEE, Jun. 2020, pp. 1–7. doi: 10.1109/HORA49412.2020.9152928.

26. M. Naderi and M. Ghanbari, "Adaptively Prioritizing Candidate Forwarding Set in Opportunistic Routing in VANETs," *Ad Hoc Networks*, vol. 140, p. 103048, Mar. 2023, doi: 10.1016/j.adhoc.2022.103048.

27. S. Zeadally, R. Hunt, Y.-S. Chen, A. Irwin, and A. Hassan, "Vehicular ad hoc Networks (VANETS): Status, Results, and Challenges," *Telecommun Syst*, vol. 50, no. 4, pp. 217–241, Aug. 2012, doi: 10.1007/s11235-010-9400-5.

28. M. Mehrtak *et al.*, "Security Challenges and Solutions Using Healthcare Cloud Computing," *JMedLife*, vol. 14, no. 4, pp. 448–461, Aug. 2021, doi: 10.25122/jml-2021–0100.

29. R. M. Califf and L. H. Muhlbaier, "Health Insurance Portability and Accountability Act (HIPAA): Must There Be a Trade-Off between Privacy and Quality of Health Care, or Can We Advance Both?," *Circulation*, vol. 108, no. 8, pp. 915–918, Aug. 2003, doi: 10.1161/01.CIR.0000085720.65685.90.

30. T. Karunathilake and A. Förster, "A Survey on Mobile Road Side Units in VANETs," *Vehicles*, vol. 4, no. 2, pp. 482–500, May 2022, doi: 10.3390/vehicles4020029.

18 COVID-19
Predicting Daily Caseload and Mortality during Multiple Waves of the Epidemic in Different Countries

M. I. M. Wahab, Azam Dekamin, Nades Palaniyar,
Mohamad Y. Jaber, and Horace Chan

18.1 INTRODUCTION

A novel severe acute respiratory syndrome coronavirus 2 (SARS-CoV-2) infection in humans causes coronavirus disease 2019 (COVID-19) (Oves et al., 2020; Jiang et al., 2020; Cascella et al., 2020). COVID-19 was first reported in December 2019 among people living in Wuhan, China (World Health Organization, 2020), and it has spread globally, infecting large portions of the population in almost every country. As of October 2022, over 628 million cases of the disease and 6.57 million deaths have been reported in multiple waves worldwide (Worldometers, 2021), including Canada, the United States, Germany, Italy, and Spain. Predicting the spread of COVID-19 is essential to prevent overloading of the healthcare system and make appropriate plans to minimize the impact of the pandemic on the economy. Current models do not satisfactorily forecast the waves for extended periods in different countries. Many early models used the data over a few months for prediction (Wu et al., 2020; Sun et al., 2020). These models may sufficiently predict the pandemic in certain countries, but they are often inadequate to predict the pandemic in many countries that experience multiple waves over several years. Therefore, models predicting multiple waves (infection and death) in various countries would be useful.

A diffusion model is used to predict the number of daily cases of COVID-19 because most epidemic curves of the spread of diseases show exponential growth and decay. The diffusion model that best explains such characteristics is the Bass diffusion model (BDM; Bass, 1969). The BDM for COVID-19 uses a concept similar to the diffusion of a new product (virus) in a market (population) where potential adapters (patients) would adapt the product (get infected) from current/past adapters (patients) via word-of-mouth (spread of virus). Others have extended the BDM to incorporate various features (Bass et al., 1994; Norton & Bass, 1987; Jiang & Jain, 2012). Certain social media platforms (e.g., Facebook) use the Prophet model to determine market diffusion (Facebook, 2020). We developed a modified model incorporating the concepts of BDM and Prophet models. Our model predicts the number of daily cases over multiple epidemic curves and the number of deaths that occur when trying to flatten the epidemic curve accurately. Hence, this chapter provides a decision tool that predicts the number of daily cases during pandemic waves and could help better manage healthcare capacity, especially in intensive care units (ICUs).

18.2 METHODS

18.2.1 DATA COLLECTION AND MODELING OF THE DAILY INFECTED CASES

We collected the number of cases from the Johns Hopkins University Center for Systems Science and Engineering, a reliable data source in the world (JHUCSSE, 2020). We adapted BDM (Bass,

DOI: 10.1201/9781003485629-18

1969) to predict multiple epidemic curves. In particular, we used the Johns Hopkins data and predicted the (i) number of daily cases, (ii) total number of cases over the whole epidemic, (iii) peak value of the number of daily cases, and (iv) percentage of the population infected during the epidemic.

18.2.2 FORECASTING THE DAILY INFECTED CASES

Let t be any day during the epidemic period. Let $g(t)$ be the likelihood of infection at time t, and $G(t)$ be the cumulative function of the likelihood of infection. The relationship between the likelihood of infection and the cumulative function of the likelihood of infection can be expressed as

$$G(t) = \int_0^t g(t)\,dt. \tag{18.1}$$

The likelihood of infection at time t given that one has not yet been infected is given by

$$\frac{g(t)}{[1 - G(t)]} = a + bG(t), \tag{18.2}$$

where a and b are positive constants. The left-hand side of Eq. (18.2) is the hazard rate. The right-hand side of Eq. (2) shows that the hazard rate is linear in the cumulative function of the likelihood of infection. Knowing $G(0) = 0$, a, and b, the solution to Eq. (18.2) can be written as

$$G(t) = \frac{1 - e^{-(a+b)t}}{1 + \left(\dfrac{b}{a}\right)e^{-(a+b)t}}, \tag{18.3}$$

and the likelihood of infection is given by

$$g(t) = \frac{d}{dt}G(t) = \frac{\left[\dfrac{(a+b)^2}{a}\right]e^{-(a+b)t}}{\left(1 + \left(\dfrac{b}{a}\right)e^{-(a+b)t}\right)^2}. \tag{18.4}$$

Reinfections within a short period of time are unusual (Wherry, 2021) and also lead to a 90% lower probability of hospitalization (Abu-Raddad et al., 2021). Hence, those infected by SARS-CoV-2 for the second time experience mild symptoms that do not burden the healthcare system, that is, rarely require ICU beds. Therefore, the number of infected cases at day t, $I(t) = mg(t)$, is given by

$$I(t) = am + (b - a)T(t) - (b/m)[T(t)]^2, \tag{18.5}$$

where $T(t)$ is the cumulative number of infected cases in the $(0, t)$ interval, and $T(t) = mG(t)$, where m is the total number of infected cases during the epidemic.

18.2.3 ESTIMATING THE PARAMETERS OF THE MODEL

The number of daily infected cases is given by Eq. (18.5). To estimate the parameters of the model, a, b, and m, the following expression is used: $I(t) = \alpha + \beta T_{t-1} + \gamma(T_{t-1})^2$, where $t \geq 2$, $I(t)$ is the number of infected cases at day t, and T_{t-1} is the cumulative number of cases through day

$t-1$. Since $\alpha=am$, $\beta=b-a$, and $\gamma=-b/m$, the coefficients of Eq. (5) can be found, where $a=\alpha/m$, $b=\beta+\alpha/m$, and $m=\left(-\beta\pm\sqrt{\beta^2-4\alpha\gamma}\right)/2\gamma$.

18.2.4 Forecasting the Number of Deaths

Given the number of daily cases, we also predicted the number of daily deaths due to COVID-19. Time series is one of the forecasting methods that analyzes the previous observations and predicts the future. The Prophet model is a nonlinear regression model that can fit daily, weekly, and yearly seasonality well using open-source analytical tools (Facebook, 2020). This flexible time series analysis can handle missing values and outliers besides predicting the future. The Prophet model uses adjustable parameters at its core, although it works well with the default values. The Prophet model can also work with multivariate and univariate datasets. We applied a multivariate Prophet model to analyze the COVID-19 time-series data. Inputs to the model were the daily number of cases and deaths, and the output was the daily number of deaths.

18.3 RESULTS

18.3.1 The First Epidemic Wave

To predict the first epidemic wave, data for the daily cases up to April 10, 2020, were obtained from the Johns Hopkins University Center for Systems Science and Engineering (JHUCSSE, 2020). The extracted data were rearranged before implementing a nonlinear regression described in Eq. (18.5). The nonlinear regression was implemented using Python. The model was applied to the daily case data obtained for several countries. Predicted epidemic curves for Italy, the United States (Figure 18.1, Table 18.1), Spain, Germany, and Canada (wave 1 peaks, Table 18.1) fitted the datasets well. Based on the predicted epidemic curve for each country, we determined the peak of the epidemic curves in which the highest predicted number of daily cases occurred (Table 18.1). The right tail of the predicted epidemic curves reliably provided the end of a particular epidemic wave. We also plotted the cumulative daily cases of the first wave based on the predicted and the actual cumulative daily cases for Italy, Spain, Germany, the United States, and Canada (Figure 18.2A–E). These analyses show that the model predicted a single wave well, and this form of the graph can also be used to predict the end of the waves.

18.3.2 Multiple Epidemic Curves

In general, the number of cases was low in the summer of 2020, representing the end of the first wave in many countries. The number of cases started to increase in the fall and winter of 2020. That was the second major wave. To predict the second wave, we collected the daily cases as of December 14, 2020, from the Johns Hopkins University Center for Systems Science and Engineering (JHUCSSE, 2020). We used the same modified diffusion model outlined in Section 18.2 to predict the subsequent waves. The periods of the first, second, and third waves vary from country to country (Table 18.2). When Canada, Germany, Italy, and Spain were in the second wave, the United States was already in the third curve.

The model predicted the peak (i.e., the dates for the highest number of daily cases) for each epidemic curve (Table 18.2). Plotting daily and cumulative datasets shows that the real data matches well with the predicted datasets (e.g., Canadian dataset; Figure 18.3A, B). The second epidemic wave shows a drop and a rise in the actual daily cases in October 2020. Spikes often indicated that the weekend data were added on Mondays. Such spikes may lead to a higher prediction of the number of cases. The cumulative curves often eliminate the spurious peaks occurring in the daily case datasets and predict the pandemic curves correctly (Figure 18.3B). The model also correctly predicted the daily cases with two waves for Italy (Figure 18.4), Spain (Figure 18.5), and Germany

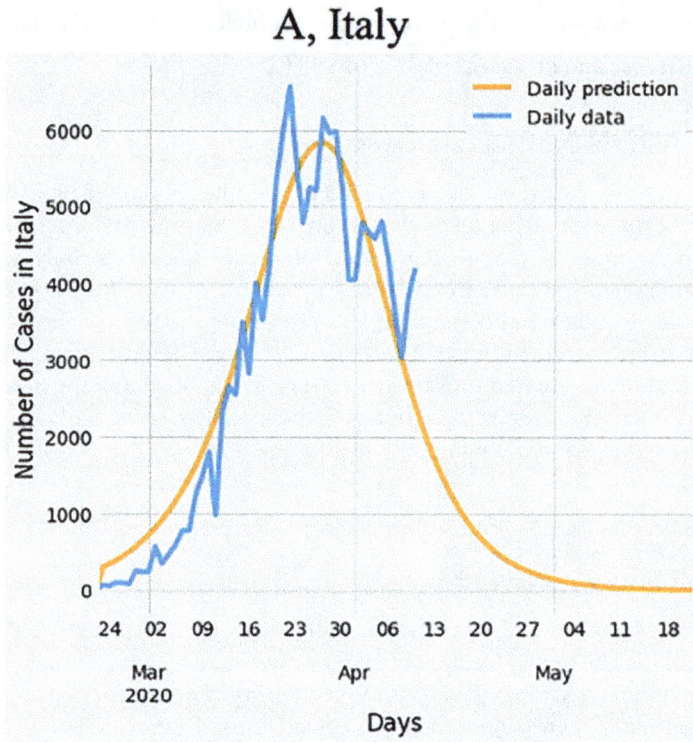

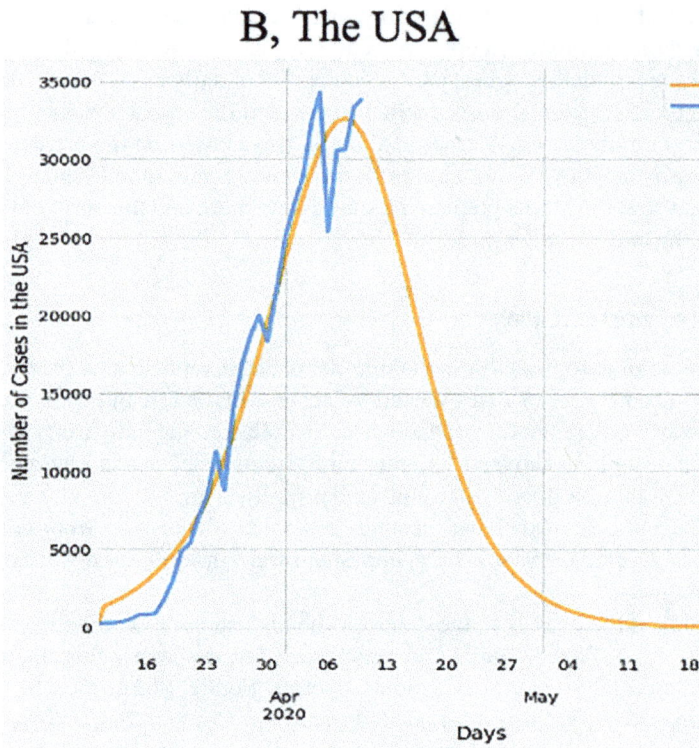

FIGURE 18.1 Actual Daily Cases for Italy and the United States as of April 10, 2020, and Their Predicted Curves of the First Wave of the Pandemic. (A) Italy. (B) The United States. Blue, actual daily cases. Yellow, predicted daily cases.

TABLE 18.1

Estimated Date for the Highest Number of Daily Cases as of April 10, 2020

Country	Peak Date
Italy	March 27, 2020
Spain	April 4, 2020
Germany	April 4, 2020
United States	April 8, 2020
Canada	April 9, 2020

TABLE 18.2

Estimated Dates of the Highest Number of Daily Cases (Peaks), Based on the Modified Diffusion Model Using the Data up to December 14, 2020

Country	First Wave	Second Wave	Second Wave peak	Third Wave	Third Wave Peak
Italy	2020-03-13 to 2020-09-30	2020-10-01 to 2020-12-14*	2020-11-16	-	-
Spain	2020-03-13 to 2020-07-01	2020-07-02 to 2020-12-14*	2020-10-30	-	-
Germany	2020-03-09 to 2020-08-22	2020-08-23 to 2020-12-14*	2020-12-01	-	-
United States	2020-03-13 to 2020-06-15	2020-06-15 to 2020-08-19	2020-07-26	2020-08-20 to 2020-12-14*	2021-03-31
Canada	2020-03-13 to 2020-08-07	2020-08-08 to 2020-12-14*	2020-12-29	-	-

*Note that * indicates the last date of the data collected for the prediction studies, but not the end of the waves.*

(Figure 18.6). Hence, the model can predict daily case numbers in the pandemic with two waves in different countries.

Based on the dataset (up to December 14, 2020), it was apparent that the United States experienced three waves in the same period (Figure 18.7A). The model correctly represented those three waves and further predicted the next peak and the extent of the third wave (Figure 18.7A, B; Table 18.2). Therefore, the modified diffusion model predicts one, two, and three waves of the COVID-19 pandemic in different countries based on the partial data available at a given time point of the pandemic.

18.3.3 PREDICTION OF DEATH RATE

We used a multivariate Prophet model to predict the COVID-19 death rates in Canada (two waves) and the United States (three waves). Daily COVID-19 deaths in Canada from March 13, 2020, to December 14, 2020, had a full wave and a partial wave (Figure 18.8A). We first tested/trained the model for a period of 15 days (June 01, 2020, to June 15, 2020), when the number of deaths was decreasing (Figure 18.8B). We next tested/trained the model for one month (from November 1, 2020, to December 1, 2020) when the death rate was increasing (Figure 18.8C). Finally, we predicted the number of COVID-19 deaths in Canada during the rest of the second wave using all the records except the periods selected for testing/training the model (from December 14, 2020, to April 15, 2021; Figure 18.8D). Based on the prediction, the cumulative number of deaths in Canada during the first two waves (from March 13, 2020, to April 15, 2021) was 21,982, and the mean absolute percentage deviation of the model-based prediction was 16.25. Therefore, the multivariate Prophet model used in this study was able to predict the death rates well in the pandemic with two waves.

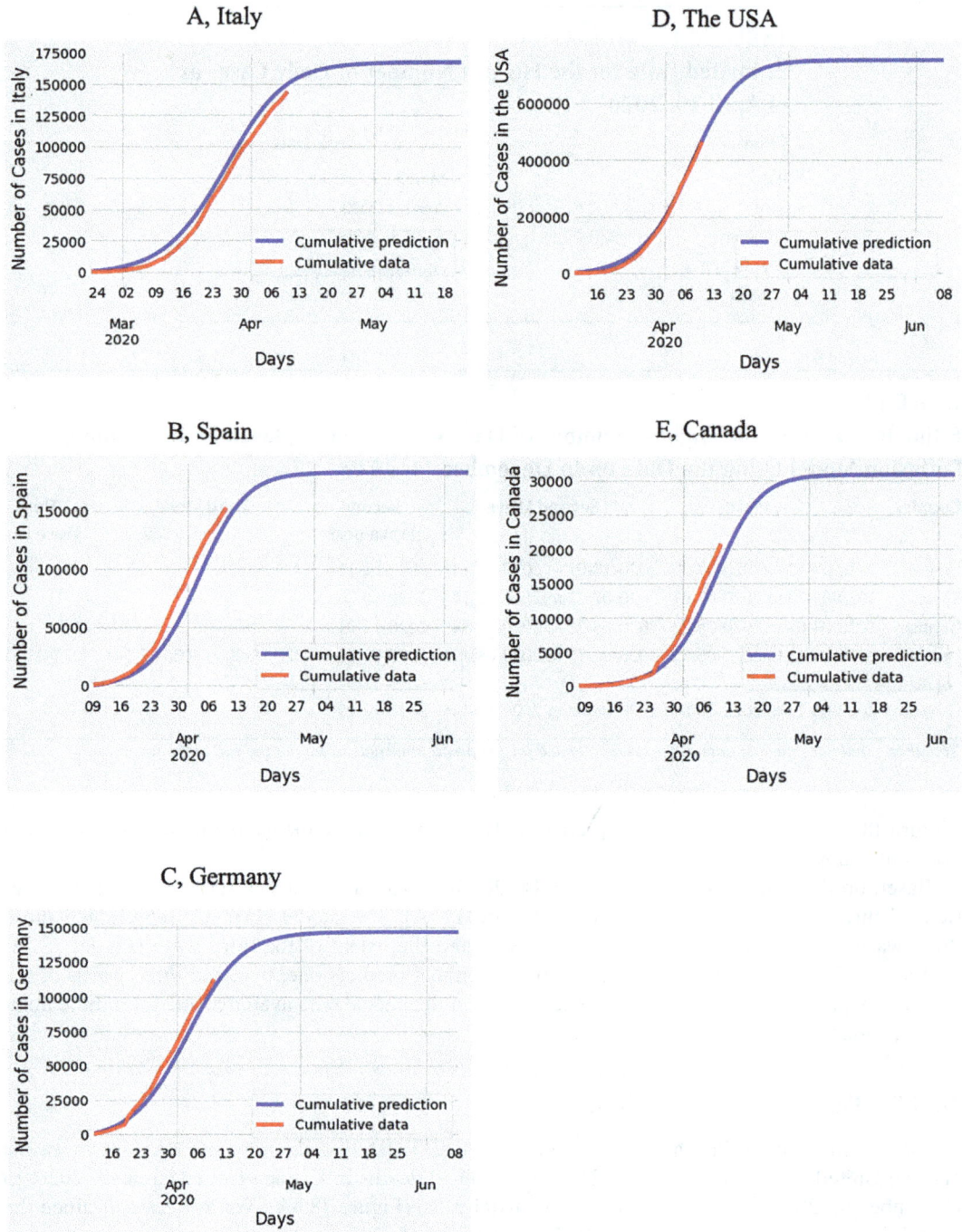

FIGURE 18.2 Observed and Predicted Cumulative Cases during the First Wave of the Pandemic in Italy, Spain, Germany, the United States, and Canada. The prediction was made based on the data collected from the beginning of the pandemic up to April 10, 2020. (A) Italy, (B) Spain, (C) Germany, (D) the United States, and (E) Canada. Red, observed cumulative cases. Blue, predicted cumulative cases.

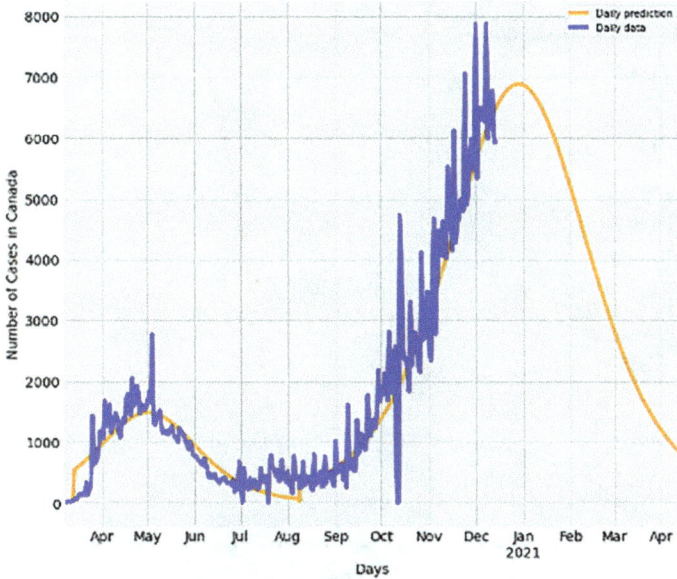

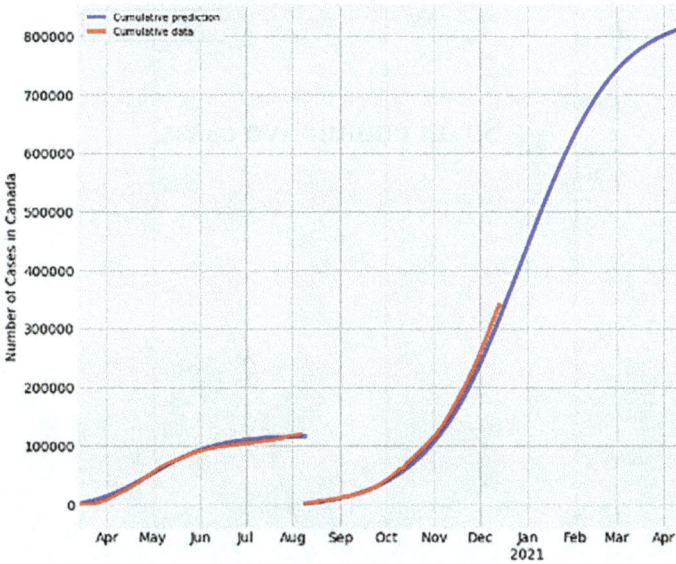

FIGURE 18.3 Actual and Predicted Daily and Cumulative Cases of the First and Second COVID-19 Waves in Canada. (A) Actual daily cases (blue) in Canada as of December 14, 2020, and predicted curve (yellow; up to April 10, 2021) during the first two waves of the pandemic. Ovals highlight the irregularities in data deposition to the database. (B) Actual cumulative data (red) for Canada based on the data from the beginning of the pandemic up to December 14, 2020, and predicted cumulative curves for waves 1 and 2, up to April 10, 2021.

Italy cumulative cases

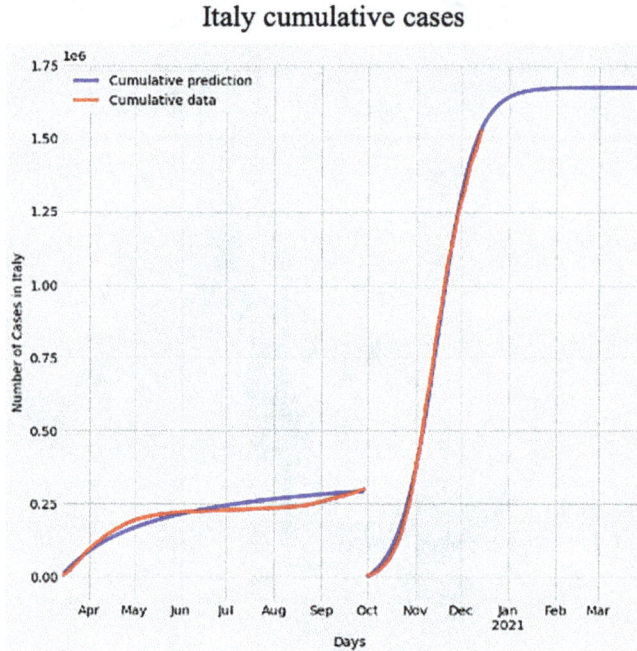

FIGURE 18.4 Cumulative Actual and Predicted Curves of Italy's First Two COVID-19 Waves. Actual cumulative cases (red) in Italy as of December 14, 2020, and predicted curves (blue) during the first two waves of the pandemic.

Spain cumulative cases

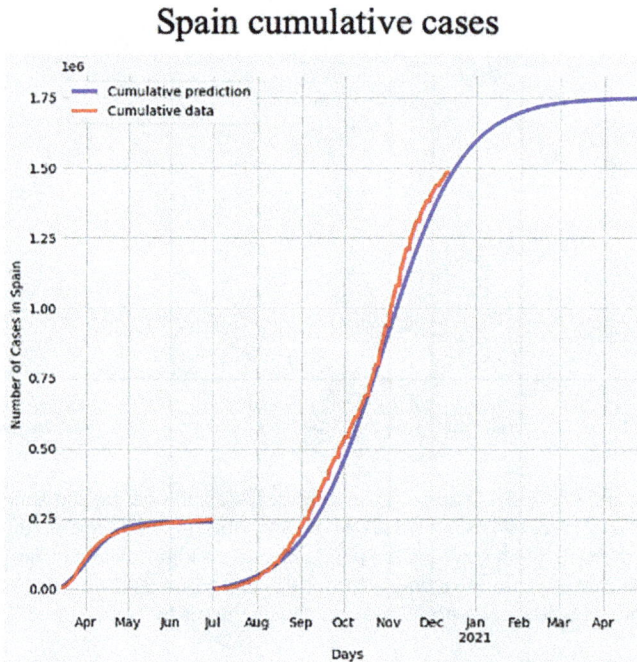

FIGURE 18.5 Cumulative Actual and Predicted Cases of Spain's First Two COVID-19 Waves. Actual cumulative cases (red) in Spain as of December 14, 2020, and predicted curves (blue) during the first two waves of the pandemic until April 10, 2021.

Germany cumulative cases

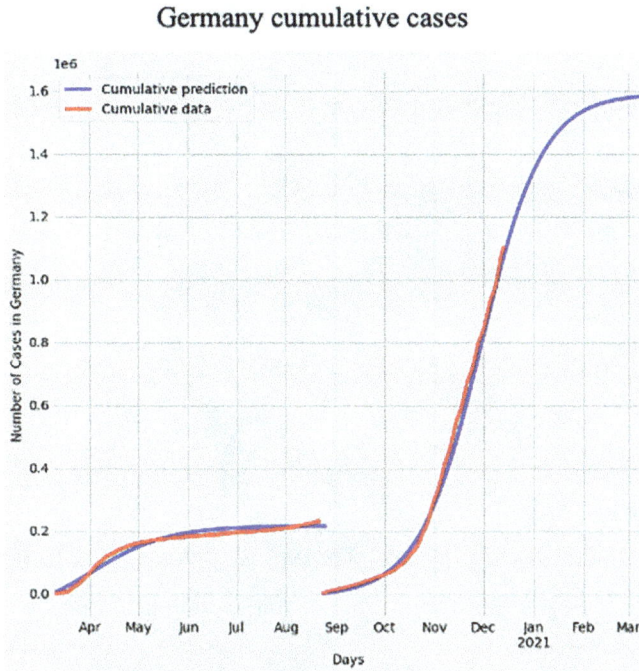

FIGURE 18.6 Cumulative Actual and Predicted Cases of Germany's First Two COVID-19 Waves. Actual cumulative cases (red) in Germany as of December 14, 2020, and predicted curves (blue) during the first two waves of the pandemic.

COVID-19 daily deaths in the United States had a large first wave, a smaller second wave, and a partial third wave (March 13, 2020, to December 14, 2020; Figure 18.9A). We first tested/trained the model for 14 days (May 11–25, 2020), when the number of deaths decreased (Figure 18.9B). We next tested/trained the model for 15 days (July 26, 2020, to August 10, 2020), when the number of deaths was not changing drastically (Figure 18.9C). Finally, we tested/trained the model for 19 days (October 11–30, 2020), when the number of deaths increased (Figure 18.9D). These three tests/ training sessions were conducted at different peaks. Using the trained model, we predicted the daily COVID-19 deaths in the United States for the next 3 months (March 14, 2020, to June 16, 2021); we used all the records for prediction, except the periods selected for testing/training the model (Figure 18.9E). The cumulative number of deaths in the United States for the entire period (March 14, 2020, to June 16, 2021) was 734,966, and the mean absolute percentage deviation was 14.62. Therefore, the multivariate Prophet model used in this study was also able to predict the death rates well in the pandemic with three waves.

18.4   FLATTENING AN EPIDEMIC CURVE WITH MITIGATION

In this section, we investigate how a country could control the number of daily cases within the available healthcare capacity—a strategy known as "flattening the curve." A graphical representation of this is depicted in Figure 18.10.

The model presented in Section 18.2 has no mitigation factor. Such models do not represent situations resulting in an overwhelming healthcare system, probably in a collapse (Díaz-Guio et al., 2020; Buheji et al., 2020). In contrast, in this section, we adopt a generalized model in Bass et al. (1994) for the case where there are efforts to flatten the curve. Let $y(t)$ be the effort by the government to mitigate the number of cases on day t. Such mitigation delays the likelihood of infection.

A, The USA daily cases

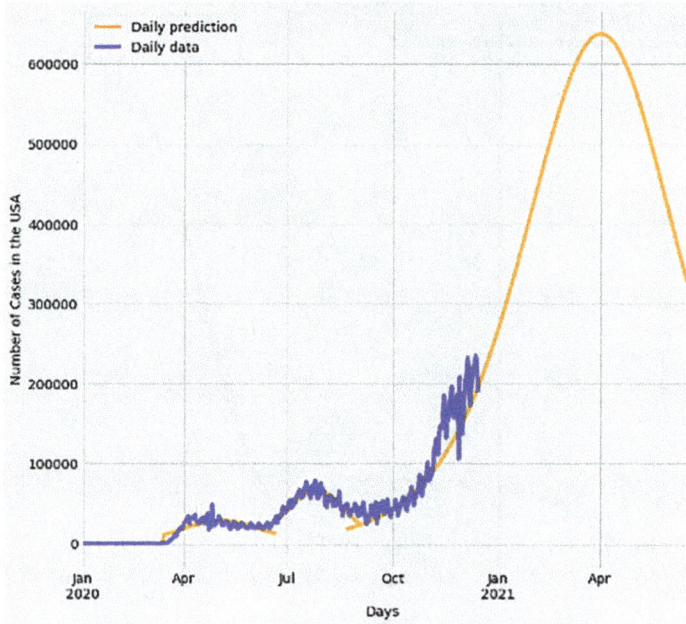

B, The USA cumulative cases

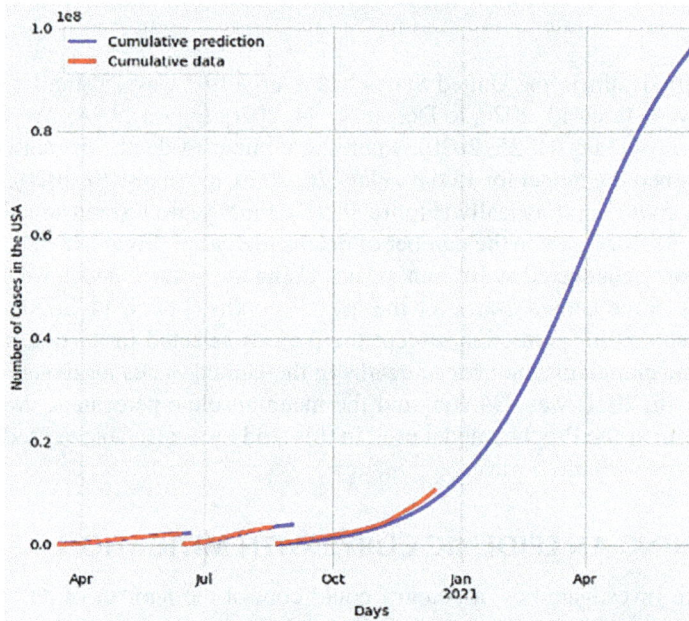

FIGURE 18.7   Daily and Cumulative Actual Cases and Predicted Curves of the United States' First Three COVID-19 Waves. (A) Observed daily cases (blue) in the United States as of December 14, 2020, and predicted curve (yellow) during the first three waves of the pandemic. (B) Actual cumulative data (red) for the United States as of December 14, 2020, and predicted cumulative curves for waves 1, 2, and 3.

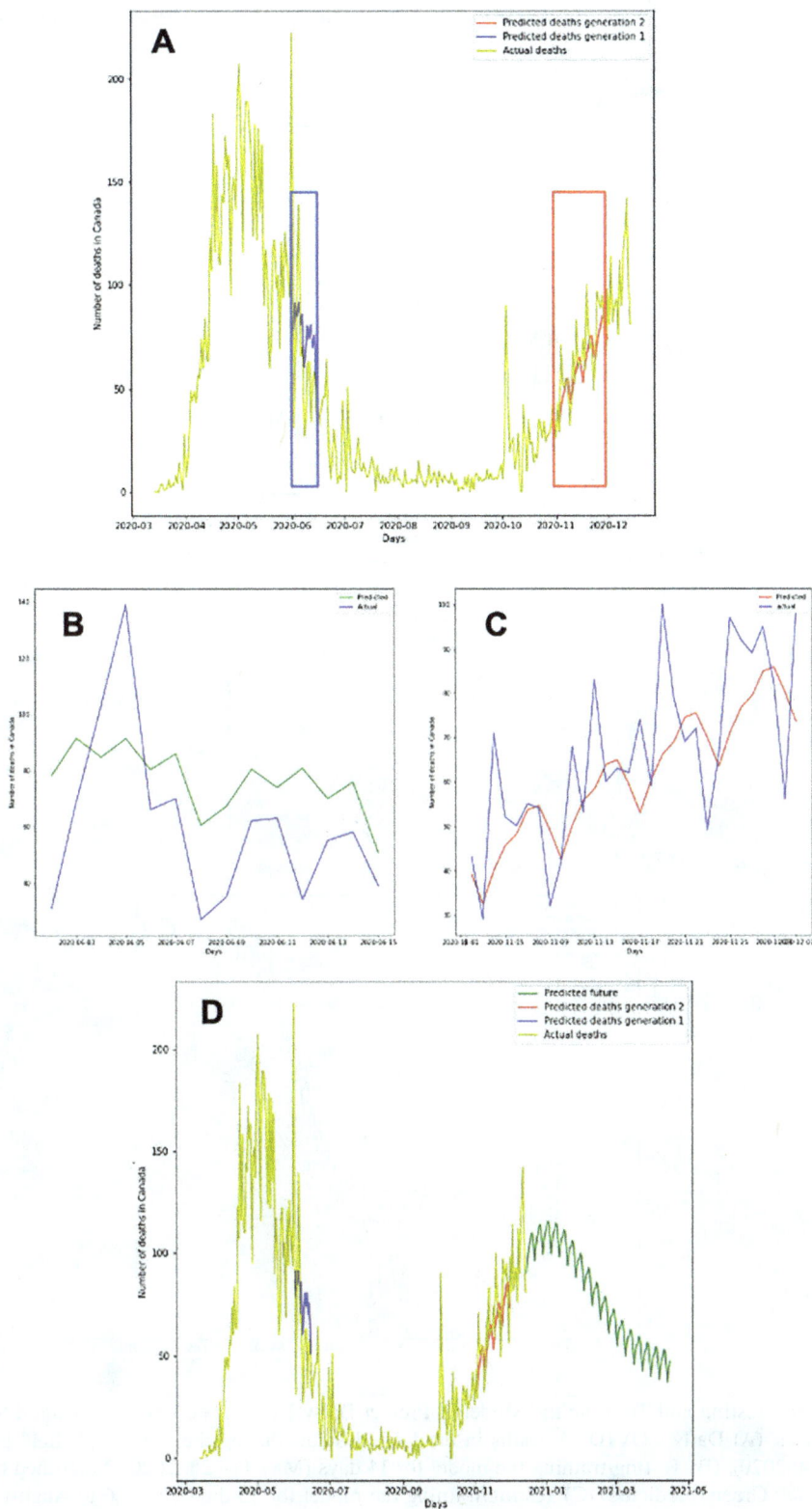

FIGURE 18.8 Testing and Training the Model to Predict Daily Death Rate Using Canadian Data for the First 2 Waves of the Pandemic. (A) Daily COVID-19 deaths in Canada during the year 2020 (light green; until December 14, 2020). (B) Testing/training the model for 14 days (June 1–15, 2020). Magnified blue box of A. Blue, actual. Green, predicted. (C) Testing/training the model for 1 month (November 1 to December 1, 2020). Magnified red box of A. Blue, actual. Red, predicted. (D) Predicted COVID-19 deaths in Canada until April 15, 2021 (green).

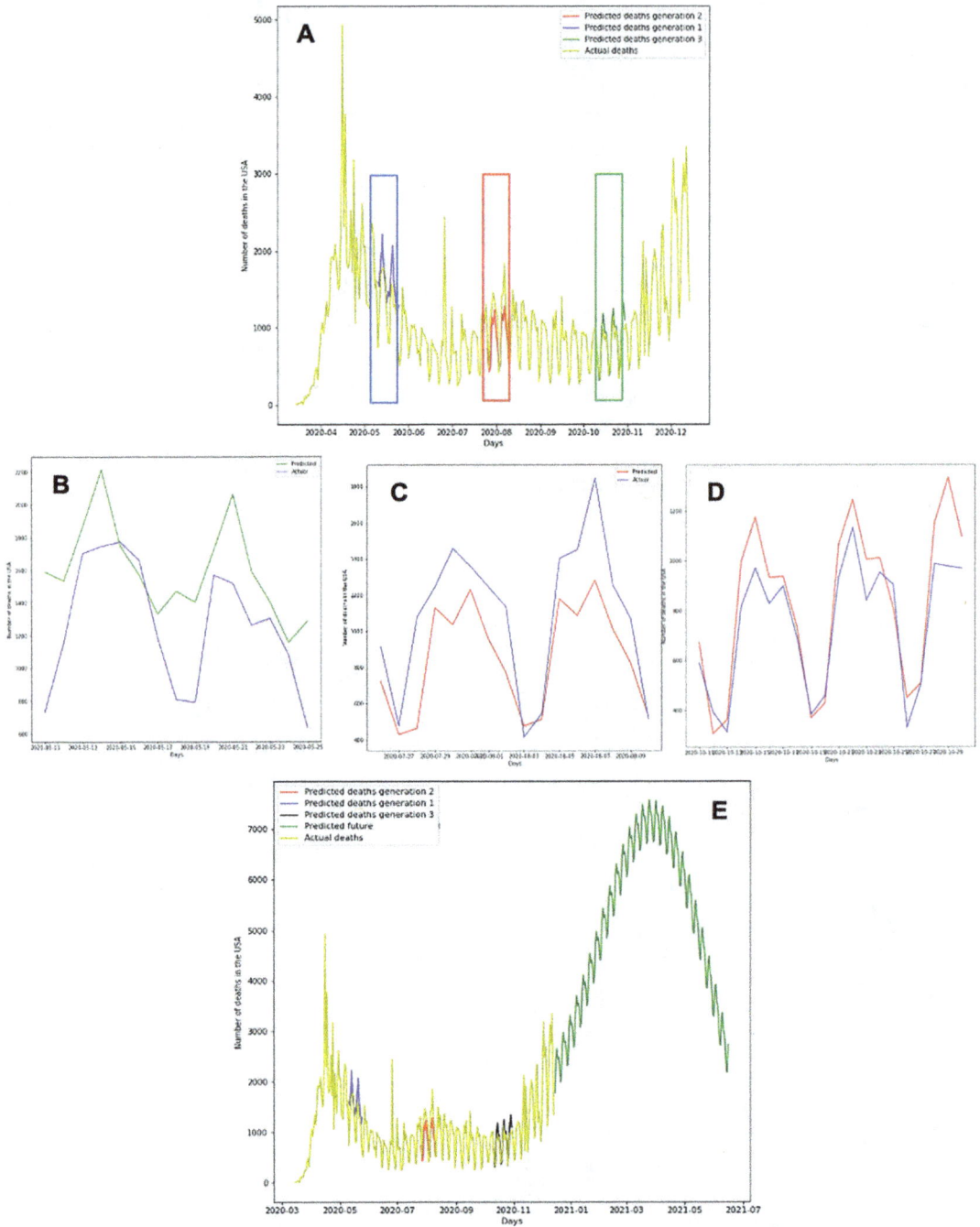

FIGURE 18.9   Testing and Training the Model to Predict Daily Death Rate Using the United States Data for three waves. (A) Daily COVID-19 deaths in the United States during the year 2020 (light green; until December 14, 2020). (B) Testing/training the model for 14 days (May 11– 25, 2020). Magnified blue box in A. Blue, actual. Green, predicted. (C) Testing/training the model for 15 days (July 26 to August 10, 2020). Magnified red box in A. Blue, actual. Red, predicted. (D) Testing/training the model for 19 days (October 11–30, 2020). Magnified green box in A. Blue, actual. Red, predicted. (E) Predicted COVID-19 deaths in the United States until June 16, 2021 (green).

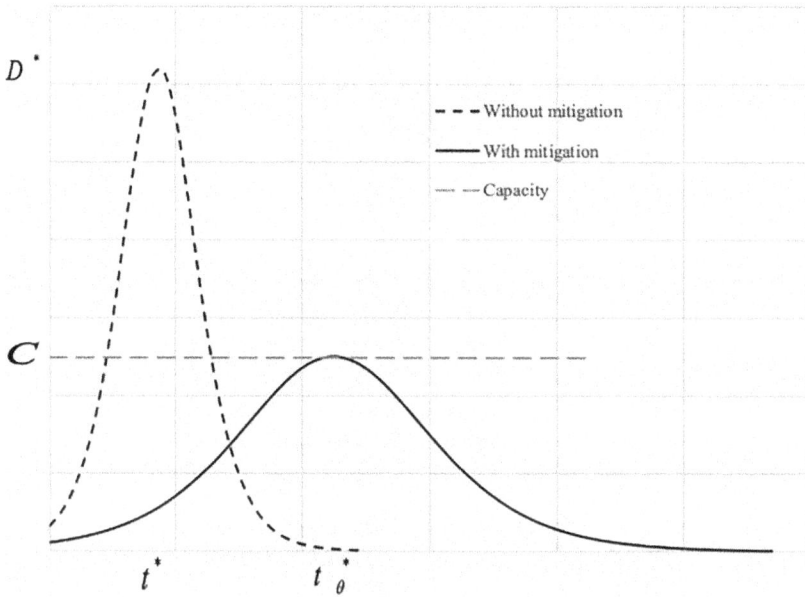

FIGURE 18.10 Flattening the Curve for a Given Healthcare Capacity.

Consequently, the likelihood of infection on day t, given that one has not yet been infected, can be expressed as

$$\frac{g(t)}{[1-G(t)]} = \{a + bG(t)\} y(t). \tag{18.6}$$

We consider the case where the government mitigates the infection at a constant rate. Accordingly, let $y(t) = \theta t$, where θ is the percentage of reduction in the daily cases the government wants to achieve so that all infected patients can be treated with available healthcare capacity, that is, the number of beds in the ICU. Now, substituting $y(t) = \theta t$ in Eq. (18.6) and assuming $y(0) = 0$, the likelihood of infection can be expressed as

$$g_\theta(t) = \frac{\left[\dfrac{\theta(a+b)^2}{a}\right] e^{-\theta(a+b)t}}{\left(1 + \left(\dfrac{b}{a}\right) e^{-\theta(a+b)t}\right)^2}. \tag{18.7}$$

In Eq. (18.7), we used $g_\theta(t)$ to indicate the likelihood function with mitigation, which delays the peak of the epidemic curve. Differentiating Eq. (18.7), we can obtain the time of the peak with mitigation as

$$t_\theta^* = \frac{\ln(b/a)}{\theta(a+b)}. \tag{18.8}$$

Substituting Eq. (18.8) into Eq. (18.7), we can obtain the peak of daily cases with mitigation, and it is given by

$$I\left(t_{\theta}^{*}\right) = \frac{\theta m (a+b)^2}{4b}. \tag{18.9}$$

Similarly, we can also obtain the time of the peak and the peak of daily cases without mitigation for the model presented in Section 18.2.1, and they are t^* and $I\left(t^*\right)$, respectively, and given by

$$t^* = \frac{ln(b/a)}{(a+b)}. \tag{18.10}$$

$$I\left(t^*\right) = \frac{m(a+b)^2}{4b}. \tag{18.11}$$

Now, from Figure 18.10, let the predicted peak daily cases be D^*, and the available healthcare capacity be C. Consequently, the following expression can be written as

$$\frac{D^*}{C} = \frac{I\left(t^*\right)}{I\left(t_{\theta}^{*}\right)}. \tag{18.12}$$

We substitute Eqs. (18.9) and (18.10) into Eq. (18.12) to determine the rate at which the government needs to mitigate the infection, $\theta = C / D^*$. To demonstrate this, for example, consider the predicted daily cases for Italy (as depicted in Figure 18.1), which has a maximum of 5,836. For example, in Figure 18.10, the epidemic curve represented by the dashed line is the predicted curve, while the epidemic curve represented by the solid line is the mitigated curve. If we assume that its ICU capacity is 4,000, Italy would have to mitigate the daily cases by 31.56%, which is 1−4000/5836 = 1−68.54%, not to overload its healthcare system. Mitigation actions could include social distancing, "work from home" orders, or other measures that inhibit the spread of the virus.

18.5 DISCUSSION

Several attempts have been made to predict the daily cases of COVID-19 and the death rate of patients. However, many models failed to predict these parameters satisfactorily. We tested, trained, and evaluated the predictive value of modified versions of BDM and Prophet using the datasets for five countries at different waves. Our approach predicted the daily cases and mortality well in single and multiple pandemic waves. Therefore, this approach could be useful for planning medical care logistics and hospital ICU bed/ventilator requirements.

Some studies focus on using models to predict the numbers of susceptible, infected, and recovered (SIR) individuals using a differential equation approach (Li et al., 2020). However, the primary advantage of the BDM is that it fits without any initial conditions and assumptions. It also does not require time-consuming parameterization, and computational time is reasonable compared to alternative models (Bass et al., 1994), making it appealing to healthcare officials and operations managers. Bass et al. (1994) show why the model presented in Bass (1969) works well without including decision variables such as price and advertising. Then, they extend the model with those decision variables. Norton and Bass (1987) incorporated both diffusion and substitution in the Bass model (Bass, 1969). Jiang and Jain generalized the Norton–Bass model to distinguish two different types of substitutions (Jiang & Jain, 2012). SIR-based models estimate the average number of people getting infected by each infected individual, incubation rate, and recovery rate. Such rates are inconsistent among multiple waves and misleading for the same disease (Eryarsoy et al. (2021). However, BDM can easily be applied to different waves as the data for those waves are fed into the model. Data for different waves can certainly be identified from figures such as Figures 18.3A and 18.7A.

For handling missing values and inconsistencies in daily and death case reports, we implemented a robust data validation procedure leveraging various data sources. In particular, we cross-referenced multiple data sources such as the World Health Organization (WHO) and Worldometer to mitigate the inconsistency and fill in missing values by applying the voting method. This systematic approach, which was instrumental in strengthening the reliability and validation process of our data, significantly improved its accuracy and performance, underscoring the value of our efforts.

The BDM can determine the likelihood of infection of a new disease at any given time. This likelihood depends on (a) the percentage of people who are independently infected by an unknown source and (b) the percentage of people who are infected by others who are known to have been infected previously.

A few studies have recently used diffusion models to predict the number of cases and fatalities during pandemics. We believe that Eryarsoy et al. (2021) is the closest to this work. They have modified the BDM to address the shortcomings in compartmental models like SIR. They developed two sub-models that work in tandem. Model 1 modifies the BDM and does not require initial conditions; the second applies a lag parameter and case fatality rate to the reported data. Similar to this chapter, they have demonstrated the model's applicability to COVID-19 pandemic data to predict the number of daily cases in different countries for the first epidemic curve. Eryarsoy et al. (2021) focused on the inaccuracy of the reported cases. However, this work differs from Eryarsoy et al. (2021). Unlike other studies, we aimed to predict multiple epidemic curves indicating the number of cases over time. We also predict the number of deaths using the Prophet model. It is a reliable and fast nonlinear regression model that can be applied to multivariate datasets. Finally, using a modified version of the Bass model, we consider the available capacity of the healthcare system to determine the percentage of reduction in the daily cases the government wants to achieve.

Modeling separately in each country provides a satisfactory prediction because many of these parameters are often specific for each country. Therefore, the approach presented in this chapter is also helpful for planning activities, personnel, and resources in hospitals, funeral homes, and other services. The number of deaths can be predicted using the model. Approaches presented in this chapter could help plan for the best treatment for the patients and ICU allocations, reduce mortality, increase recovery, reduce the cost of the system, and lower the economic impact.

18.6 LIMITATIONS

Based on recorded data from reputable sources, our statistical analysis and modeling were limited to daily cases and mortality reports from April 2020. Nevertheless, our models predict these parameters accurately based on the data obtained from the initial parts of each wave in specific countries. However, there are several limitations in this study.

First, underreporting cases and incomplete data stem from the burden on front-line health providers and limited accessibility of healthcare in certain areas during the pandemic, which could impact the prediction's daily case and death rate performance.

Second, the lack of detailed information on public health interventions and safety measures for each country plays a pivotal role in virus transmission patterns that could affect the curve and mortality rates. Non-pharmaceutical interventions (NPIs), including mask mandates, civic actions, and hand hygiene protocols, varied significantly across countries during the pandemic. Civic actions (e.g., lockdowns, restriction on indoor gatherings, remote work, and social distancing), critical factors in reducing COVID-19 transmission rates, were not accessible in this research. Additionally, pharmaceutical interventions (PIs) such as vaccines and public health safety measures such as quarantine policies that were highly effective in controlling COVID-19 were assumed to be consistent in diverse countries due to the unavailability of country-specific information.

Third, a simplified model assuming a uniform population was used due to the insufficient detailed information regarding different segments of the individuals within a population. However, each sub-group of individuals segmented in similar geographical locations, age groups, occupational sectors, and socioeconomic levels had different exposure risks and interacted at varying levels, which could change the accuracy of the prediction.

Fourth, our model did not incorporate the lack of precise data on COVID-19 virus mutations, including Delta and Omicron variants, which caused fluctuations in spread, hospitalization, and mortality patterns that could potentially improve prediction accuracy.

Therefore, more comprehensive data, including patient demographic features, public health interventions, and virus mutations, could strengthen the evidence base for improving the results, which may assist in shaping preventative care policies for future unpredictable pandemics.

18.7 CONCLUSION

A diffusion model that fits the data without decision variables is employed to predict the number of daily cases of COVID-19. The predicted epidemic curves show the highest number of daily cases during the epidemic and its occurrence time. The right tail of the epidemic curve indicates the end of the epidemic. The results also show that the predicted cumulative number of daily cases is close to that of the actual data. We extend the analysis to more than one epidemic curve. The results are also consistent for different countries. An extended version of the diffusion model was also employed to determine the rate of mitigating daily cases. The results show the level of mitigation necessary for the government to keep the number of cases within the available ICU capacity. The approach presented in this study could help predict daily caseload and mortality rates in different countries at different waves and better manage the pandemic.

REFERENCES

Abu-Raddad LJ, Chemaitelly H, Bertollini R. Severity of SARS-CoV-2 reinfections as compared with primary infections, *The New England Journal of Medicine* (2021) 385:2487–489. doi: 10.1056/NEJMc2108120

Bass FM. A new product growth model for consumer durables, *Management Science* (1969)15:215–27. https://www.jstor.org/stable/2628128

Bass FM, Krishnan TV, Jain DC. Why the Bass model fits without decision variables, *Marketing Science* (1994) 13:203–23. https://www.jstor.org/stable/183674

Buheji M, Shorrab AA, Bragazzi NL, Buhiji A. Re-inventing the intensive care units capacity in response to COVID-19 pandemic second wave. *International Journal of Management* (2020) 11(10):914–23

Cascella M, Rajnik M, Aleem A, Dulebohn SC, Di Napoli R. Features, Evaluation and Treatment Coronavirus (COVID-19). https://www.ncbi.nlm.nih.gov/books/NBK554776/. (accessed Apr. 19 2020).

Díaz-Guio DA, Villamil-Gómez WE, Dajud L, Pérez-Díaz CE, Bonilla-Aldana DK, Mondragon-Cardona A, Cardona-Ospina JA, Gómez JF, Rodríguez-Morales AJ. Will the Colombian intensive care units collapse due to the COVID-19 pandemic? *Travel Medicine and Infectious Disease* (2020) 38:101746. doi: 10.1016/j.tmaid.2020.101746

Eryarsoy E, Delen D, Davazdahemami B, Topuz K. A novel diffusion-based model for estimating cases, and fatalities in epidemics: The case of COVID–19. *Journal of Business Research* (2021) 124:163–78. doi: 10.1016/j.jbusres.2020.11.054

Facebook (2020). https://towardsdatascience.com/time-series-analysis-with-facebook-prophet-how-it-works-and-how-to-use-it-f15ecf2c0e3a (accessed Jan. 5, 2020).

JHUCSSE (2020). Johns Hopkins University Center for Systems Science and Engineering https://github.com/CSSEGISandData/COVID–19. (accessed Apr. 10, 2020).

Jiang S, Shi Z, Shu Y, Song J, Gao GF, Tan W, Guo D. A distinct name is needed for the new coronavirus. *The Lancet.* (2020) 395:949. doi: 10.1016/S0140–6736(20)30419–0

Jiang Z, Jain DC. A generalized Norton-Bass model for multigeneration diffusion, *Management Science* (2012) 58:1887–97. doi: 10.1287/mnsc.1120.1529

Li Q, Guan X, Wu P, Wang X, Zhou L, Tong Y, Ren R, Leung KSM, Lau EHY, Wong JY, Xing X, Xiang N, et al. Early transmission dynamics in Wuhan, China, of novel coronavirus-infected pneumonia. *The New England Journal of Medicine* (2020) 382:1199–207. doi: 10.1056/NEJMoa2001316

Norton JA, Bass FM. A diffusion theory model of adoption and substitution for successive generations of high-technology products, *Management Science* (1987) 33:1068–86. doi: 10.1287/mnsc.33.9.1069

Oves M, Ravindran M, Rauf MA, Omaish Ansari M, Zahin M, Iyer AK, Ismail IMI, Khan MA, Palaniyar N. Comparing and contrasting MERS, SARS-CoV, and SARS-CoV-2: prevention, transmission, management, and vaccine development. *Pathogens*. (2020) 9(12):985. doi: 10.3390/pathogens9120985

Sun J, Chen X, Zhang Z, Lai S, Zhao B, Liu H, Wang S, Huan W, Zhao R, Ng MTA, Zheng Y. Forecasting the long-term trend of COVID-19 epidemic using a dynamic model. *Scientific Reports* (2020) 10:21122. doi: 10.1038/s41598-020-78084-w

Wherry J. COVID reinfections are unusual—but could still help the virus to spread. *News Article, Nature*, (14 January 2021). doi: 10.1038/d41586-021-00071-6

World Health Organization (2020), Pneumonia of unknown cause—China: disease outbreak news. https://www.who.int/csr/don/05-january-2020-pneumonia-of-unkown-cause-china/en/ (accessed Apr. 19 2020).

Worldometers (2021) https://www.worldometers.info/coronavirus/ (accessed Jun. 16, 2021).

Wu JT, Leung K, Leung GM. Nowcasting and forecasting the potential domestic and international spread of the 2019-nCoV outbreak originating in Wuhan, China: a modelling study. *The Lancet*. (2020) 395(10225): 689–97. doi: 10.1016/s0140–6736(20)30260-9

Index

Note: Page numbers in *italics* indicate a figure, and page numbers in **bold** indicate a table on the corresponding page.

3D optical transfer function, *148*, 149; 2D optical transfer function, *148*
23andMe, 184

A

access
    AI and service, 60
    to healthcare, Canada, 5, 31
    to patient health information, Canada, 69
    patients' to technology, Canada, 76
    to telehealth, 35–36
access controls, 163, 180, 187, 189, 210
access to training *see* training
accident prevention, 244
accountability, 17, 49, 62, 70, 184, 191, 217
accuracy, 49
    AI in COVID-19 patient management, 46
    AI/ML models, 48
    of ANNs, 44
    data, 2, 3, 36
    enhanced diagnostic accuracy, 48
    in psychological assessment, 59–60
activity of daily living (ADL), 85, *85*, 91–92
    distribution of outcomes, 88, **88**
    trajectories of, *86*, 86–87, *93*, *94*, **96**, *96*
adaptability, 5, 44, 72, 146, 163
adaptation, 50, 72, 129, 135, 193
addiction consult service (ACS), 31
administrative burden, 73, 74, 75, 84, 185
advanced attack strategies, 228
Advanced Encryption Standard (AES), 189
advanced persistent threats (APTs), 207, 228, 234
aging infrastructure, 208
AI *see* artificial intelligence
air pollution, 244
algorithmic bias, 49, 57, 155, 185, *see also* bias
alternating direction method of multiplier (ADMM), 151
alternative strategies, data breaches, 221
ambulance tracking system, 245, *246*, **247**
ANN *see* artificial neural network
Anthem Inc., data breach, 188
API interactions, 252
artificial intelligence (AI), 2, 4–5, 12–13, 41–51, 55–57
    algorithmic bias in healthcare, 185
    associated technology and, 241
    benefits in post-pandemic healthcare, 48–49, 103
    in business operations, 218–219
    contributions of, 60–61
    cyberattacks (CAs), 233
    enhanced capabilities, 228
    ethical consideration in, 50
    healthcare transformation, 182, 191
    in-house challenges during pandemic, 41–43
    innovations during pandemic, 44

    limitations in post-pandemic healthcare, 49–50
    mental health diagnosis, 59–60, 62–63
    opportunities and challenges, 215–217
    overview, 215
    in post-pandemic healthcare, *50*
    practical applications of autonomous, 217–218
    predictive analytics, 255
    predictive technologies, 113
    racial bias in dermatology, 185
    role during pandemic, 44–46
    role in post-pandemic healthcare, 47–48
    service accessibility, 60
    social/community challenges, 43
    use and proliferation of, 240
artificial neural network (ANN), 44
Australia
    Digital Health Literacy Project, 34
    Indigenous Telehealth Project, 36
    legislation and reporting requirements, 209
    National Broadband Network (NBN), 33
    outpatient telehealth test, 14
    primary care in, 19
    telehealth, 26
authentication, 13
    access controls and, 189
    strong security measures and, **212**
    trust and, 256
    zero trust architecture (ZTA), 229
autonomy, 50, 183, 191
awareness, 210
    lack of, **205**
    need for, 256
    situational, 249
    training and, 202
    vulnerability, 221

B

beneficence, 61, 183
best practices
    for developing vaccines, 129–130
    healthcare informatics, 192–193
bias
    algorithmic, 49, 57, 155, 185
    data, 49
    fairness and, 191
    in predictive analytics, 185
    racial bias in dermatology, 185
big data analytics (BDA), 113, 122, 126, 128, 182
billing codes, 73
black market, 203, 205, 212, 231
broadband infrastructure, 33, 163
budget limitations *see* limited budget
Bundesamt fur Sicherheit in der Informationstechnik (BSI), 223
burnout *see* clinician burnout

C

California Telehealth Network (CTN), 36
Cambridge Analytica scandal, 188
Canada, *265*
    accessibility of patient health information, 69
    COVID-19 deaths in, 263, *269*
    digital care in, 68
    electronic medical record (EMR), 71
    health systems centralization, 16
    implementing change in, 70
    interoperability issues in digital health, 69
    issues in physician remuneration, 73–74
    medical school program, 168
    patient data, secondary uses of 70
    predicted epidemic curves, 261
    primary care for vulnerable populations, 19
    surgical procedures, restriction on, 24
    Telehealth Education for Seniors, 34
    telehealth in, 26, 29, 30, 33, 65
Canadian Interprofessional Health Collaborative (CIHC),
        65, 68
case studies
    23andMe, 184
    bias in predictive analytics, 185
    continuum of care in Canada, 71–72
    EHR usability and clinician burnout, 185–186
    genetic discrimination, 184–185
    medication errors due to EHR transcription error, 185
    racial bias in dermatology AI, 185
    vehicular ad hoc networks (VANETs), 248
    Virtual Hallway platform, 74–75
cellular vehicle-to-everything (C-V2X), 250–251
Centers for Disease Control and Prevention (CDC), 9–11,
        25, 28
    CDC Social Vulnerability Index (CDC-SVI), 15
centralized dispatch system, 250
ChatGPT-4, 233; ChatGPT-4o, 234
citation relevance analysis, 120, *120*
clinical decision-making, 2, 4, 13, 17, 20, 47, 166
clinician burnout, 185–186
cloud computing, 44, 181, 252
Clustered Regularly Interspaced Short Palindromic
        Repeats (CRISPR), 99, 101
COBIT (IT standard), 222
cognitive behavioral therapy (CBT), 55, 57, 58, 61
collaboration, 20, 193
    with cybersecurity experts, 222
    data sharing and, 19
    for expansion of broadband infrastructure, 33
    between healthcare providers and HCs, 112
    innovation and, 126
    interdisciplinary, 50, 73, 125, 128
    international/cross-border, 10, 110, 111, 127, 165
    international data sharing and, 101
    interprofessional, 75
    patient engagement and, 72
    strategic, 122
    in vaccine distribution, 130
    in virtual care, 73
collaborative care, lack of incentives for, 73
collaborative
    innovation ecosystems, 193
    practice, 68

collision avoidance, 249
communication with infrastructure, 249
compliance
    corporation, 235
    cyberattacks (CAs), 231–232
    cybersecurity, 223
    with data privacy regulations, 4
    issues with, 231–232
    regulatory, 190, 210, 221, 222
    with technical regulations, 137
computational deconvolution algorithms, 151–153,
        153, 154
computational imaging techniques
    in fluorescence microscopy, 149–150
    in healthcare informatics, 155
computer security incidence response team (CSIRT),
        225, 226
confidentiality, 183
    breaches, 186
Consensus 2.0, 233
consent, 20, 35, 191, *see also* informed consent
contactless healthcare service, 47–48
contact tracing, 17, 44, 45
containment, 224, 225, 226
contextual training, 168, 173
continuous
    evaluation, 192
    improvement, 49, 130, 192
    learning, 49, 169, 172, 193
continuum of care, 70–72, *71*
control objectives (COs), 222
convolutional neural network (CNN), 45, 150, 152
cooperation, 241
cost(s), 208
    complexity and, 228
    of cyberattacks, 238, 241
COVID-19 pandemic, 1, 41, 129, 135, **206**, 259–274
    AI assisting healthcare workers during, 44–46
    challenges in post-pandemic, 3–5
    contactless services, 47–48
    curve flattening, 267–272
    data analytics, 16–18
    data collection and modeling of daily infected cases,
        259–260
    data security and privacy in, 12–14
    declared as pandemic by WHO, 27
    detection through medical imaging, 45
    drug and vaccine development, 46
    effects on maternal and newborn health, 42
    estimating parameters of the model, 260–261
    first epidemic wave, 261, *262*, **263**, *264*
    fluorescence microscopy, 145–146, 156
    forecasting daily infected cases, 260
    forecasting number of deaths, 261
    HC behavior, 128
    HC preferences, 116
    health disparities, 43
    health informatics and, 9–11, 18–20, 160, 162
    human life loss worldwide, 83
    industrial collaboration, 111
    innovations in AI during, 44
    limitations, 273–274
    material shortage for frontline workers, 42
    mental health challenges, 55, 58–59

misinformation and infodemic, 43, 46
multiple epidemic curves, 261–263
overview, 259
physician burnout, 75
prediction of death rate, 263, **264–267**, 267
prevention of, 124
privacy and security of telehealth during, 32
remote patient monitoring (RPM), 14–16
research methods, 259–261
research results, 261–267, *262*, **263**, *264–267*
stresses of healthcare providers, 172
telehealth utilization during, 19, 27–28, 33
treatment monitoring, 45–46
vaccine distribution, 116, 128
vulnerabilities in international healthcare, 24
critical infrastructure, 203, 205, 229, 235
cross-border data transfers, 187
cryptography, vulnerability of, 228
customer purchase behavior, 125–126
cyberattacks (CAs), 205–207, **206–207**, 231–242
    artificial intelligence (AI), 233
    background, 231
    compliance, 231–232
    cost of, 238
    cybersecurity, 239–241
    data breach, 235–238, **236, 238**
    defined, 232
    evolution, 242
    frequency, severity, and evolution, 235
    governance and regulation, 242
    healthcare breaches, **239**
    healthcare organizations, 241
    impact on healthcare, 238, **239**
    research and development, 241–242
    sophistication of, 228–229
    transparency, 232
    true cost, 241
    types and purpose of, 235
cybercriminals, 84, 199, 203, 205, 209, 232
cyber incident breakdown, **200**, *201*
Cyber Incident Reporting for Critical Infrastructure Act of
    2022, 235
cyber resilience, 208–211
    action plan for, 211
    healthcare sector-wide, 211
cyber roadmap, 211
cybersecurity, 198–213, 221
    application, 211, **212**
    attacks *vs,* attempts, 240
    breaches, 221–222, **225**
    challenges, **204–205**, 205–208, **206–208**, 240–241
    cyberattacks (CAs), 239–241
    cyber resilience, 208–211
    digitalization in healthcare, 198
    experts collaboration, 222
    future of healthcare, 227–229
    healthcare organizations, 200–205
    human factors in, **204**
    imperative for healthcare, 210–211
    implications and opportunities, 219–222
    infrastructure, 222
    laws, 223–224
    measures, 252–253
    posture in health, 198–199

standards, 223
statistics and trends, 199–200, 229
target for attacks, 200–205
threat, 220–221
training for healthcare staff, 227
Cybersecurity and Infrastructure Security Agency
    (CISA), 224
cybersecurity attacks, 200–205, *201*, 240
cybersecurity frameworks (CSFs), 215, 222–223
cyber threats, 188–189, 190

D

data accountability, 193
data analytics, 104, 182, *see also* big data analytics
    capabilities to track and manage virus, 165
    COVID-19 pandemic, 16–18
    theoretical frameworks and, 125
data bias, 49, 122, 126
data breaches, 186, 207–208, **208**, 234, 235
    Anthem Inc., 188
    cyberattacks (CAs), 235–238, **236, 238**
    healthcare, 228
    horizontal analysis, 237, 238
    vertical analysis, 237, **238**
data collection
    autonomy and informed consent, 183
    lack of standard for, 16
    during the pandemic, 17
    risks, 186
data-driven approach, 83–94
    activity of daily living (ADL), 85, *85*
    research methods, 85–87
    research results, 88–93, **89–92**
data encryption, 222, 223
data exchange, 10–11, 64, 181
data extraction, 58
data governance, 193
data integrity, 12, 170, 184, 205, 228
data minimization policies, 193
data misuse, 186
data privacy, 5, 180
    breaches, 188
    ethical challenges, 17
    ethical considerations, 20
    regulations, 4
    in telehealth, 34, 35
data processing, 17, 181, 187, 252
data protection, 222
    by design/default, 187
    measures, 84, 163, 164
    patient rights and, 162
    principles and requirements, 187
    regulations, 255
data quality, 12, 49
data retention policies, 193
data safety/security, 49, 184, 256
    in healthcare informatics (HI), 12–14
    ransom payments, 221
    strategies, 14
data sharing, *see also* information sharing
    collaboration and, 126
    international, 101
    network infrastructure, 164

privacy concern in, 13
protocols, 5
qualitative assessment study, 14
for research and innovation, 191
success of remote patient monitoring (RPM) in, 11
data storage, cloud computing for, 252
data subject rights, 187
dedicated short-range communication (DSRC), 250
deep learning (DL), 44, 151–152
deficient training, 166
deployment
    costs, 256
    in cross-sectoral networks, 122
    data security and, 61
    of digital health tools and technologies, 20
    of predictive technologies, 126, 127
    process to ensure infrastructure local needs, 33
dermatology AI, racial bias in, 185, *see also* artificial
        intelligence (AI)
detailed control objectives (DCOs), 222
detection, incident response plan, 224–225
deterioration of healthcare, 244
device security, 210
DHTs *see* digital health technologies
diagnostic accuracy, 48
digital contact tracing, 45
digital disruption, 136
digital healthcare
    in Canada, 68
    equitable access to, 5, 31
    expansion of, 28
    patients' access to technology, 76
    privacy challenges in, 186–188
    transition, 165
    trends in, *51*
    trust and integrity, 193
digital health revolution, 181–182
digital health technologies (DHTs), 65–79
    continuum of care, 70–72, *71*
    digital care in Canada, 68
    digital technology, 67–68
    ethical and legal considerations, 69–70
    evidence to support virtual care, 66–67
    funding and payment, 69
    health data management, 69–70
    implementing change in Canada, 70
    interoperability, 70–72
    patient leading role, 75–77
    stakeholders, 75–77
    team-based care, 67–68
    virtual care, 67–68
    workflow change, 72–75
digital investments, 136
digitalization, 60, 136, 137, 142, 182, 198
digitalized psychometric assessments, 59–60
digital
    platforms, 56, 60, 62, 70, 130
    technology, 56, 66, 67–68, 72, 112, 136
    transformation, 65, 136, 209
disease
    forecasting, 44, 45
    testing challenges, 42–43
distributed denial of service (DDoS), **204**, 205, **206**
double extortion, 221

driver health monitoring, *248*, 248–249
    challenges and future directions, 249
    emergency communication, 249
    emergency response, 249
    integration in vehicles, 248
    platform, 248
    real-time health assessments, 248
drug development, 46, 49, 101, 104
drug discovery, 45–46, 49
dynamic routing, 250

E

economic pressure, 240
economics, 165–166
educational materials development, 72
electronic health record (EHR), 3, 11, 13, 102, 198, 239
    errors and patient safety, 185
    integration, 251
    medication errors due to transcription error, 185
    usability and clinician burnout, 185–186
electronic medical record (EMR), 48, 71, 72, 75, 84,
        136, 239
electron multiplying charge-coupled devices
        (EMCCDs), 150
emergency medical services (EMS), 243, 248, 256, 257
    vehicles, 249–250
emergency vehicle management system (EVMS), 249
emergency vehicle signal coordination (EVSC), 249
emerging technologies, 5, 36–37, 193, 257
employee
    awareness, 222
encryption, 189, 210, 222, 223, 228
equity, 184
    accessibility in telehealth, 35–36
eradication strategies, 226
errors, electronic health records (EHRs), 185
ethics/ethical, 256
    consideration in AI, 50, *see also* artificial intelligence
    digital health technologies, 69–70
    dilemmas in healthcare informatics, 184–185
    ethics-by-design approach, 191
    frameworks, 191
    guidelines, 191
    in healthcare informatics, 180, 183–186, 190–192
    principles in healthcare data and technology, 183
    standards, 191–192
    strategies for integrating, 192–193
    trade-offs, 190–191
experimental analysis, 153–155, *153–155*

F

facilitation, 72
fairness and bias, 191, *see also* bias
Fast Healthcare Interoperability Resources (FHIR), 251
fee-for-service model, 73
financial cost-saving, 30–31, *see also* cost(s)
fleet management systems, 254–255
fluorescence microscopy, 2, 145–156
    computational deconvolution algorithms in, 151–153
    computational imaging techniques in, 149–150
    experimental analysis, 153–155, *153–155*
    image estimation, 150

imaging drawbacks in, 146–149
modeling image formation in, 149–150
in pandemic-related research, 145–146
fraudulent billing, 203
frontline workers, lack of materials support for, 42
funding and payment, 69
future-oriented approaches, 193

G

General Data Protection Regulation (GDPR), 20, 35, 192, 220, 226
    data protection and privacy, 180, 186–187
    financial penalties, 202
    fines for noncompliance, 188
    patient data protection, 186
generalized inverse accelerating inverse alternating minimization (GILAM), 151, 154
genetic
    discrimination, 184–185
    testing and privacy, 184
genome-wide association studies (GWAS), 98, 101
genomics, 98–102, *see also* personalized medicine
    advancement, 104–106
    challenges, 104–106
    overview, 98–99, *99, 100*
geographic information system (GIS), **247**, 251, 253–255
global cyberattacks, *see also* cyberattacks
    history, 234–235
    overview, 233
    purpose and scope of, 233
    trends, 234–235
global positioning system (GPS), **247**, 250, 251
Google Health data partnership, 188
governance, lack of, 240
green fluorescent protein (GFP), 145

H

hardware, 181, *see also* device security
healthcare (HC) behavior, 110–117, 122, 126–127
healthcare, *see also* healthcare informatics
    betterment of, 244
    cybersecurity, **204–205**, 205, 210–211
    deterioration of, 244
    ethical principles for technology, 183
    genomics in, 98–102, *99, 100,* 104–106
    guidelines for providers, 192
    information, 203
    personalized medicine (PM), 102–106, *103*
    stakeholders, 202
    transport and, *254*
healthcare data, 203, **204–205**
    ethical principles in, 183
    management, 188–190
healthcare industry, security of, 209–210
healthcare informatics (HI), 1–6, 145–156, 160–174, 180–193
    acceptance of training, 168–169
    background, 162–166
    best practices, 192–193
    challenges in post-pandemic, 3–5
    computational imaging techniques, 155
    COVID-19 pandemic and, 1, 9–11, 18–20

data security and patients' information privacy in, 12–14
deficient training, 166
economic fallout from crisis, 165–166
ethical concerns in, 180, 183–186
ethical difficulties in data collection and analysis, 17
ethical dilemmas in, 184–185
ethical principles, 20
ethics and privacy of technology in, 190–192
evolution of, 181–183
fluorescence microscopy, 145–156
fragmented training, 167, 173
health policy, 163–164
health program curricula, 167
health worker groups, 169
health workforce training challenges, 166–169
infrastructure, 164–165
in-house challenges faced during pandemic, 41–43
insufficient contextual training, 168
legislation, 162–163, 165–166
literature review, 2–3
medical informatics, 145
mixed health worker reception, 168–169
overview, 160–162, 180–181
privacy challenges in digital healthcare, 186–188
recommendations, 192–193
remote patient monitoring (RPM), 14–16
research methodology, 166
security necessities in healthcare data management, 188–190
unequal access to training, 169
workforce training challenges, 169–173
healthcare organizations, 200–205
    AI and associated technology, 241
    clinical decision-making for patients, 47
    cooperation, 241
    cyberattacks (CA), 241
    health information management (HIM), 47
    training, 241
healthcare professionals (HCPs), 111, 112
healthcare sector-wide cyber resilience, 211
healthcare service
    fleet management systems, 254–255
    GIS, 254
    technologies for assisting, 253–255
healthcare services, 42, 70, 72, 210, 229, 248, 250–255
    accessing, 9, 31, 48, 57, 131, 198
    cellular vehicle-to-everything (C-V2X), 250–251
    cloud computing for data storage and processing, 252
    cybersecurity measures, 252–253
    dedicated short-range communication (DSRC), 250
    electronic health record (EHR) integration, 251
    GIS, 251
    GPS, 251
    high-quality, 137
    interagency collaboration framework, 253
    moral determinant of health, 217
    online transition, 13
    patient-centered, 37
    RPM in accessibility of, 15
    sensor networks, 251–252
    telemedicine integration, 252
    vehicle-to-everything communication, 250

healthcare workers, 5, 168, 172, 217
    burnout, 185–186
    diversity, 172–173
    groups, 169
    motivation of, 141
    reception, 168–169, 172
    shortages, 42
    training, 166–169, 277
    workload reduction, 46
health data management, 69–70
health inequities, 43
health information management (HIM), 47
health information technology (HIT), 11–12
Health Insurance Portability and Accountability Act
    (HIPAA), 12, 14, 35, 164, 180, 183, 187–188,
    190, **204**, 209, 220, 223
Health Level Seven International (HL7), 251
health policy, 163–164
health program curricula, 167, 171
health sector threat, 199–200
horizontal analysis, data breaches, 237, 238
hospital security, 202–203
human factors, 10, 18, 190, 227
    in cybersecurity, **204**
Human Genome Project (HGP), 99–100
hypertext transfer protocol (HTTP), 252, 253

I

identity theft, 199, 203, **207**, 212, 228
imaging drawbacks, 146–149
incentives, 73
incident
    attribution, 225
    recovery, 224–227
    response, 210, 221, 222, 224–227
India
    ambulance services available *vs.* required in, 245,
        245
    COVID-19 pandemic's indirect effects, 42
    healthcare consumerism in, 137
    implementation of VANETs in, 248
    need of healthcare informatics in, 20, 160
    traffic congestion in, 243
Industry 4.0, 245
Industry-Related Standard, 223
infectious disease testing, 48
infodemic, 43, 46
information and communication technologies (ICT), 25,
    47, 48
information sharing, 20, 25, 161, 193, 203, **204**, *see also*
    data sharing
informed consent, 35, 50, 69, 161, 168, 183, 191, 192
infrastructure, 164–165
    communication with, 249
    cybersecurity, 222
    requirements, 256
innovation management, 135–143
    hypothesis testing, 141–142
    limitations and scope for research, 142–143
    literature review, 136–139
    managerial implications, 142
    overview, 135–136
    research findings, 140–141

    research methodology, 139–140
    research results, 139–140
insider leak/threat, 186, 189, **207**
insurance fraud, 203
integration, 182–183
    electronic health record (EHR), 251
    strategies, 192–193
    telemedicine, 250
intellectual property theft, 228
intelligent agent *see* artificial intelligence
intelligent transportation systems (ITS), 3, 243–257
    challenges, 255–256
    driver health monitoring for safe driving, *248*,
        248–249
    healthcare services, 250–255
    impact of road traffic management on health, 243–244
    mobility of EMS vehicles, 249–250
    overall impact, 244–245
    overview, 243
    research, 256
    solutions in, 255
    VANETS in healthcare, *245–246*, 245–248, **247**
interagency collaboration framework, 253
Internet of Medical Things (IoMT), 180, 203, 245
Internet of Things (IoT), 3, 5, 44, 200, **204**
    attacks, **207**
    vulnerability, 228
    wearable technology and, 253–254
interoperability, 5, 10, 171, 182–183, 251, 255
    computational imaging, 155
    continuum of care, 70–72
    efficiency of healthcare delivery, 3
    hinderance in HI, 161
    issues between providers in Canada, 69
    issues in quantum-resistant solutions, 228
    legislative bills on, 163
    of manufacturer, 16
    risk of data breaches, 13
interpretability, 49
interprofessional education (IPE), 68
interprofessional education and collaborative practice
    (IPECP), 65, 68
interprovincial licensure compacts, 74
investment, 190, 213
    benefits of, 21
    in chatbot technologies, 48
    in technology, 73, 127, 165
    in telehealth, 28
    in workforce development, 165
ISO/IEC 27000, 223
IT professionals, 202
    ethics, 192
    guidelines, 192
    role in mitigating cyber vulnerabilities, 219
    training challenges, 166

K

Kazakhstan, 135–143, *see also* innovation management
    adapting digital interventions, 137
    digitalization in medicine, 137
    healthcare and innovative practices, 135
    innovation in healthcare in, 139
    managerial implications, 142

medical industry in, 140–141
strategy, 138

L

learning and improvement, 49, 169, 172, 193, *see also* training
legal
    challenges, 49, 183
    compliance, 221, 222
legislation/laws, 209
    cybersecurity, 223–224
    healthcare informatics (HI), 162–163, 165–166
license, 7, 170, 217
    in Canada, 74
long-term health effects, 43
Long Term Plan, UK, 28–29

M

machine learning (ML), 4, 5, 49, 219, 227, **247**
    in AI, 36, 44, 161
    benefits of, 37
    blind deconvolution of 3D microscopy, model, 151
    in misinformation, 46
    healthcare industry, 182, 185
    in pandemic, 2
    importance of telehealth, 33
    infectious disease diagnostics, 48
    in medical industry, transformation 191
    in optimizing patient care, 47
    predictive technologies, 47, 113, 126
    sentiment analysis, 59
    social medical injustice and, 216–217
    Vaxign-ML, 46
managerial dynamic capabilities (MDC), 110, 111–112, *121*, 129–130
mapping, 250
medical devices, 202
    informed consent and autonomy, 50
    interconnected, **204**
    portable, 138
    protection, **212**
    QSR role in safety of, 223
    regulatory and legal challenges, 49
    role in telehealth, 14
    security, 239
    vulnerabilities, 199, 202
medical Internet of Things (MIoT), 1, 228
medical records, 29
    tampering with, 228
    targeted by cybercriminals, 84
    virtual telemedicine, 72
medication errors, 185
microscopy *see* fluorescence microscopy
misinformation, 43, 112
    preventing spread of, 45, 46
misuse of data *see* data misuse
ML *see* machine learning
mobile health (mHealth), 182, 198
mobility of EMS vehicles, 249–250
modeling image formation, 149–150
modern technologies, 136–138, 172, 198, 202
multiagency healthcare delivery, 208–209

multidimensional technology acceptance model (MDTAM), 122
multi-factor authentication (MFA), 189, 200, 202, 211
My Health Records Act 2012, 209

N

National Institute for Health and Care Excellence (NICE), 66
natural language processing (NLP), 61
navigation assistance, 250
network
    containment, 226
    security, 210, **212**
    stability, 256
next-generation sequencing (NGS), 98, 100–101, 104
NIST CSF, 222–223
NMEA 0183, 251
noise reduction, 244
nuclear pore complex (NPC), 145, 154

O

online risks, 202, *see also* cybersecurity
outbreak detection, 45

P

pandemic *see* COVID-19 pandemic
pandemic-related research, 145–146
patient
    access to technology, 74
    behaviors, 59
    and provider satisfaction, telehealth, 29–30
patient-centric care, 182–183
    enhanced, 190–191
patient data/information, 202, 231
    data breaches, 186
    privacy and security, 34–35
    privacy in healthcare informatics, 12–14
    privacy principles, *70*
    protection, 187, 188, 209, **212**
    risk due to disruption and downtime, **204**
    threat to confidentiality, 186
    transfer of, 251
patient dignity, 183–184
patient emotions, 59
patient leading role, 75–77
patient mental health impact, 43
patient privacy, 49
    regulatory frameworks for, 186–188
patient rights, 183–184, 187–188
penalties, 187, 188
personal health information (PHI), 187, **207**, 212, 219–221, 227
personal identifiable information (PII), 203, 219–220, 227
personalized medicine (PM), 98–100, 102–104, *103*, 182, *see also* genomics
    advancement and challenges, 104–106
    overview, 98–99, *99*
personalized treatment plans, 48
pharmaceutical industry, 228
pharmacogenomics, 103–104
phishing, 189, **206**

physical containment, 225
physical inactivity, 244
physician remuneration, 73–74
point spread function (PSF), 146, 149, 154
Poisson–Gaussian probability density, *150*
policy-level barriers to workflows, 73–74
policymakers guidelines, 192
political influence, in acceptance of vaccines, 111–112
population health, prediction of, 47
population mental health impact, 43
post-COVID syndrome, 43, *see also* COVID-19 pandemic
post-incident activities, 227
post-pandemic healthcare
    AI role during, 47–48, *50*
    benefits of AI in, 48–49
    limitations in AI, 49–50
post-pandemic mental health challenges, 55–63
    AI-enhanced service delivery and accessibility, 60
    AI in detection and treatment, 59–60
    assistive contributions of AI, 60–61
    data extraction, 58
    ethical and regulatory considerations, 61–62
    exclusion criteria, 58
    impact of COVID-19 on, 58–59
    inclusion criteria, 57–58
precision medicine, 47, *see also* personalized medicine
predictive analytics, 48, 182
    artificial intelligence (AI), 255
    bias in, 185
predictive modeling, 48, 59, 62, 104, 164, 166, 252
predictive techniques, for vaccine selection, 120, *120*
predictive technologies, 110, 116–118, 126
    challenges, 122
    efficacy of, 131
    forecasting of vaccine demand, 127
    in healthcare institutions, 123
    ML algorithms in development of, 113
    in pharmaceutical companies, 123
    research and development, 113
    in vaccine distribution, 111–112, 118, 128
    in vaccine preference strategies, 121
    in vaccine selection, 120
Problem-Oriented Medical Record (POMR), 181
Project Nightingale, 188
protected health information (PHI), 187
protein structure prediction, 46
public communication, 127, 226

Q

quality of communication, 256
quality system regulation (QSR), 223
quantum computing, 160, 220, 227–228
quantum-resistant cryptography, 228

R

racial bias, in dermatology AI, 185
ransom payments, 221
ransomware, 220
    attacks, 32, 188–189, 199, 205, **206**, 208, **212**, 213, 221, 223
    Change Healthcare attack, 221
    resilience against, 222

    threats, **212**
    trust issues with, 221
recovery
    planning, 222
    strategies, 227
regulatory
    agencies, 231–232
    challenges, 4, 49
    compliance, 190, 210, 221, 222
    frameworks, 4, 49, 62, 163, 186–188, 191, 199
reimbursement rates, 73
remote
    data access, 202
    monitoring, 48–49
remote patient monitoring (RPM), 11–12, 78
    during COVID-19 pandemic, 14–16
    healthcare informatics (HI), 14–16
reporting agencies, 231–232
reporting requirements, 208, 209, 231, 233
representational state transfer (REST), 252, 253
resistance co-occurrence analysis, 119, *119*
resource constraints, 190, 213
risk
    cloud transition, **204**
    healthcare entities, 203
    pharmaceutical industry, 228
road traffic
    accidents, 244
    management, impact on health, 243–244

S

scalability, **204**, 250, 252, 256, 257
screening challenges, 42–43
secure data sharing protocols, 193
secure real-time transport protocol (SRTP), 252
Secure Sockets Layer/Transport Layer Security (SSL/ TLS), 189
security-by-design, 211
security operation center (SOC), 224
sensitive medical data, 186
sensor networks, 251–252
sentiment analysis, 59, 62
severe acute respiratory syndrome coronavirus 2 (SARS-COV-2) *see* COVID-19 pandemic
signal-to-noise ratio (SNR), 152
simple object access protocol (SOAP), 253
single-molecule localization microscopy (SMLM), 152
situational awareness, 249
smart hospital systems, 228
social/community challenges, 43
social engineering, 189, 190, 202, **206**, 227
software, 181
stakeholder
    access, **212**
    collaboration, 191
    engagement, 191
standardization, 160, 171, 256
    of health technologies, 170
    of HI training, 166
    of information, 164
    interoperability and, 16, 161
Standard of Good Practice (SoGP), 223

stimulated emission depletion (STED), 146
stress, 58–59, 145, 170, 244, 248
structured illumination microscopy
        (SIM), 146
supply chain disruption, 42, 228
susceptible, infected, and recovered (SIR), 272
synchronous telehealth, 25

T

team-based care, 65, 67–68
technology
        adoption, 190–191
        changes, 241
        ethical standards and, 191–192
        limited patient access to, 74
technology acceptance model (TAM), 122, 125
Technology Informatics Guiding Educational Reform
        (TIGER) initiative, 170
telecommunication networks, 198
telehealth, 24–37, **27**, 198
        advantages, 29–31
        asynchronous, 25
        in Australia, 26
        in broadband infrastructure, 33
        in Canada, 29
        challenges and barriers to, 31–32
        classifications, 25
        data privacy in, 34, 35
        defined, 25
        emerging technologies impact on, 36–37
        equity and accessibility, 35–36
        evolution of, 26
        financial cost-saving, 30–31
        history of, 26
        impact of innovations on, 36–37
        investment in, 28
        literature review, 24–25
        medical devices role in, 14
        outpatient test, 14
        patient and provider satisfaction with, 29–30
        patient data privacy and security, 34–35
        recommendations, 32–37
        synchronous, 25
        travel, consultations during, 253
        in United Kingdom, 28–29
        in United States, 27–28
        in user digital literacy, 33–34
        utilization during COVID-19, 19, 27–28, 33
telemedicine, 25, **27**, 28, 165, 182, 198
        as benefits of AI, 48–49
        integration, 250, 252
        standardized guidelines and regulations, 74
        workflows, 72–73
teletherapy, 15, 31, 60
Theory, Context, Characteristics, and Methods (TCCM),
        116, 123–126
        characteristics and factors, 124–125
        customer purchase behavior, 125–126
        literature review, 124
        predictive technology, 126
        theory development, 123–124
theory of planned behavior (TPB), 125
threats

to confidentiality, 186
cybersecurity, 220–221
to data integrity, 228
health sector, 199–200
insider, 186, 189, **207**
timeliness in psychological assessment., 59–60
traffic management, 243–245, 249
training, 210
        acceptance of, 168–169, 172
        access to, 172–173
        awareness and, 202
        challenges faced by health workers, 166–169
        challenges faced by IT professionals, 166
        contextual, 168, 173
        deficient, 166
        delivery approaches, 170
        employee, 222
        fragmented, 167, 173
        healthcare organizations, 241
        healthcare workers, 227
training challenges, 169–173
        acceptance of training, 172
        approaches to training delivery, 170
        customization, 171–172
        health worker reception, 172
        diversity and access to training, 172–173
        integration into health program curricula,
                171
        strengthening, 170–171
        sustainable solutions to, 169–170
trajectories
        of activity of daily living (ADL), 86, *86*, *94*
        T-programs for, 96–97, **97**
transcription error, 185
transmission control protocol (TCP), 252,
        253
transparency, 118, 219
        accountability and, 61, 70, 180, 184
        cyberattacks (CAs), 232
        integrity of vaccine development and, 112
        lacking in AI algorithms, 4, 49, 50
        to maintain public trust, 20
transparent data practices, 193
transport layer security (TLS), 252–253
treatment plans, personalized, 48

U

United Kingdom, 18–19
        surgical procedures restrictions, 24
        telehealth in, 28–29
        telemedicine usage, 33
        virtual consultation methods, 76
United States, 9, 12, 188, *268*, *270*
        COVID-19 deaths in, 267
        data collection standardization lacking, 16
        data privacy policies, 35
        frontline workers, 42
        Health Insurance Portability and Accountability Act
                (HIPAA), 35, 183, 186–187
        restriction in surgical procedures, 24
        Rural Digital Opportunity Fund (RDOF) in, 33
        telehealth in, 27–29, 32, 33
        telemedicine in, 26

usability, EHR, 185–186
user digital literacy, telehealth in, 33–34
Uzbekistan–Azerbaijan Health Decade, 138–139

V

vaccines, 110–132
    analysis, 116–123
    best practices for developing, 129–130
    citation relevance analysis, 120, *120*
    conceptual mapping, *114*
    descriptive analysis, 118–121, *119*
    development, 46
    distribution, 111
    findings, 126–130
    HC behavior, 111
    limitations, 130–131
    managerial dynamic capabilities (MDC), 111–112,
        121, *121*, 129–130
    methodological approach, 113–116, *115*
    overview, 110–111
    political influence in acceptance of, 111–112
    predictive techniques for selection, 120, *120*
    predictive technologies in distribution, 111–112
    recommendations, 130–131
    research, 121–123
    resistance co-occurrence analysis, 119,
        119
    selection frequency, 120, *120*
    TCCM, 116, 123–126
    trust in acceptance of, 111–112
vehicle communication, 246–247, 250
vehicular ad hoc networks (VANETs), *245–246*, 245–248,
        247, 256
    case study, 248
    challenges and benefits of, 247

vendor
    management, 222
    risk management, 210
virtual care, 67–68, 77–78
    evidence to support, 66–67
    licensure, 74
virtual containment, 226
Virtual Hallway platform, 74–75
VosViewer software, 117
vulnerability
    awareness, 221
    of cryptography, 228
    of IoT devices, 228
vulnerable populations, 18, 19, 32, 35, 43, 173

W

wearable technology, 253–254
whole exome sequencing (WES), 100
whole-genome sequencing (WGS), 100, 101, 104
workflows, 48, 72–75
    license regulations, 74
    operational and policy-level barriers, 73–74
    telemedicine, 72–73
    Virtual Hallway platform, 74–75
workload reduction, 46
World Health Organization (WHO), 11, 25, 273
    1978 Alma-Ata Declaration, 138
    on deaths due to COVID-19, 41
    declaring COVID-19 as pandemic, 9, 27, 41
    digital transformation of healthcare, 65
    on mental health due to COVID-19, 55

Z

zero trust architecture (ZTA), 229

For Product Safety Concerns and Information please contact our EU
representative GPSR@taylorandfrancis.com
Taylor & Francis Verlag GmbH, Kaufingerstraße 24, 80331 München, Germany

* 9 7 8 1 0 3 2 7 7 9 6 9 0 *